DATE DUE

JY 30 98		
DE 18 98		
FE 17 99		
MR 31 99		
MY 24 00		
MY 27 99		
MY 3 00		
DE 8 00		
AG 8 02		
JE 11 03		
SE 6 07		

DEMCO 38-296

Aerobic Fitness & Health

Roy J. Shephard, MD, PhD, DPE
University of Toronto

Human Kinetics Publishers

loging-in-Publication Data

Shephard, Roy J.
    Aerobic fitness and health / Roy J. Shephard.
        p.   cm.
    Includes bibliographical references (p.) and index.
    ISBN 0-87322-417-5
    1. Physical fitness.   2. Exercise.   3. Health.   I. Title.
    QP301.S468   1994
    613.7--dc20   93-457
                                                     CIP

ISBN: 0-87322-417-5

Copyright © 1994 by Roy J. Shephard

Managing Editor: Julia Anderson
Assistant Editors: Julie Lancaster, Dawn Roselund, and John Wentworth
Copyeditor: Dianna Matlosz
Proofreader: Kathy Bennett
Production Director: Ernie Noa
Typesetting and Text Layout: Julie Overholt
Text Design: Keith Blomberg
Cover Design: Jack Davis
Interior Art: Jim Hampton
Printer: Braun-Brumfield

Printed in the United States of America

10 9 8 7 6 5 4 3 2 1

Human Kinetics Publishers
Box 5076, Champaign, IL 61825-5076
1-800-747-4457

Canada: Human Kinetics Publishers, P.O. Box 24040,
Windsor, ON N8Y 4Y9
1-800-465-7301 (in Canada only)

Europe: Human Kinetics Publishers (Europe) Ltd.,
P.O. Box IW14, Leeds LS16 6TR, England
0532-781708

Australia: Human Kinetics Publishers, P.O. Box 80,
Kingswood 5062, South Australia
618-374-0433

New Zealand: Human Kinetics Publishers,
P.O. Box 105 231, Auckland 1
(09) 309-2259

Contents

Preface

This book was conceived as a successor to *Endurance Fitness* (Shephard, 1977a). Rather than attempting to prepare a new edition of the earlier work, I decided to discuss possible interactions between aerobic fitness and health anew, focusing on the developing consensus without obscuring it with dated ideas. Nevertheless, I have adopted a similar philosophy to the one that guided the earlier book: presenting current knowledge with a simplicity that should make it accessible to a broad range of health professionals while avoiding the missionary enthusiasm of the fitness fanatic. Most of the ideas I advance have a broad basis of scientific support, which is rigorously documented. Where an idea needs further research, I have indicated the extent of uncertainty and the reasons I believe more investigation is warranted. The book should thus appeal particularly to those who are active in fitness, health promotion, and sports medicine and who seek an overview of the current situation.

The opening chapter facilitates discussion by reviewing the nature and validity of the distinctions that have recently been drawn between physical activity and exercise, the classic index of aerobic fitness (maximal oxygen intake, or aerobic power) and its apparent synonym (aerobic capacity), and health-related versus performance-related increments of fitness. I then offer a simple model linking physical activity, aerobic fitness, and health.

Chapter 2 looks at the physiological determinants of aerobic fitness, bringing into a contemporary focus the continued debate on the importance of a peripheral versus a central limitation of prolonged rhythmic exercise. I comment on current levels of physical activity and aerobic fitness in chapter 3. Because the interpretation of available data is still limited by problems of sampling and disagreements on methodology, I critique established and new procedures for measuring human activity patterns and resulting levels of fitness before looking at demographic information on the effects of growth, aging, gender differences, socioeconomic gradients, and secular trends.

As the next logical step, chapter 4 explores the potential for improving current levels of aerobic fitness by increasing habitual activity. I assess the current status of the "nature versus nurture" debate and describe an optimal training regimen for developing aerobic fitness, with adaptations of the standard prescription proposed for childhood, pregnancy, old age, and ill health. The response of sedentary individuals is compared with that of endurance athletes, and I note potential problems of overtraining and the loss of physical condition with detraining.

The study of aerobic fitness has many intrinsic rewards. For the exercise scientist, it provides a fascinating example of the integrating capacity of the body, because many organ systems are linked to meet the oxygen demands of the active tissues. But for many fitness professionals and sports medicine specialists, the greatest attraction of aerobic fitness remains its potential impact on the health of the exerciser. Chapter 5 examines this area in depth. *Health* is defined in its broadest sense. Although there are occasional hazards of overenthusiastic exercise—ranging from a minor muscle or tendon injury to the precipitation of myocardial infarction or cardiac arrest—I argue that the overall health impact of regular and moderate aerobic activity is very favorable. There is now strong evidence that such exercise is helpful, both in preventing many forms of disease and in speeding the recovery process. An even stronger reason for encouraging regular physical activity is enhancement of the quality of life. The benefits range from an immediate elevation of mood to a prolongation of independent living in old age.

Aerobic Fitness and Health not only provides a compact scientific account of interactions between aerobic exercise and health, it also offers hard evidence of health benefits that can be advanced to persuade the general population to engage in regular physical activity. Information in the exercise sciences is now distributed over a vast body of literature, but I hope that the extensive bibliography given here will allow eager graduate students to undertake in-depth reviews of topics of particular interest.

My own process of education in this discipline has been ongoing for some 30 years now. It has involved interactions with an enormous number of faculty colleagues, postdoctoral fellows, graduate assistants, undergraduate students, and participants in exercise programs, not only in Toronto but in many parts of the world. I would certainly like to acknowledge all of the wonderful individuals who have contributed to my understanding of aerobic fitness, but I fear the tally of debts has become much too large to print. I can merely express my deep and collective gratitude to you all. I hope that this synthesis of your wisdom will hold some of the same fascination for you that it has for me.

Credits

Chapter 1

Figure 1.1 and Table 1.1 are from "Exercise, Fitness, and Health: The Consensus Statement" in *Exercise, Fitness, and Health* (pp. 5, 6) by C. Bouchard, R.J. Shephard, T. Stephens, J.R. Sutton, and B.D. McPherson (Eds.), 1990, Champaign, IL: Human Kinetics. Copyright 1990 by Human Kinetics Publishers, Inc. Reprinted by permission.

Table 1.2 is from "Factors Affecting Body Density and Thickness of Subcutaneous Fat" by R.J. Shephard, G. Jones, K. Ishii, M. Kaneko, and A.J. Olbrecht, 1977, *American Journal of Clinical Nutrition*, **22**, pp. 1182-1183. Copyright © Am. J. Clin. Nutr. American Society for Clinical Nutrition. Reprinted by permission.

Table 1.3 is from *The Well-Being of Canadians. Highlights of the 1988 Campbell's Survey* (p. 51) by T. Stephens and C. Craig, 1990, Ottawa: Canadian Fitness and Lifestyle Research Institute. Copyright 1990 by Canadian Fitness and Lifestyle Research Institute. Reprinted by permission.

Table 1.4 is from *A New Perspective on the Health of Canadians* (p. 20) by M. Lalonde, 1974, Ottawa: Health and Welfare Canada. Copyright 1974 by Health and Welfare Canada. Reproduced with permission of the Minister of Supply and Services Canada 1992.

Table 1.5 is from "Geriatric Benefits of Exercise as an Adult" by R.J. Shephard and W. Montelpare, 1988, *Journal of Gerontology: Medical Sciences*, **434**, p. M88, July 1988. Copyright © 1988 by The Gerontological Society of America. Reprinted by permission.

Chapter 2

Figure 2.1 is from "The Use of Fuels for Muscular Work" by R.W. McGilvery. In *Metabolic Adaptations to Prolonged Physical Exercise* (Proceedings of the 2nd International Symposium on Biochemistry of Exercise [WSM 7]) (p. 16) by H. Howald and J.R. Poortmans (Eds.), 1975, Basel, Switzerland: Birkhäuser Verlag AG. Copyright 1975 by Birkhäuser Verlag. Adapted by permission.

Figures 2.3-2.5, 2.8-2.10, and Tables 2.1 and 2.3 are from *Endurance Fitness* (2nd ed.) by R.J. Shephard, 1977, Toronto: University of Toronto Press. Copyright 1977 by University of Toronto Press. Reprinted by permission.

Figure 2.7 is from "Exercise and Physical Fitness" by R.J. Shephard, 1968, *Ontario Medical Review*, **35**, p. 77. Reprinted with the permission of the Ontario Medical Association.

Figure 2.11 is from "Exercise and Stress Testing Workshop Report, National Conference on Exercise in the Prevention, in the Evaluation and in the Treatment of Heart Disease" by S.M. Fox and W. Haskell, 1969, *The Journal of the South Carolina Medical Association*, **65**(Suppl. 1), p. 77. Copyright 1969 by *The Journal of the South Carolina Medical Association*. Reprinted by permission.

Table 2.2 is from "Limitations of Exercise by Dyspnea" by K.J. Killian, 1987, *Canadian Journal of Sport Sciences*, **12** (Suppl.), p. 57S. Copyright 1987 by and reprinted with permission from the *Canadian Journal of Sport Sciences*.

Chapter 3

Figure 3.1 is from "The Canadian Home Fitness Test: 1991 Update" by R.J. Shephard, S. Thomas, and I. Weller, 1991, *Sports Medicine*, **11**, p. 359. Reprinted by permission.

Figure 3.2 is from "Progress and Problems in the Promotion of Physical Activity" by K.E. Powell, T. Stephens, B. Marti, L. Heinemann, and M. Kreuter. In *Sport for All* (p. 64) by P. Oja and R. Telama (Eds.), 1991, Amsterdam: Elsevier. Copyright 1991 by Elsevier Science Publishers B.V. Reprinted by permission.

Figure 3.3 is from *Fitness and Health of an Inuit Community: 20 Years of Cultural Change* by A. Rode and R.J. Shephard, 1992 (unpublished report). Reprinted by permission of Roy J. Shephard.

Figure 3.4 and Table 3.19 are from "Activity Patterns of the Canadian Eskimo" by G. Godin and R.J. Shephard. In *Polar Human Biology* (pp. 199, 207) by O.G. Edholm and E.K.E. Gunderson (Eds.), 1973, London: Butterworth-Heinemann Limited. Copyright 1973 by Butterworth-Heinemann Limited. Reprinted and adapted by permission.

Figures 3.5, 3.6, 3.8, and Table 3.22 are from *Endurance Fitness* (2nd ed.) by R.J. Shephard, 1977, Toronto: University of Toronto Press. Copyright 1977 by University of Toronto Press. Reprinted by permission.

Figure 3.7 is from "A Simple Method to Assess Exercise Behavior in the Community" by G. Godin and R.J. Shephard, 1985, *Canadian Journal of Applied Sport Sciences*, **10**, p. 146. Copyright 1985 by and reprinted with permission from the *Canadian Journal of Sport Sciences*.

Figure 3.9 is from *Body Composition in Biological Anthropology* (p. 13) by R.J. Shephard, 1991, London: Cambridge University Press. Copyright 1991 by Cambridge University Press. Reprinted by permission.

Tables 3.2 and 3.11 are from *Human Physiological Work Capacity* (pp. 17, 83) by R.J. Shephard, 1978, London: Cambridge University Press. Copyright 1978 by Cambridge University Press. Adapted and reprinted by permission.

Table 3.7 is from "Seasonal Differences in Aerobic Power" by R.J. Shephard, H. Lavallée, J-C. Jéquier, R. LaBarre, M. Rajic, and C. Beaucage. In *Physical Activity Assessment: Principles, Practice and Applications* (p. 202) by R.J. Shephard and H. Lavallée (Eds.), 1978, Springfield, IL: Charles C Thomas. Adapted courtesy of Charles C Thomas, Publisher, Springfield, Illinois.

Tables 3.8 and 3.25 are from A. Rode and R.J. Shephard, "Fitness of the Canadian Eskimo: The Influence of Season," *Medicine and Science in Sports,*

5(3), pp. 170-173, 1973, © by The American College of Sports Medicine. Adapted and reprinted by permission.

Table 3.9 is from "Current Developments in Europe" by G. Rose. In *Atherosclerosis II* (p. 311) by R.J. Jones (Ed.), 1970, Berlin: Springer Verlag. Copyright 1970 by Springer Verlag. Adapted by permission.

Table 3.13 is from *The Well-Being of Canadians. Highlights of the 1988 Campbell's Survey* (p. 74) by T. Stephens and C. Craig, 1990, Ottawa: Canadian Fitness and Lifestyle Research Institute. Copyright 1990 by Canadian Fitness and Lifestyle Research Institute. Reprinted by permission.

Table 3.14 is from *Fitness and Lifestyle in Canada* by Canada Fitness Survey, conducted by Canadian Fitness and Lifestyle Research Institute (formerly known as Canada Fitness Survey), 1983, Ottawa: Canadian Fitness and Lifestyle Research Institute. Copyright 1983 by Canada Fitness Survey. Adapted by permission.

Table 3.15 is from *Canadian Standardized Test of Fitness (CSTF) Operations Manual* (3rd ed.) by Fitness Canada, 1986, Ottawa: Fitness Canada. Adapted by permission.

Table 3.16 is from *Aerobics* by K.H. Cooper, 1983, New York: Bantam. Reprinted by permission.

Chapter 4

Figure 4.1 is from R. Paffenbarger, "Contributions of Epidemiology to Exercise Science and Cardiovascular Health," *Medicine and Science in Sports and Exercise*, 20(5), pp. 426-438, 1988, © by the American College of Sports Medicine. Adapted by permission.

Figure 4.3 is from *Endurance Fitness* (2nd ed.) by R.J. Shephard, 1977, Toronto: University of Toronto Press. Copyright 1977 by University of Toronto Press. Reprinted by permission.

Figure 4.4 is from K.H. Sidney and R.J. Shephard, "Frequency and Intensity of Exercise Training for Elderly Subjects," *Medicine and Science in Sports*, 10(2), pp. 125-131, 1978, © by The American College of Sports Medicine. Adapted by permission.

Figure 4.5 is from "Urinary Catecholamine Excretion and Lactate Concentrations in Competitive Hockey Players Aged 11 to 23 Years" by C.J. Blimkie, D.A. Cunningham, and F.Y. Leung. In *Frontiers of Activity and Child Health* (p. 316) by H. Lavallée and R.J. Shephard (Eds.), 1977, Québec: Editions du Pélican.

Figure 4.6 is reprinted by permission of Greenwood Publishing Group, Inc., Westport, CT, from *Physiology and Biochemistry of Exercise* by R.J. Shephard. Copyright by Praeger Publishers and published in 1982 by Praeger Publishers.

Figure 4.7 is from "Time Course of Loss of Adaptations After Stopping Prolonged Intense Endurance Training" by E.F. Coyle, W.H. Martin, D.R. Sinacore, M.J. Joyner, J.M. Hagberg, and J.O. Holloszy, 1984, *Journal of Applied Physiology*, 57(6), pp. 1857-1864. Copyright 1984 by The American Physiological Society. Adapted by permission.

Figure 4.8 is from "Effects of Detraining on Responses to Submaximal Exercise" by E.F. Coyle, W.H. Martin, D.R. Sinacore, M.J. Joyner, J.M. Hagberg, and J.O. Holloszy, 1985, *Journal of Applied Physiology*, **59**, pp. 853-859. Copyright 1985 by The American Physiological Society. Reprinted by permission.

Table 4.3 is from "Endurance Training and Body Composition of the Elderly" by K.H. Sidney, R.J. Shephard, and J. Harrison, 1977, *American Journal of Clinical Nutrition*, **30**, p. 329. Copyright © American Society for Clinical Nutrition. Reprinted by permission.

Chapter 5

Figure 5.1 is from "Influence of Exercise and Lifestyle Variables Upon High Density Lipoprotein Cholesterol After Myocardial Infarction" by T. Kavanagh, R.J. Shephard, L.J. Lindley, and M. Pieper, 1983, *Arteriosclerosis*, **3**, p. 255. Copyright 1983 by the American Heart Association. Adapted by permission of the American Heart Association, Inc.

Figure 5.2 is from "Acute Exercise and Immune Function: Relationships Between Lymphocyte Activity and Changes in Subset Counts" by S. Shinkai, S. Shore, P.N. Shek, and R.J. Shephard, in press, *International Journal of Sports Medicine*. Reprinted by permission.

Figure 5.3 is from "Physical Fitness and All-Cause Mortality: A Prospective Study of Healthy Men and Women" by S.N. Blair, H.W. Kohn, R.S. Paffenbarger, D.G. Clark, K.H. Cooper, and L.W. Gibbons, 1989, *Journal of the American Medical Association*, **262**(17), p. 2399. Copyright 1989 by the American Medical Association. Reprinted by permission.

Table 5.2 is from "Health Hazard Appraisal—The Influence of an Employee Fitness Programme" by R.J. Shephard, P. Corey, and M.H. Cox, 1982, *Canadian Journal of Public Health*, **73**, p. 185. Copyright 1982 by the *Canadian Journal of Public Health*. Reprinted by permission.

Table 5.7 is from "Exercise in the Tertiary Prevention of Ischemic Heart Disease: Experimental Proof" by R.J. Shephard, 1989, *Canadian Journal of Sport Sciences*, **14**, pp. 79-80. Copyright 1989 by and reprinted with permission from the *Canadian Journal of Sport Sciences*.

Table 5.8 is from I. Vuori, L. Suurnakki, and T. Suurnakki, "Risk of Sudden Cardiovascular Death (SCVD) in Exercise," *Medicine and Science in Sports and Exercise*, **14**(2), pp. 114-115, 1982, © by The American College of Sports Medicine. Reprinted by permission.

Table 5.9 is reprinted with permission. "Response to Exercise After Bedrest and After Training: A Longitudinal Study of Adaptive Changes in Oxygen Transport and Body Composition" by B. Saltin, G. Blomqvist, J.H. Mitchell, R.L. Johnson, K. Wildenthal, & C.B. Chapman, 1968, Circulation 38: VII-1 to VII-78. Copyright 1968 American Heart Association.

1
Chapter

Physical Activity, Aerobic Fitness, and Health

Physical activity, fitness, and health have very different meanings for different investigators. It is thus vital to begin with a brief review of terminology, clearly defining the basic concepts of physical activity, fitness, and health.

Physical Activity

Physical activity may be regarded as any body movement produced by muscular contraction that leads to a substantial increase in a person's energy expenditure. Whereas a single burst of movement can be developed anaerobically, if the movement pattern is carried out repeatedly for several minutes, the main source of energy then becomes aerobic metabolism, and a corresponding increase in the consumption of oxygen develops over 20 to 30 s.

Attempts to distinguish several components of physical activity were initiated by Caspersen, Powell, and Christenson (1985) and were developed further by Bouchard, Shephard, Stephens, Sutton, and McPherson (1990). Potential categories include occupational activity ("work"), domestic chores, required programs of physical education, and leisure activity (exercise, sport, training, dance, and play).

Energy Expenditure

The energy expenditure of the body includes the metabolic cost of physical activity, together with basal metabolism, the thermal effects of feeding, lactation, and the synthesis of new tissue. The liberation of heat may be expressed as an absolute value (watts, W, or kilojoules per min, kJ/min), or as a ratio to the body surface area potentially available for heat loss (W/m^2) or as a ratio to total of lean tissue mass (W/kg). Methods of standardizing the data for interindividual differences of body size are discussed further in the appendix.

The body conforms to the Newtonian principle of the conservation of energy. Thus, if observations are made carefully over an adequate period of time (1-2 weeks), any changes in tissue mass reflect an imbalance between the energy value of food ingested and the energy cost of the various demands for energy expenditure. Physical activity is both the largest and the most variable element. Depending on the individual's fitness level, a 5- to 20-fold increase over resting metabolism can be developed in a few minutes of vigorous exercise, and a healthy young adult can sustain a 5- to 8-fold increase of metabolism throughout an 8-hour working day. If an ultra-long-distance athlete is involved in an event such as the Tour de France, energy expenditures may total as much as 30 to 40 MJ/day. In contrast, the total daily energy expenditure of a frail elderly person (6 MJ/day) is only a little greater than the basal metabolism.

The basal metabolic rate (BMR) averages about 2.8 kJ/min per m² of body surface area, or about 7.3 MJ/day in a man and 5.7 MJ/day in a woman of average size. The BMR thus accounts for a substantial fraction of the total daily energy expenditure in all except well-trained athletes. If data are expressed per unit of body surface area or per unit of body mass, basal readings show a small but progressive decrease with age. Values are low in obese subjects, because in such individuals an increased proportion of the total body mass is attributable to metabolically inert stored fat.

The ingestion of food leads to a small immediate increase of the resting energy expenditure, this being greatest after a fatty meal (the so-called specific dynamic action of fat). The magnitude of the thermic effect is modified by the availability of food, habitual activity patterns, and obesity (Molé, 1990; Rothwell & Stocks, 1983; Tremblay, Coté, & LeBlanc, 1984). Small (10%-15%) but more permanent increases in BMR are induced by ingesting a plethora of food (the so-called Luxuskonsumption; Rothwell & Stocks, 1983). Conversely, restriction of food intake reduces the BMR by 10% to 15%, complicating the treatment of obesity. Metabolism may also show a small increase for some hours following prolonged bouts of physical activity (Molé, 1990), and more persistent increases in resting metabolism contribute to acclimation to very cold climates (Shephard, 1985a).

Nursing mothers incur additional energy expenditures associated with the secretion of milk. Depending on the age of the nursing infant, the demand may amount to 1 to 2 MJ/day. Increased energy is also required during synthesis of new tissue (e.g., healing, training, growth, and pregnancy). For example, at term, the resting metabolism of a pregnant woman is increased by about 1.5 MJ/day.

Occupational Activity

Some authors, including Knuttgen and Kraemer (1987), argue that the term *work* should be limited to its Newtonian definition (force × distance), with values reported in joules or kilojoules. However, many people continue to refer to the activities undertaken during paid employment as *work*. On the basis of worksite observations, J.R. Brown and Crowden (1963) suggested gross energy expenditures ranging from 8 kJ/min during light work to 31 or more kJ/min for very heavy work.

Early investigators studying the apparent epidemic of cardiovascular disease (J.N. Morris, 1951) focused on occupational physical activity (J.N. Morris, Heady, Raffle, G. Roberts, & Parks, 1953; Paffenbarger, 1977), arguing that such activity was particularly likely to have a favorable influence on both aerobic fitness and cardiovascular health because an individual's classification (active or sedentary) was likely to be sustained for 30 to 40 years of working life. However, such studies could make only a crude classification of occupational activity. Because of seniority or the onset of symptoms of cardiovascular disease, a worker was sometimes transferred to a less demanding task without a change in his or her official job description. Moreover, any effect from work-related classifications of habitual activity was often confounded by differences of ethnic group, socioeconomic status, and personal lifestyle. In part because they were less tired and had a higher socioeconomic status, individuals classed as having sedentary jobs commonly adopted more active leisure pursuits than those who reported that they were engaged in heavy occupational activity (Canada Fitness Survey, 1983).

There still remain occasional occupations with a high energy demand, for instance, the postal carrier who must carry heavy loads over long distances and up many steps (Shephard, 1983c). However, mechanization and automation have greatly complicated job classification by reducing the energy cost of some supposedly heavy jobs to the point that they demand little more physical activity than light work. Thus, in terms of the primary index of aerobic fitness, the maximal oxygen intake, Allen (1966) observed only minor differences between those who were engaged in heavy and those engaged in light employment, even after standardizing data for leisure pursuits.

For all of these reasons, epidemiologists have found *work* progressively less useful as a basis of categorizing an individual's level of habitual physical activity, and irrespective of the type of employment, most people must now seek to maintain or improve their personal fitness during their leisure time, rather than relying on the vigor of their occupational activities.

Domestic Chores

In the developed western world, changes in domestic furnishings, the introduction of power equipment (such as washing machines and vacuum cleaners), and the increased use of disposable items have reduced the cost of most domestic chores far below the classic figures cited by Durnin and Passmore (1967). Most housework now involves only light physical activity, the one exception being the care of dependents. Both play with young children and the nursing of elderly relatives can still make quite heavy physical demands on caregivers. Other householders sometimes boost their daily energy expenditure more or less deliberately by such activities as gardening or do-it-yourself home improvement projects.

In less developed societies, normal household duties (including the cultivation of food for the family, the carrying of water, and the search for firewood) remain a substantial segment of the total daily energy expenditure for the majority of the population. Cycling or walking to and from the place of work or education is also an important source of regular physical activity in some countries.

Physical Education

Physical education may connote either a voluntary or a required program of physical activity, taught within a school (or sometimes a university) system. In Canada, primary school students receive one to five 30- to 45-min periods of physical activity each week. At this age, instruction is typically given by the ordinary classroom teacher. Specialists usually teach the 3 to 4 years of required programs and the final 2 to 3 years of optional programs in high school, and through university.

Physical educators have stridently argued the need for a quality, required daily program of instruction, taught by specialists, throughout the child's years of schooling (Bailey, 1974; Shephard, 1982a). Nevertheless, many instructors fail to bring students to an adequate intensity of aerobic activity for more than a few minutes of the supposed exercise period, and it remains uncertain whether the usual school program has any impact on either the immediate aerobic fitness of children (Goode et al., 1976; Pate & Shephard, 1989; Shephard, 1992a) or their exercise behavior after leaving school.

Traditionally, physical education programs have been heavily influenced by Swedish gymnastics and military drill, which emphasize rhythmic calisthenics. Many students heartily detest such programs and often adopt very sedentary lifestyles immediately after leaving school (Ilmarinen & Rutenfranz, 1980). Some U.S. schools place a heavy emphasis on competitive team sports such as American football and basketball. These programs also have a high drop-out rate during adolescence and early adult life. Defections begin with students who fail to develop an appropriate body build for their chosen sport at adolescence (Shephard, Lavallée, & LaRivière, 1978). And perhaps because of difficulties in finding suitable teams or discouragement caused by declining performance levels, holders of major athletic "letters" at U.S. universities often become less active by early middle-age than their "nonathletic" peers (Montoye, Van Huss, Olson, Pierson, & Hudec, 1957).

Recently, physical educators have shifted their emphasis to teaching activities that are likely to improve immediate health and to carry over into adult life: family-oriented pursuits such as walking, cycling, canoeing, and swimming (Shephard, 1982a). It has further been recognized that program content should change progressively with the age of the student. In the first 2 years of primary school, the focus should be on learning basic motor skills. From the age of 8 to 10 years, activities that develop cardiorespiratory function and muscular endurance should be added. In early adolescence, the student can explore a variety of sports and active leisure pursuits to discover those for which he or she has a special aptitude.

In later adolescence, students' motivation may be sustained and enhanced by linking the required activity to exploration of the natural environment (Telama, 1978, 1991), through such pursuits as hiking, canoeing, and cross-country skiing. Finally, at all ages it is important to link physical activity instruction with teaching on other aspects of personal lifestyle.

Leisure Activity

The average person in developed societies has 3 to 4 hr of free, leisure, or discretionary time each day (Hanke, 1979; Stundl, 1977). Wide interindividual variations in free time reflect corresponding differences in the duration of paid work (including overtime and "moonlighting"), the travel time to and from work, the number and age of any dependents, the division of labor within the home, and the economic need for self-sufficiency activities, such as the cultivation of crops or maintenance and repair of the home. Leisure activity is undertaken in discretionary time and can potentially lead to a significant increase in daily energy expenditure. Options include exercise, sport, training, dance, and play.

EXERCISE. The term *exercise* implies that leisure activity is being undertaken for a specific purpose, such as an improvement of health or an increase of personal fitness. Often, a physician or an exercise specialist carefully prescribes the regimen, specifying the mode of activity, its intensity, frequency, and duration, and the recommended temporal pattern (continuous or intermittent activity; American College of Sports Medicine, 1990; see chapter 4). Sometimes, a subject may feel compelled to conform to the recommendation and suffer a sense of guilt or failure if unable to do so.

The health-seeking motivation of the participant has particular importance when examining the relationship of physical activity to personal lifestyle. Some large national surveys of physical activity have found little association between abstinence from cigarettes and regular physical activity (Norwegian Confederation of Sport, 1984; Perrier, 1979; Shephard, 1986c, 1989b). However, if health-seeking activity is distinguished from activity that has other motives (social interaction, excitement, competition, vertiginous stimulation, esthetics, or the quest for the body beautiful; Kenyon, 1968), then an association between health-seeking physical activity and abstinence from cigarettes can be demonstrated (Perrier, 1979; Shephard, 1986c, 1989b).

SPORT. Europeans have used the word *sport* to describe all forms of recreational activity, not only competitive games, but also individual, health-related aerobic pursuits such as walking and jogging (McIntosh, 1980; Oja, 1991). The English might even be tempted to add to their definition of sport such pursuits as hunting, fishing, and shooting. However, for our present purpose, it seems preferable to retain the North American concept of sport as vigorous physical activity that is pursued in a quest for such pleasures as social interaction, excitement, competition, danger, and vertiginous stimulation. Required school sport is conveniently categorized with physical education, and professional sport (for simplicity) is not discussed.

The elements of excitement, competition, and danger immediately introduce psychological factors that modify the physiological and biochemical reactions to a given intensity of effort (Blimkie, Cunningham, & Leung, 1977). For example, the secretion of catecholamines is much greater when a person plays a hockey game than when performing an equivalent intensity of aerobic exercise on a cycle ergometer. In consequence, apparently equal doses of these two types of physical activity may have substantially different effects on health.

TRAINING.   Training implies participation in a program of regular and vigorous physical activity with the primary intention of improving either physical performance or health through the development of some component of fitness, such as cardiovascular function or muscular strength. Attempts to combine programs of cardiorespiratory and muscular conditioning often limit the response in one or both domains (see chapter 4).

If the focus of the program is on the development of cardiovascular function, variables influencing the individual's response include the intensity of the required activity relative to the initial physical condition of the individual, the frequency and duration of individual training sessions, and the total length of the training program. It is generally agreed that the first of these variables is the most important (American College of Sports Medicine, 1990; Shephard, 1968b). The precise dose-response relationship for the enhancement of aerobic fitness and the optimization of related aspects of health is less certain (American College of Sports Medicine, 1990; Haskell, 1991). However, there is growing evidence of a gradual response of both variables to sustained bouts of quite moderate aerobic exercise (S.N. Blair, Kohn, Paffenbarger, Clark, Cooper, & Gibbons, 1989). An excessive amount of training can actually impair cardiorespiratory function, suppressing many elements of the immune system and exposing the individual to an increased risk of acute infections (Fry, Morton, & Keast, 1991; Niemann, Johanssen, Lee, & Arabatzis, 1990).

DANCE AND PLAY.   Dance involves rhythmic movements of both the body and the limbs, generally to music. With the possible exception of aerobic dance classes, dance is not usually viewed as an important source of physical conditioning. The quest is rather for social interaction or the esthetics of body movement. Nevertheless, participation in an evening of dance can demand both a substantial intensity of physical activity and an appreciable total energy expenditure. Dancing is a particularly attractive form of physical activity for older people, because, in addition to opportunities for social interaction, the rhythm of the music can be selected to regulate the intensity of effort, and the variety of movement provides a greater source of motivation than stereotypical exercise programs.

Play is a category of leisure activity in which the primary motivation is a semispontaneous détente. Some forms of play are largely sedentary, but particularly in young children, spontaneous play can also involve quite vigorous physical activity, typically in short bursts.

Patterns of Physical Activity

A broad distinction may be drawn between rhythmic, dynamic movements where there is little increase of muscle tension and strongly opposed efforts where there is little movement. Dynamic contractions tend to develop cardiorespiratory function, whereas opposed contractions develop muscular performance. A dynamic contraction may involve a shortening or a lengthening of the muscle. Such efforts are termed *concentric* and *eccentric* contractions, respectively. One form of aerobic exercise with a substantial eccentric component is the task of running downhill on a laboratory treadmill. Such activity places a heavy load on the muscles that are involved, and they may be sore for several days following an exercise session.

If the activity is intermittent rather than continuous, it is important to specify the duration of both active and recovery phases. Short bursts of intensive aerobic activity can be sustained by local oxygen stores in the blood and myoglobin, but if the active phase lasts for 30 s or longer, there is a progressive increase of blood lactate that must be metabolized during the recovery intervals (I. Åstrand, P.O. Åstrand, Christensen, & Hedman, 1960).

Finally, it is necessary to consider the volume of active muscle and body posture. Repetitive large-muscle movements are generally limited by cardiorespiratory function (see chapter 2), but if only a few smaller muscles are involved in the activity, then the task becomes increasingly dependent on peripheral factors (Shephard, Bouhlel, Vandewall, Monod, 1988a). If the active body parts are held above heart level (e.g., a person who is painting a ceiling with a small brush), gravitational forces are also likely to limit the local delivery of oxygen to the working muscles (I. Åstrand, 1971).

INTENSITY.   The intensity of physical activity may be expressed as an absolute rate of working, for example, the external power output in watts measured on a cycle ergometer. The difficulty with this approach is that the physiological strain imposed on the subject varies with the size of the individual and the mechanical efficiency with which he or she can convert chemical energy into the measured form of external work. Some tasks such as cycling, stepping, and walking have a fairly consistent mechanical efficiency, with an interindividual variation of only 5% to 10% about the mean value for a given age. But if the power output were to be measured in a technically demanding sport such as swimming, then the mechanical efficiency could vary by as much as 400% between a champion competitor and an indifferent recreational swimmer.

The oxygen consumption provides an alternative measure of the intensity of physical activity. It may be expressed in L/min or mmol/s under standard dry-gas conditions of temperature and pressure (STPD; see the appendix). This approach eliminates problems arising from interindividual differences of mechanical efficiency, but there remains a fourfold difference of peak oxygen intake between a well-trained endurance competitor (4.5 mmol/s; 6 L/min) and a typical sedentary older person (1.1 mmol/s; 1.5 L/min). Thus, the determination of oxygen consumption during a bout of submaximal exercise provides little information about the physiological load that a given task imposes on a particular individual.

A third option is to class the intensity of effort in terms of the oxygen cost of the task per unit of body mass (μmol/[kg·s]; ml/[kg·min]). This is a very convenient method of data standardization for many activities (see the appendix), because the oxygen cost of tasks that involve a displacement of body mass varies almost directly with that mass (Godin & Shephard, 1973a). An analogous approach is to express all observations as ratios of resting metabolism (METS), usually assumed to average 2.6 μmol/(kg·s) or 3.5 ml/(kg·min). MET units have become quite popular among clinicians, particularly as a simple means of prescribing activities in rehabilitation programs. Although mass standardization is generally quite an effective means of both expressing and regulating the intensity of effort, in weight-supported activities such as cycling, rowing, and swimming, a heavy individual operates at a lower relative stress than a person whose body mass is below average.

A final possibility is to express the observed intensity of activity relative to some index of the individual's peak aerobic power. The calculation may be based on the observed maximal oxygen intake, the peak power output, the observed heart rate relative to the corresponding peak value, the fraction of the heart rate reserve that is being utilized (observed heart rate/[peak heart rate − resting heart rate]), or a rating of perceived exertion (on the original scale of Borg, 1971, the perceived exertion ranges from 6 units at rest to 18-20 units in peak effort). There are two practical obstacles to such approaches: (1) the individual's peak oxygen intake, peak power output, peak heart rate, and peak rating of exertion differ somewhat even between such standard laboratory tasks as uphill treadmill running, cycle ergometry, and bench stepping (Shephard et al., 1968a), and (2) in any given set of circumstances an adverse environment or a transient illness may substantially modify peak values relative to the figures measured or assumed for optimal conditions (Wright, Sidney, & Shephard, 1978).

Concepts of what is intense effort vary widely from one discipline to another. The nutritionist is concerned with the subject's average food intake a week; energy expenditures of 7 to 10 MJ/day may thus be classed as sedentary, and expenditures of 14 to 16 MJ/day as very vigorous activity. The industrial physician considers the performance that can be sustained over a 7- to 8-hr day. Based on brief measurements of oxygen consumption using a Kofranyi-Michaelis respirometer (see chapter 3), J.R. Brown and Crowden (1963) classed occupational activities demanding less than 8.4 kJ/min as light work, 8.4 to 13.8 kJ/min as light to moderate work, 13.8 to 20.9 kJ/min as moderate to heavy work, 20.9 to 31.4 kJ/min as heavy to very heavy, and more than 31.4 kJ/min as very heavy work. In evaluating the industrial classification, it is important to recognize that peak intensities of occupational activity are rarely sustained over the entire working day, and that observations may have been biased upwards because recording periods were short. The person prescribing aerobic exercise takes a third perspective; interest is usually focused on bouts of exercise that last for only 15 to 30 min. Potential intensities for a young adult show a very wide range, from 5 kJ/ min at rest to perhaps 75 kJ/min or more in maximal aerobic effort. Table 1.1 summarizes the type of intensity categorization used in exercise prescription, expressing all values in METS, and taking account also of the expected decrease in peak aerobic performance with age.

FREQUENCY.   Many activities, both occupational and recreational, are seasonal in nature. It is usual to ask individual subjects about the frequency of participation over the past week or month, but attempts to elicit longer periods of recall lead to increasingly inaccurate assessments. It is thus helpful to question different segments of a population sample at different times throughout an entire year.

Frequency is usually reported as the number of activity sessions undertaken in a typical week, although some surveys (e.g., the Canada Fitness Survey, 1983) have also noted activities performed at least once a month or once a year. If prompt cards are used, a surprising number of occasional activities may be elicited. Usually, this will tend to exaggerate the extent of the individual's overall involvement in physical activity, but for some purposes it may be important to know about occasional very intense occupational or recreational activities.

DURATION.   The duration of a typical activity session is reported in minutes. Commonly, the duration is overstated, and it is important that the respondent *exclude* the time spent in travel, socializing, changing, and other preparations for a given activity.

DOSE-RESPONSE RELATIONSHIP.   What is the form of the dose-response relationship linking the amount of physical activity that a person undertakes

Table 1.1
Perceived Intensity of Physical Activity

Semantic intensity	Relative intensity (% max. aerobic power)	Absolute intensity (METS)			
		Young	Middle-aged	Old	Very old
Rest	7-25*	1.0	1.0	1.0	1.0
Light	<35	<4.5	<3.5	<2.5	<1.5
Moderate	<50	<6.5	<5.0	<3.5	<2.0
Heavy	>50	<9.0	<7.0	<5.0	<2.8
Very heavy	>75	>9.0	>7.0	>5.0	>2.8
Maximum	100	~13	~10	~7	~4

Note. Reprinted from Bouchard et al. (1990) by permission.

*The percentage of maximal aerobic power corresponding to a resting state varies with the age and the fitness of the individual.

(some combination of intensity × frequency × duration), and any biological response (assessed by gains of aerobic fitness or health)? It seems likely that there is a threshold dose of physical activity below which no adaptation occurs, a zone of increasing effect, and a ceiling beyond which there is no further improvement of either aerobic fitness or health. Excessive training may even lead to signs of overdosage, such as poor compliance, long-lasting fatigue, musculo-skeletal injuries, an increased incidence of cardiac problems, and an impaired immune response (see chapter 4; also Fry, Morton, & Keast, 1991; Shephard, Verde, Thomas, & Shek, 1991a). Details of the dose-response relationship are unclear (Haskell, 1991) but probably depend on the type of activity undertaken, the type of benefit sought, the age and initial fitness of the individual, and constitutional factors. Aging seems to narrow the margin between an effective and an excessive dose of exercise, requiring a more careful prescription of physical activity (Shephard, 1990b, 1991c). The effects of a single dose of exercise, both positive and negative, may persist for several days. Further detailed study of the interactions between intensity, frequency, and duration of physical activity is needed to establish a basis for safer and more effective prescription of exercise.

Physical Fitness

When I was a student, my professor thought the term *physical fitness* so vague that he resolutely prohibited its use. H.E. Johnson (1946) wrote,

> Quantitative assessment of physical fitness is one of the most complex and controversial problems of applied physiology. This situation arises in part from lack of general agreement on what constitutes fitness for withstanding various types of stress, and in part from lack of agreement on what measurements allow valid comparisons to be made among different individuals exposed to the same stress. (pp. 535-536)

An expert committee of the World Health Organization struggled with seven successive drafts for a definition of fitness, finally agreeing that fitness was "the ability to perform muscular work satisfactorily" (Shephard, 1968b). This conclusion, hardly earth-shattering, was reached largely because the time available for discussion had been exhausted! Others have conceived fitness as "a capacity for living" (E.C. Davies, Logan, & McKinney, 1961), embracing physical, social, and psychological well-being—the broad field of human ecology (Shephard, 1977a). The fit person is well adapted to the demands of a particular task (Hollmann, 1991), be it athletic competition, the performance of physical or mental work in industry and commerce, participation in hunting, gathering, or cultivating crops, or survival in the face of congenital disorders, infections, metabolic disorders, or neoplasia. Such adaptation may be either inherited or acquired (as a result of training).

Social and psychological adjustments are distinct issues, and this book is concerned mainly with the physical component of fitness, the matching of physical characteristics to environmental demands.

Darwinian Fitness

One of the original hypotheses of the Human Adaptability Project of the International Biological Programme (IBP) (Weiner, 1964; Worthington, 1978) was that a high level of physical fitness might offer a Darwinian advantage to a particular ethnic group colonizing an adverse habitat. This would be the case if fitness increased a people's chances of survival to the age of reproduction or influenced their success in mating, childbirth, and child-rearing. For instance, a fit person might be perceived as a more attractive marriage partner or might be more successful in providing adequate food and shelter for a family under harsh environmental conditions.

However, a detailed evaluation of aerobic power and other components of fitness in a number of hunter-gatherer cultures has not offered much support to the original IBP hypothesis (see chapter 4; also Shephard, 1978). Although in the past groups such as the Inuit of the Canadian Arctic worked long hours in their quest for food, the intensity of the required effort was quite moderate, below the commonly accepted threshold for aerobic training. Moreover, many indigenous populations have lived at the boundaries separating several widely differing eco-systems, and the traditional hunter-gatherer exploiting such habitats faced a correspondingly wide variety of daily physical challenges. In such a situation, no one type of fitness could confer a clear competitive advantage. Indeed, the success of both hunting and survival has often depended more on intelligence and a capacity for technical innovation than on a high level of either aerobic fitness or physical strength. In consequence, interindividual differences of fitness have had little selective effect.

Age, Gender, and Perceptions of Physical Fitness

Members of developed societies show large interindividual differences in their perceptions of physical fitness, depending on their age, gender, and socioeconomic status. The typical male undergraduate at age 20 years seeks a type and level of fitness that will earn him a place on the varsity team. By the age of 30, his objective becomes control of a bulging waistline or a greater sense of physical well-being. At 40, the same person may know several colleagues who have suffered myocardial infarctions, and he now wants a level of fitness that will minimize his own risk of developing overt cardiovascular disease. As the aging process continues its apparently inexorable course, a new problem appears: working capacity shrinks to the point that many formerly simple tasks become quite formidable. Our subject now hopes merely to maintain sufficient fitness to meet the daily demands of the factory and home without undue fatigue, while leaving him some measure of energy both to enjoy his leisure and to cover occasional emergencies.

Bailey, Shephard, Mirwald, and McBride (1974) noted that whereas Canadian men had a perception of their current fitness that accorded fairly well with laboratory measurements of cardiorespiratory function, there was little correlation between a woman's rating of her physical condition and laboratory assessments of aerobic fitness. They hypothesized that in response to the North American sociocultural norms of that era, urban Canadian women were evaluating their physical condition in terms of a good figure, good posture, and good body carriage.

The social changes of the past two decades have done much to equate male and female perceptions of fitness, and perhaps as a consequence, Canadian studies have shown substantial (10%-20%) gains in the aerobic performance of adolescent girls and young women over this period (R. Gauthier, Massicotte, Hermiston, & MacNab, 1983).

Athletic Fitness

Many authors have conceived physical fitness primarily in terms of athletic performance. P.O. Åstrand and Rodahl (1970) implicitly accepted this view when they wrote "physical performance or fitness is determined by the individual's capacity for energy output (aerobic and anaerobic processes), neuromuscular strength (muscle strength and technique) and psychological factors (e.g., his [sic] motivation and tactics)" (p. 6).

The fitness of any competitor is highly task-specific. Through a combination of initial endowment and repeated practice, the athlete attains a level of fitness that has a potential for excellence in a particular event. Thus, endurance competitors are marked by an outstanding development of aerobic function (peak aerobic power output and maximal oxygen intake), but their muscle strength is less than that of competitors in power events. There are two immediate corollaries of the specificity of athletic fitness: (1) any testing of such fitness must be equally specific to the competitor's event (e.g., a swimmer must be evaluated in a pool or a swimming flume; Dal Monte, Faina, & Menchinelli, 1992; Holmér, 1974), and (2) the price of excellence in one type of competition may be an impairment of other aspects of body function (e.g., a marathon runner may actually show a loss of lean tissue from the chest and the arms during prolonged training). Critical factors for success in aerobic competition are the extent to which the peak aerobic performance observed on a treadmill can be reproduced or exceeded when a person is involved in competition or exercising on a sport-specific ergometer, and the efficiency of technique whereby the athlete translates the available, sport-specific aerobic power into propulsion of the body along the track or across the pool.

Endurance athletes often seek and achieve a much higher standard of aerobic fitness than is demanded or even needed by *homo sedentarius*, the ordinary citizen of a large metropolis. The discipline of undertaking many hours of physical training each day undoubtedly builds some aspects of the competitor's character, but the relentless pursuit of an Olympic goal by a teenager can also lead to a serious neglect of normal social and psychological development. Further, interest in a healthy lifestyle may be lost quite rapidly when the age of peak athletic performance has passed (P.O. Åstrand et al., 1963; Montoye et al., 1957).

Performance-Related Fitness

The fitness of children enrolled in school programs of physical education has traditionally been evaluated by a battery of performance tests, such as a 50-meter sprint and the number of sit-ups performed in 1 minute (American Alliance for Health, Physical Education, Recreation and Dance [AAHPERD], 1980; Conger, Quinney, Gauthier, & Massicote, 1982). Moreover, the achievement of individual students relative to population norms for such tests has provided a criterion for motivational awards such as those offered by the President's Council on Physical Fitness and Sports (1985).

However, it has long been recognized that the scores on such tests are heavily influenced not only by the genetic endowment of the individual and by training, but also by body size, motivation, opportunities for practice of the required skills, and immediate environmental conditions (G.R. Cumming, 1971; Drake, White, & Shephard, 1969; Shephard & Lavallée, 1978). Recently, the trend has been to modify performance test batteries by including such items as skinfold thicknesses and a distance run of 1.0 to 2.4 km (Pate & Shephard, 1989), with claims that the revised test battery measures health-related fitness (AAHPERD, 1980).

Occupational Fitness

Karpovich and Sinning (1971) suggested that physical fitness is "the degree of the ability to execute a specific physical task under specific ambient conditions." If the concern at hand is for a high level of immediate worksite productivity rather than long-term health, then both the type and the level of fitness required will vary greatly with a person's occupation. The mental efficiency of a civil service clerk or a production-line worker may be impaired by a combination of boredom and a low level of habitual physical activity, but the impairment can probably be corrected by either a brief burst of arousing exercise or some other diversion from normal duties (LaPorte, 1966; Shephard, 1986a, 1986b, 1989a).

In contrast, there can be a substantial loss of physical working capacity if a miner or a lumberjack has an inadequate level of aerobic fitness. Those who are employed in physically demanding occupations find difficulty in returning to a full normal working day if their aerobic fitness and muscle strength have been impaired by bed rest following illness or injury, and they show corresponding benefit from an occupationally specific fitness program (Fried & Shephard, 1969, 1970). Many physically active occupations call for general endurance associated with a large peak power output and maximal oxygen intake, but in other tasks local training is needed. Thus, a house painter may benefit from specific strengthening of the wrist and shoulder muscles (I. Åstrand, 1971).

Pravosudov (1978) claimed that in the Soviet factories of the 1970s, worker athletes produced 4% to 10% more than their sedentary peers. However, the selection of "premium employees" with high motivation could have accounted for both athletic involvement and greater productivity (Baun, Bernacki, & Tsai, 1986). Danielson and Danielson (1982) reported that Canadian forest firefighters who had participated in an aerobic training program were able to cut a longer firebreak in one day than untrained controls, but the superiority of the trained workers was apparent only when it was necessary to fight a fire under the added cardiovascular stress of very hot and arduous conditions. Because automation has progressively reduced the physical demands of most industrial tasks, it is now much less common to find a cross-sectional association between a measure of aerobic fitness, such as maximal oxygen intake, and the productivity of a healthy individual. On the other hand, many worksite fitness programs continue to claim small (1%-3%) gains of productivity for employees who participate in their activities (Shephard, 1986a, 1986b, 1989a).

Because aging leads to a progressive decline in oxygen transport and muscle strength, one might anticipate that deteriorating fitness would increasingly limit the occupational performance of older employees. In practice, complaints of inadequate fitness and resultant fatigue are rare among older workers, in part because daily involvement in tasks with a heavy physical demand has conserved the appropriate facets of fitness, and in part because the older worker has effectively reduced the demands of the job through promotion, delegation of duties, or adoption of a slower working pace (Shephard, 1990a).

In extreme old age, the continuing deterioration of function may reduce oxygen transport to perhaps 9 to 10.5 μmol/(kg·s), 12 to 14 ml/(kg·min), a level where the completion of normal household duties becomes fatiguing (Shephard, 1990b, 1991c). At this stage, a training program that restores endurance fitness will add materially to an individual's independence and thus to quality of life.

Health-Related Fitness

Certain physiological and biochemical characteristics, whether inherited or acquired, have a better prognosis than others. In this sense, we may speak collectively of an individual's health-related or physiological fitness, and link this to both activity patterns and health outcomes. Among the variables contributing to health-related fitness, the traditional markers of aerobic fitness (i.e., peak aerobic power, aerobic capacity, and anaerobic threshold) are all important. Other significant items include cardiopulmonary variables (resting heart rate, the blood pressure at rest and during exercise, the electrocardiographic response to exercise, and static and dynamic lung volumes), body composition (the body mass in relation to height, the percentage and distribution of body fat, muscle mass, and tendon and bone structure) and biochemical indices (blood sugar, lipid profile, and measures of immune function).

Aerobic Fitness

The traditional index of aerobic fitness is the maximal oxygen intake, or aerobic power. It may be defined as the plateauing of oxygen intake observed when a subject performs to exhaustion a progressive, large-muscle exercise, such as uphill treadmill running, step climbing, or cycle ergometry. A plateau is commonly defined as an increase in oxygen intake of less than 150 ml/min (i.e., 112 µmol/s) or less than 2 ml/(kg·min) (i.e., 1.5 µmol/[kg·s]) in response to a further substantial increase in the rate of working. Subsidiary evidence of a maximal aerobic effort (Shephard, 1982b) includes a heart rate close to the anticipated peak value for the subject's age (Fox & Haskell, 1968), a respiratory gas exchange ratio greater than 1.15, and an increase of blood lactate that is appropriately large (8-11 mmol/L) relative to the subject's age. The duration of the test is 9 to 11 min, so that no more than a few minutes of peak aerobic effort are required during the measurement. (The physiological determinants of aerobic power are discussed in chapter 2.)

Aerobic power is not synonymous with health-related fitness, though this has sometimes been supposed. Nevertheless, a large aerobic power is one of the most important physiological indicators of good physical condition. It is necessary in many forms of strenuous occupational activity, and the maintenance of aerobic power makes a major contribution to quality of life in old age. Some measure of aerobic power is thus included in any test battery that purports to measure health-related fitness.

Some authors have called a person's peak aerobic power *aerobic capacity*, but this is dimensionally incorrect. Aerobic power corresponds to a rate of working rather than the completion of a specified quantity of work. The aerobic capacity is properly defined as the amount of aerobic effort that can be sustained over a specified period, for example, 30 min. The physiological determinants of aerobic capacity differ somewhat from the factors limiting aerobic power (see chapter 2). In general, aerobic power is better sustained in a fit than in an unfit individual, or (expressed in another way), the fit person can operate at closer to peak aerobic power than a sedentary subject if exercise is required for a prolonged period.

If a subject performs a progressive exercise test, a point is reached at perhaps 70% of maximal oxygen intake when the blood flow to some of the more vigorously contracting muscles fails to meet the local oxygen requirement. Lactate then diffuses into the bloodstream more rapidly than it can be metabolized or excreted, and it accumulates in the peripheral blood (where it can be detected by serial measurements). The physiology of the process is complex (Shephard, 1992c), but the data provide a further index of aerobic function without the necessity of demanding an all-out effort from the subject. Note is taken of the steady work rate or oxygen consumption when the blood lactate concentration reaches an arbitrary plateau value of 2 mmol/L (the so-called *ventilatory threshold*) or 4 mmol/L (the *anaerobic threshold*). Alternatively, approximate values for these two break-points can be derived from the associated changes of ventilation; as work rate increases, the subject's ventilation increases disproportionately to oxygen consumption, and subsequently there is a rapidly increasing elimination of carbon dioxide (McLellan, 1987).

There is usually a fair correlation between aerobic power and the various measures of lactate threshold in any given subject. The determination of breakpoints is particularly useful in evaluating the aerobic fitness of the elderly and patients with clinical disorders, where maximal testing is either impracticable or dangerous, and the normal relationship between submaximal heart rate and oxygen consumption has been distorted by disease (e.g., the sick sinus syndrome) or medication such as beta-blocking drugs.

Cardiopulmonary Variables

Given that the resting cardiac output is relatively constant in individuals of similar body size, a slow resting heart rate implies a large cardiac stroke volume and thus a good myocardial contractility, with a large reserve of cardiac function to meet the demands of aerobic exercise. This usually implies that the individual is well trained. Aerobic fitness is also associated with a low heart rate at any given submaximal rate of working on a standard ergometer (Shephard, 1982b).

A large pulse pressure is commonly a sign of a large cardiac stroke volume and is thus positively associated with aerobic fitness. On the other hand, a high resting blood pressure or an above-average rise of blood pressure during exercise (Guerrera et al., 1991) must be considered indices of poor health-related fitness. Commonly, these findings are linked to obesity, muscle weakness, an adverse lipid profile, and an inadequate level of habitual physical activity, with an increased risk of developing ischemic heart disease, cerebrovascular catastrophe, and renal failure. An excessive rise of blood pressure during exercise may also be an early warning of subsequent hypertension (Jetté, Landry, Sidney, & Blümchen, 1988). Before diagnosing that the resting blood pressure is high, careful attention must be paid to the conditions of measurement, because the anxiety associated with a formal medical examination can in itself increase the resting blood pressure by about 10 mm Hg (Shephard, Cox, & Simper, 1981; M.A. Young, Rowlands, Stallard, Watson, & Littler, 1983). Relaxed values in excess of 160/90 mm Hg are regarded as undesirable.

The finding of a below-average resting blood pressure does not necessarily carry any disadvantage for health, provided that the individual in question can withstand a sudden change of posture without dizziness. However, a failure to maintain the blood pressure on moving from a supine to a vertical posture seems associated with poor venous tone and a low level of aerobic fitness (Holmgren, 1967a). During a progressive exercise test on a treadmill or a cycle ergometer, the transition from a rising to a falling blood pressure is a particularly ominous sign; it usually signals that the left ventricle is failing, secondary to myocardial oxygen lack.

Adverse electrocardiographic findings during a progressive exercise test include substantial horizontal or downsloping ST segmental depression (e.g., a negative voltage of greater than 0.1 mV 80 ms after the main QRS complex), and frequent or polyfocal premature ventricular contractions (PVCs) occurring early during the ventricular repolarization cycle. In a statistical sense, such changes are frequently associated with myocardial ischemia. Although there are also a substantial proportion of subjects who show false positive records (Shephard, 1981), the person with an abnormal exercise electrocardiogram has at least a twofold increase in the risk of succumbing to a myocardial infarction or sudden death within 5 to 10 years (Shephard, 1981) and must thus be considered as having poor health-related fitness.

Lung volumes such as vital capacity were once considered an important indicator of a subject's fitness (Dreyer, 1920). In the young adult, it is now recognized that aerobic fitness is determined much more by cardiovascular than by respiratory function (see chapter 2). Nevertheless, a large vital capacity may give the advantage of added buoyancy to an endurance swimmer. It is also undeniably better for anyone to have a large rather than a small vital capacity, and low values may reflect such hazards as exposure to cigarette smoke and industrial dusts. Moreover, if an older person develops chronic obstructive lung disease, the unpleasant breathlessness associated with using more than 50% of the vital capacity can become the key factor limiting aerobic activity.

Body Composition

A person with a good level of health-related fitness should show a body mass that is close to the actuarial ideal value, with a low percent body fat, an adequate muscle mass, strong but flexible tendons, and bones with an adequate mineral content.

Actuarial tables (Metropolitan Life Insurance Company, 1983; Society of Actuaries, 1959) judge the "ideal" body mass in a person of specified height from its association with a minimal mortality over a specified period subsequent to purchase of an insurance policy or with a maximization of the individual's life expectancy. Recent tables (Metropolitan Life Insurance Company, 1983) make small interindividual adjustments to the specified optimum mass in terms of frame size judged from biacromial breadths. In general, an excess body mass has a negative impact on health-related fitness. It is linked statistically to an increased risk of dying from such medical conditions as ischemic heart disease, diabetes, renal problems, and the complications of surgery. But much depends on the nature of the excess mass in a given individual (fat, muscle, or bone). A low body mass is also disadvantageous from the viewpoint of life expectancy; this reflects in part an association between cigarette smoking and leanness. Nevertheless, some adverse effect of suboptimal mass persists even after adjusting data for current smoking habits, perhaps because of the long-term effects of smoking on the health of former smokers, and perhaps because a lightly muscled person has a greater rise in blood pressure when attempting unaccustomed heavy physical work. For reasons that are not yet well understood, the ideal body mass shows a small increase as a person becomes older (Andres, 1990).

It is easy to progress from the concept of an ideal body mass to the parallel concept of an ideal fat mass that maximizes health-related fitness. Body fat content has traditionally been expressed as a percentage of total body mass.

Values corresponding to the ideal total body mass are then about 14% fat in men and 18% fat in women (although in practice, the discrepancy between male and female values in a sedentary population is usually larger than 4%). A substantial fraction of body fat is distributed subcutaneously. It is thus possible to specify corresponding ideal values for the thickness of a double fold of skin and subcutaneous fat (see Table 1.2).

Any excess of subcutaneous fat is undesirable, but the impact on cardiovascular prognosis seems particularly adverse if there is a masculine rather than a feminine distribution (an accumulation on the abdomen instead of at the hips and thighs; Lapidus et al., 1984; Reichley et al., 1987). This aspect of fitness is assessed by expressing either skinfold readings or body circumferences as a waist-hip ratio (Forbes, 1990).

A person may have weak muscles and an inadequate lean tissue mass as a consequence of constitution, the protein lack associated with malnutrition or excessive dieting, prolonged steroid administration, or the inactivity associated with chronic disease and prolonged bed rest. Local weakness may develop as a response to prolonged aerobic training that has been limited to another region of the body, to specific neuromuscular lesions, or to immobilization of a limb. In all such instances, health-related fitness is less than optimal. For such individuals, a task that would otherwise be a well-tolerated, aerobic form of activity may become anaerobic in type. Difficulty in perfusing the weakened muscles leads to a rapid rise of systemic blood pressure, limitation of the activity by local muscular fatigue (Kay & Shephard, 1969), and an increased risk of catastrophic myocardial ischemia. Moreover, measures to strengthen the affected muscles may greatly improve endurance performance in such individuals (Kavanagh, Lindley, Shephard, & Campbell, 1988; Kavanagh, Yacoub, Mertens, Kennedy, & Campbell, 1988; Mertens, Shephard, & Kavanagh, 1978).

Table 1.2
Skinfold Readings (Mean ± SD) Corresponding
to Actuarial Ideal Body Mass in Young Adults

Skinfold site	Male (mm)	Female (mm)
Chin	5.8 ± 8.7	7.1 ± 2.8
Triceps	7.8 ± 4.1	15.6 ± 6.2
Chest	12.0 ± 7.9	8.6 ± 3.7
Subscapular	11.9 ± 5.1	11.3 ± 4.2
Suprailiac	12.7 ± 7.0	14.6 ± 8.0
Waist	14.3 ± 8.2	15.3 ± 7.5
Suprapubic	11.0 ± 6.4	20.5 ± 8.2
Knee (medial)	8.6 ± 4.1	11.8 ± 4.2
Average (8 folds)	10.4 ± 4.9	13.9 ± 5.1

Note. Adapted from Shephard et al. (1969) by permission.

An excessive increase of body mass, such as is often seen in body builders, wrestlers, and players in contact sports, also seems disadvantageous for overall health (Shephard, 1981). The heavier the torso, the greater the amount of work that must be performed when displacing the body's center of mass; this has negative conseqences for endurance performance and, by increasing the cardiac work rate, may predispose athletes to premature death.

A change in the structure of collagen in the tendons and ligaments (e.g., an increased cross-linkage of fibrils; Shephard, 1987a) leads to a progressive structural weakening and a loss of flexibility. The latter imposes an important limitation on the overall function of older subjects (Shephard, 1990b, 1991c). The awkwardness resulting from impaired mobility increases the energy cost of many tasks, reducing potential performance for a given level of aerobic power. The affected joints also become more vulnerable to injury during aerobic activity, and ultimately limitations in the range of motion at major joints threaten both independence and the quality of life (Shephard, 1991c). Flexibility of the joints is thus an important element of health-related fitness.

Weakened bones are susceptible to both falls and overuse injuries, and the resultant musculoskeletal problems have a negative impact on long-term interest in physical activity and thus endurance fitness. Therefore, the maintenance or increase of bone density is a significant component of programs to improve health-related fitness. Regular weight-bearing or resisted activity apparently has such an effect (E.L. Smith, Raab, Zook, & Gilligan, 1989). However, if aerobic training, such as distance running, is pursued to the point of lean tissue loss and a reduction in blood levels of reproductive hormones (most obvious in the female, because of an associated athletic amenorrhea), there is usually some decrease of bone density (Drinkwater, Nilson, Ott, & Chesnut, 1986).

Biochemical Indicators

There is an optimum range of blood sugar readings for health. High values either at rest or after ingestion of a standard quantity of glucose imply an increased risk of developing diabetes. In general, aerobic training leads to an improvement in both values. At the opposite extreme, very low resting or exercise blood glucose levels (<3mM) can lead to fatigue and impaired cerebral function during sustained endurance activity (Niinimaa, Wright, Shephard, & Clarke, 1977).

Good health is also associated with a favorable lipid profile, including a low total-cholesterol concentration, a high ratio of HDL-cholesterol to total-cholesterol (particularly the subfraction, HDL-2-cholesterol), and high plasma concentrations of the associated Apo-protein A-I (Haskell, 1984, 1991; Kottke et al., 1986; Rifkind & Segal, 1983). Again, the person with a high level of aerobic fitness commonly has a favorable lipid profile, but it is less certain that aerobic fitness must be increased in order to optimize blood lipids.

The last 10 years have seen increasing investigation of the interaction between physical activity and immune function. A number of measures, such as immunoglobulin concentrations, the ratio of helper to suppressor T-cells, and the response of peripheral blood monocytes to specific mitogens, show that moderate aerobic training enhances resting immune function (Shephard, Verde, S.G. Thomas, & Shek, 1991). Beneficial consequences such as a greater resistance to infection, a lower risk of developing a neoplasm, and a lower incidence of autoimmune diseases might be suggested (Mackinnon, 1992), although the quantitative health significance of the immune changes has yet to be evaluated. On the other hand, the dose of exercise seems critical for the immune system, and excessive aerobic training is associated with at least a temporary depression of immune function (Mackinnon, 1992; Shephard, Verde, Thomas, & Shek, 1991). Newsholme (1990) hypothesizes that glutamine is an important substrate for the genesis of lymphocytes and that the adverse effects of excessive exercise may therefore be linked to reduced migration of glutamine from the overworked muscle into the bloodstream.

Aerobic Fitness and the Duration of Physical Activity

No single, compact definition of fitness could encompass all the ideas of Darwinian, athletic, performance-related, occupational, aerobic, and health-related fitness that we have discussed. However, it is possible to narrow the search for descriptors of a well-adapted individual if we arbitrarily distinguish the period of activity for which fitness is sought.

In brief efforts (i.e., activities with a duration of less than 1 min), a good performance depends on muscular strength, coordination, agility, flexibility, swift reaction times, and a high level of motivation. Moreover, the subject must tolerate a large accumulation of lactate and hydrogen ions in the active tissues. In activities of moderate duration (1 min to 1 hr), fitness is still influenced by almost all of these factors, but they become progressively subordinate to the ability of the body to transfer oxygen from the atmosphere to the working muscles. In protracted activities (longer than 1 hr), fitness becomes increasingly dependent on the extent and availability of energy reserves in the active tissues (intramuscular glycogen and fat) and on the subject's ability to replenish these stores from the diet, from glycogen and fat deposits elsewhere within the body, and from the hepatic synthesis of glucose (the process of gluconeogenesis). The dissipation of heat and the establishment of an appropriate balance between the intake of water and its loss in sweat and exhaled gas also assume an increasing importance if the duration of activity is extended beyond a few minutes.

Many athletic events demand quite brief efforts. At the opposite extreme, the marathon cyclist, the Inuit hunter, and the soldier on a forced march may all be interested in the type of conditioning that facilitates several days of continuous exercise. But the great mass of ordinary citizens, if they are interested in fitness at all, are concerned with the ability to undertake vigorous activity of moderate duration, what we may term *aerobic fitness*. Aerobic fitness is the main physiological determinant of success in completing any projects in the home or the factory that demand sustained heavy work. Moreover, if we are to show a relationship between the fitness of the individual and such aspects of health as obesity and cardiovascular disease, it will likely reflect the striking of a suitable balance between the intake of food and the performance of regular, moderate aerobic exercise of the type likely to improve aerobic fitness.

Aerobic fitness is not synonymous with the ability to carry large quantities of oxygen from the atmosphere to the working tissues. The body fat content, the strength of key muscles, and the performance of the heart while under load are also important determinants of the ability to undertake long periods of moderate, rhythmic exercise. Nevertheless, the primary factor limiting the performance of such activity is undoubtedly *aerobic power*, the ability of the cardiorespiratory system to transport oxygen from the atmosphere to the working muscles (see chapter 2).

The person with a high level of aerobic fitness has three basic characteristics (Darling, 1946):

1. An ability to maintain the various processes involved in metabolic exchange close to the resting state during strenuous but submaximal, dynamic exercise
2. An ability to reach and sustain a high peak rate of working
3. An ability to restore promptly all equilibria that have been disturbed when the activity is halted

Ideally, testing is based on the second characteristic (the maximal oxygen intake, or the peak power output observed during several minutes of all-out effort). However, if the facilities available to the investigator are limited, it may also be inferred from the first characteristic (as the heart rate or perceptual response to a standard bout of submaximal exercise), or from the third characteristic (as the speed of recovery of heart rate, respiratory minute volume, or blood pressure following a standard bout of submaximal exercise; see chapter 3). If any reliance is to be placed on the responses observed during submaximal or recovery tests, the task must be as fully learned as possible, in order to avoid complications from interindividual differences of anxiety and clumsiness during testing (Shephard, 1969).

It is often helpful to supplement a basic cardiorespiratory fitness evaluation by testing other body systems, but we may note that the person who is obese or who has weak muscles generally scores poorly on the various tests of aerobic fitness. The cardiorespiratory component of the test battery thus gives a good overall index of the person's ability to perform sustained physical work in industry and the home.

Health

The World Health Organization (1948) has defined health not as the mere absence of disease, but rather as a state of "complete mental, physical and social well-being." Each of the mental, physical, and social dimensions of health is characterized by positive and negative poles. Positive health is associated with an optimum lifestyle, a comfortable level of stress, a feeling of well-being, a capacity to enjoy life, and a tolerance of environmental challenges, whereas negative health is associated with increases in various measures of morbidity and premature mortality.

A person's lifestyle includes many individual behaviors that can affect health status. Favorable attributes include the taking of regular meals, physical activity of appropriate intensity, frequency, and duration, and adequate periods of sleep (an average of 7-8 hr each night). Among quite a long list of potential adverse habits are smoking and the consumption of excessive quantities of alcohol or other drugs. There is some tendency to a linkage between these various behaviors, with some people showing a more prudent overall lifestyle than others (Shephard, 1989b).

Selye (1978) has associated what he terms a eustress condition with optimal health. For example, in a boring, repetitive job, the normal level of stress is less than optimal. An individual holding such a job is said to be underaroused. A regimen of vigorous exercise can then be helpful in augmenting arousal to a eustress level, with an associated improvement in the individual's overall health. At the other extreme, the performance of mentally demanding jobs with a high level of responsibility or unclear managerial expectations can impose an excessive stress on a worker, resulting in manifestations of poor health such as peptic ulcers and a clinical anxiety state. For such people, vigorous, aerobic exercise would tend to increase arousal and would thus be contraindicated. On the other hand, light, relaxing exercise might reduce arousal to a level optimizing both worksite performance and health (Shephard, 1988c).

Traditional measures of illness do not provide a good assessment of the broad concept of health and well-being proposed by WHO. More appropriate indicators of health status include (1) self-reports on a Likert-type scale that links perfect health with overt illness, (2) objective measures of the individual's societal contribution, such as worksite productivity and absenteeism, and (3) the individual's demand for medical services, including office visits, hospital admissions, and the purchase of prescribed and nonprescribed drugs.

In the context of the WHO approach, morbidity may be defined as any departure, subjective or objective, from a state of complete mental, physical, or social well-being. Potential indices of population morbidity include (1) the number of persons per unit of population who report an illness during a given year (incidence), (2) the number of persons per unit of population found to be ill on any given date (prevalence), (3) the incidence or prevalence of specific conditions (e.g., the annual incidence of an indicator of ischemic heart disease, such as anginal pain or ST segmental depression), (4) the average duration of specific conditions (e.g., the average period of work lost when a person aged 40-50 years suffers a myocardial infarction), and (5) the cumulative years of positive health lost over a person's lifespan, or an equivalent, quality-adjusted lifespan (e.g., Kaplan, 1985, argues that the quality-adjusted lifespan is only about 50% of the observed calendar value if the remaining years of life must be spent in a wheelchair).

Mortality, though unfortunately ignoring the quality of life enjoyed by survivors, is more easily measured than other indices of health status. It is commonly expressed as the observed death rate for an age- and gender-specific sample of the population. Alternative measures of mortality include the typical life expectancy at a given age, the loss of productive years per unit of population due to death before the normal age of retirement, or (when a prediction of future mortality is made from current lifestyle) the calculation of an appraised age based on the chances of dying from the 12 most common conditions over a specified period, such as the next 10 years of the individual's life (Spasoff, McDowell, Wright, & Dunkeley, 1980).

Interactions Between Physical Activity, Aerobic Fitness, and Health

The basic model linking physical activity, fitness, and health is illustrated in Figure 1.1. The American Medical Association (AMA, 1966) notes that ''physical fitness depends on the individual's state of health, constitution, and present and previous physical activity.'' An increase of physical activity may be expected to increase various components of the individual's fitness, and any improvements in the aerobic component are in turn likely to improve his or her health. An increase of physical activity may also influence health less directly, by modifying some intervening variable; for example, it may reduce the risk of colonic cancer simply by speeding the passage of potential carcinogens through the gastrointestinal tract (Shephard, in press-b). Reciprocal effects may be anticipated. The model is further complicated by uncertainties regarding the dose-response relationships at each of the potential sites of interaction. Finally, many intervening variables modify the observed health responses to a given dose of activity or a given level of aerobic fitness.

Reciprocal Effects

Lack of aerobic fitness has many negative consequences for habitual physical activity. The sedentary or obese individual finds physical activity less pleasant than a more active person. Personal appearance may discourage wearing shorts or a swimsuit, and attempts at vigorous activity may lead to unfamiliar breathlessness or rapid overheating of the body. There may also be difficulty in meeting the expectations of a young and vigorous program leader, with a lack of the positive feedback that a fitter person would gain from a successful performance of the required activities.

A poor state of health, whether perceived by the individual or objectively observed, is even more likely to lead to a low level of physical activity. Negative consequences of perceived or diagnosed ill-health include personal fears about the adverse effects of exercise, activity restrictions imposed by a parent or physician, the development of unpleasant symptoms such as dyspnea when exercise is attempted, and pathological changes in the oxygen transport system that

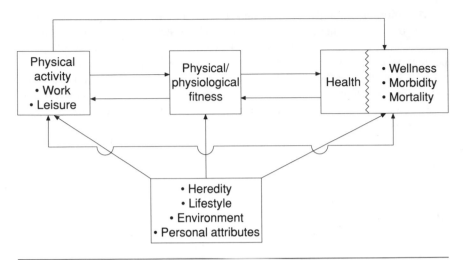

Figure 1.1   Model illustrating potential interactions between physical activity, fitness, health, and intervening variables. *Note.* Reprinted from Bouchard et al. (1990) by permission.

set an unusually low ceiling to aerobic activities. Limitation of activity by some pathological disorders may induce a vicious cycle of loss of aerobic fitness and muscle strength, worsening symptoms and restricting still further any habitual physical activity.

Intervening Variables

Personal attributes (e.g., age and gender), socioeconomic status, personality type, heredity, and environment are important intervening variables that can modify the interactions between physical activity, aerobic fitness, and health.

Increasing age is usually associated with a decrease in habitual activity (see chapter 3). It is not clear how far the reduction of physical activity is socially conditioned, but in view of the wide distribution of the phenomenon across species other than humans, it seems at least in part an inherent expression of aging. There is also a substantial gradient of aerobic fitness with age (see chapter 3). It is uncertain how far this is a true reflection of aging such as an impairment of regulatory systems (leading to a lesser exercise-induced increase of heart rate and myocardial contractility) or a deterioration of key organs (e.g., an ischemic limitation on the peak pumping ability of the left ventricle), and how far it is merely a secondary consequence of the decrease of habitual physical activity (Shephard, 1988a). Certainly, aging is associated with an increase in the prevalence of chronic disease, with inevitable consequences for both participation in physical activity and resulting levels of aerobic fitness (Canada Health Survey, 1982; Shephard, 1987b).

Gender-related differences in physical activity and levels of aerobic fitness first appear at adolescence (see chapter 3). Until recently, girls have been much less encouraged to pursue an active lifestyle than have boys, and it is thus unclear whether the observed differences have a social or a biological basis. There are some physiological reasons why women might have a lower level of aerobic fitness than men; for instance, females have a greater proportion of body fat and a lower average hemoglobin level (Drinkwater, 1984). On the other hand, as social roles have changed, the differences in endurance performance between men and women have narrowed greatly, both in the laboratory (Gauthier et al., 1983) and on the track (O'Brien, Davies, & Daggett, 1982).

Socioeconomic status and educational levels have a major impact on patterns of physical activity (Canada Fitness Survey, 1983; Stephens & Craig, 1990; also see Table 1.3), and these variables are thus likely to influence aerobic fitness status. Poorer and less well-educated individuals are less active, in part because of social conditioning and in part because physical barriers (such as lack of a car, a baby-sitter, or funds for club membership, clothing, and equipment) restrict their participation in fitness programs (Canada Fitness Survey, 1983; Stephens & Craig, 1990).

Personality type influences the psychological response (positive or negative) to a given type of physical activity; for example, the extrovert is attracted to group exercise programs and the introvert to solitary types of activity (Massie & Shephard, 1971). External motivation from a class leader, a physician, or even a coparticipant has a marked influence on early participation in and response to an exercise program, particularly among individuals with an external locus of control. But the ultimate objective of the fitness leader must be to develop a lasting, internal motivation in all class members (Shephard, 1986b).

Inheritance may be cultural or genotypic. Cultural inheritance is not mediated directly by any specific group of genes, but rather is transmitted from parents

Table 1.3
Association Between Level of Education and
Habitual Daily Leisure Energy Expenditure

	Daily energy expenditure percentage (kJ/kg)		
Educational level	High (>12.5)	Moderate (6.3-12.4)	Low (0-6.2)
Less than high school	27	21	52
High school	32	25	43
Some post-high school	34	24	42
University	41	27	33

Note. Reprinted from Stephens and Craig (1990) by permission.

to children by the commonality of educational standards, diet, opportunities for exercise, and other domestic and environmental circumstances that are shared by those who live together. Genetic inheritance is dependent on the transmission of nuclear DNA from parents to their offspring. The resulting interindividual differences of DNA influence both the observed phenotype (e.g., the level of habitual activity adopted and the maximal oxygen intake developed in response to that level) and the extent of adaptive responses to changes in environment such as a decreased intake of food energy or an increase of aerobic activity (Bouchard, 1990, 1992; Lortie et al., 1984).

Local or regional differences in the physical and chemical environment can influence both physical activity patterns and aerobic fitness, with resultant implications for health (McPherson & Curtis, 1986). For example, a climate with high temperatures and a high relative humidity discourages an active lifestyle, but at the same time there is an interaction between heat acclimatization and tolerance of aerobic exercise (InBar, Gutin, Dotan, & Bar-Or, 1978). Likewise, exposure to cold increases the mobilization of fat during aerobic exercise (O'Hara, Allen, & Shephard, 1979; Shephard, in press-c). Maximal oxygen intake is reduced during exposure to low ambient pressures (Shephard, 1982b) and certain types of air pollutants (Folinsbee, 1990). Finally, the social, cultural, political, and economic milieu (including an individual's friendships and the attitudes of his or her community toward a healthy lifestyle) can all affect physical activity patterns, aerobic fitness, and health.

The Practical Importance of Aerobic Fitness

Many scientists still maintain that the practical, social value of physical fitness—or, indeed, the immediate social value of any other topic of scientific inquiry—is unimportant to them. The discovery of truth is its own reward. Certainly, the study of aerobic fitness provides some elegant intellectual challenges, such as understanding the beautifully matched sequence of integrated adaptations that ensure an appropriate increase in the delivery of oxygen to the working muscles at the onset of exercise (Shephard, 1982b), with the fascinating attendant puzzles posed by long transmission lines and the complicated feedback mechanisms that control the body's response.

Scientists are rightly cautious in restricting themselves to ad hoc investigations. National research expenditures on physical activity patterns, fitness, and resulting changes in health remain very small relative to the purchase of such "necessities" as nuclear weapons, cigarettes, and alcohol. Nevertheless, taxpayers increasingly demand to see some practical rationale for all government-sponsored research projects. Moreover, the topic of aerobic fitness offers some exciting opportunities for studies that explore an intermediate ground between the esoteric and the ad hoc. The investigator can conserve the rigor of scientific design that will add to the sum of human knowledge, while answering important practical questions with great relevance to human health and happiness.

The economics of physical fitness is one such area of research (Shephard, 1989a, 1989c; in press-a). In many countries, Canada included, the budgets of federal departments of health and welfare are sadly out of balance. Enormous sums are devoted to high technology medical care, while only a minute fraction of the available funds is directed to the promotion of physical fitness and positive health, measures that could reduce spiralling medical costs. But it is encouraging that the imbalance of funding is now recognized, and that Canadian federal and provincial governments are moving to redirect funds from traditional medical treatment to primary preventive care (Epp, 1986; Evans, 1987; Spasoff, 1987). Plainly, changes in many aspects of personal lifestyle could have a favorable influence on community health. Paffenbarger and associates have argued (Paffenbarger, 1988; Paffenbarger, Hyde, Wing, & Hsieh, 1986) that an increase of habitual activity would be the most effective preventive tactic for North Americans, given the widespread prevalence of a sedentary lifestyle, and its role as a major cause of population morbidity and mortality.

There can be little disagreement that, from an anthropological and evolutionary perspective, humans are designed to undertake regular bouts of moderate physical activity (Weiner, 1964; Worthington, 1978). Equally, there is growing evidence that the majority of people who live in large cities are currently very sedentary (Shephard, 1986c; also see chapter 3). The most vigorous exercise of many office workers is the daily walk from car-to-elevator in the morning and from elevator-to-car in the evening. Much of the physical work in traditional, heavy industries is now carried out by machines, and it is rare to find employees who are operating at an average of more than two or three times their resting energy expenditure. For the rapidly diminishing rural population, the arduous 16-hr day of the primitive homestead has given place to small-town life; work typically involves no more than an 8-hr stint in the padded comfort of an air-conditioned combined harvester. Even arctic hunters now spend long hours watching television, their occasional journeys being made by snowmobile and power boat rather than by dogsled or canoe (Rode & Shephard, 1992). Moreover, the sedentary lifestyle is extending to ever younger ages; children who once spent their leisure time playing active games now watch television for 30 to 35 hr a week (Alderson & Crutchley, 1990; Shephard et al., 1975; Sherif & Rattray, 1976; Tucker, 1990). The long-term developmental effect of such inactivity during the years of growth poses a vital and unanswered question.

The last five decades have seen the development and subsequent waning of a major epidemic of ischemic heart disease (J.N. Morris, 1951; Shephard, 1981). In Canadian men, ischemic heart disease is the primary cause of premature death (Table 1.4). Physical inactivity has undoubtedly contributed to this epidemic (Paffenbarger, 1988; Shephard, 1981; Paffenbarger et al., 1986). Unfortunately, there are major social and economic repercussions (Shephard, 1989c), because those dying of heart attacks tend to be the most hard-driving, productive members of society at the most fruitful time in their careers. To the sobering total of premature deaths must be added the further social burden of those seriously incapacitated by nonfatal attacks. There remains a need for well-controlled studies

Table 1.4
Annual Loss of Productive Years Due to Premature
Deaths of Canadians Between Ages 1 and 70 Years

Cause of death	Males	Females
Motor vehicle accidents	154,000	59,000
Ischemic heart disease	157,000	36,000
Other accidents	136,000	43,000
Respiratory diseases	90,000	50,000
Suicide	51,000	18,000
Total	588,000	206,000

Note. Reprinted from Lalonde (1974) by permission.

of the economic effectiveness of preventive campaigns, but there seems a potential for major economic benefits through an increase in population levels of aerobic fitness (Shephard, 1986a, 1989a, 1989c, in press-a).

There is also an urgent need for research on the social consequences of workplace automation. Despite periodic recessions, in many developed countries it still seems that during much of the economic cycle too many jobs chase too few workers. However, certain by-products of automation are increasingly making themselves felt. The number of hard-core, permanently unemployed is rising in postindustrial societies as labor-intensive occupations are moved to third-world countries. Many of those who are presently without jobs lack either the intelligence or the personality to cope with the remaining opportunities for employment. Pessimists suggest that in the future such individuals never will find full-time employment. Yet even if people have no prospect of working, they still deserve a meaningful leisure rather than a lifetime of impoverished "welfare." How far can an active recreational program satisfy their needs?

An increasing number of companies are adopting compressed working weeks, in part to spread available employment among a larger number of workers and in part to maximize use of the physical plant. Employees put in 3 or 4 very long (10-12 hr) working days and then 3 or 4 "weekend" days (pursuing some do-it-yourself activity or even a second job). The pattern of physical fitness demanded by such a schedule is likely very different from that needed to complete the traditional five 8-hr working shifts a week.

Another current trend is the growth of service industries and the associated reliance on expendable consumer goods. This has eliminated such pursuits as mending the family shoes, repairing the car or bicycle, and tending the garden, all important sources of physical activity for earlier generations. Men, in particular, have been robbed of their traditional physical role around the home. Women have to work faster to complete domestic tasks and serve as a second breadwinner, but power equipment has reduced the energy cost of most of their tasks also. There is thus much scope for voluntary physical activity to make the life of the city-dweller more satisfying and to preserve the capacity for return to a simpler labor-intensive lifestyle, if this becomes necessary because of the current wastage of nonrenewable resources.

Another major concern in many nations is the rapid increase in the proportion of old and very old people. Typically, the elderly spend 10 years of life with some form of chronic disability and are almost totally dependent for the final year of their lives (Canada Health Survey, 1982). However, there have been suggestions that regular endurance exercise could reduce the biological age of active individuals by 10 to 20 years (Shephard, 1991c; see also chapter 4) with a correspondingly decreased likelihood of becoming dependent when a senior (Shephard & Montelpare, 1988; see Table 1.5) and an enormous improvement in the quality of the final years of life.

Finally, fitness researchers must determine the most effective method of persuading someone who has become accustomed to a sedentary life to undertake regular aerobic exercise. Is it better to suggest a modest, easily fulfilled exercise prescription or a more challenging regimen? If the sedentary individual persists with a progressive, demanding exercise regimen, will the result be a level of aerobic fitness similar to that observed in champion endurance athletes? And are large gains in aerobic fitness needed, or is the key to improved health modest but regular physical activity?

Table 1.5
Influence of Reported Physical Activity on Level of
Dependency During Retirement

Activity at age 50 yrs (arbitrary units*, mean ± SD)	Level of disability
9.3 ± 9.8 (n = 286)	None
8.1 ± 8.9 (n = 126)	Minor
7.7 ± 9.4 (n = 173)	Major
4.1 ± 6.6 (n = 25)	Extreme (subject institutionalized)

Note. Reprinted from Shephard and Montelpare (1988) by permission.

*Arbitrary units of exercise dose based on combination of frequency, duration, and intensity of exercise (see article cited for details).

2
Chapter

Physiological Determinants of Aerobic Fitness

This chapter first establishes the centrality of oxygen transport to the regeneration of adenosine triphosphate (ATP) and thus the sustained performance of physical activity, then considers in more detail individual determinants of the oxygen transport process.

Centrality of Oxygen Transport and ATP Regeneration

The immediate basis of human movement is the chemical energy stored in the high energy bonds of a phosphagen compound, ATP. This energy is used to induce a coupling of the contractile proteins of skeletal muscle (actin and myosin); the formation of cross-bridges between the two molecules causes the two protein chains to slide over one another, shortening the activated muscle. The quantity of ATP stored in resting human muscle is small, about 7 mmol/kg of wet tissue, or in a person with 28 kg of muscle, about 200 mmol. Stores of creatine phosphate (CP) and other high energy phosphate compounds bring the total usable phosphagen reserve to about 30 mmol/kg of wet muscle (McGilvery, 1975; Shephard, 1983a). Depending on the pH of the tissue, about 46 kJ of energy is liberated for each mole of phosphagen that is hydrolyzed.

Normally, any ATP that is broken down to adenosine diphosphate (ADP) and phosphate is immediately resynthesized by the breakdown of creatine phosphate to creatine (Henriksson, 1992a, 1992b; McGilvery, 1975), so that the observable response to vigorous exercise is a depletion of CP rather than ATP (see Figure 2.1). Chemical energy is transferred between the two reactions (see Figure 2.2) with a thermodynamic efficiency of about 85% (Shephard, 1982b). However, in part because additional energy is used in such reactions as the pumping of calcium ions through the muscle's sarcoplasmic reticulum (Rall, 1985), only about 40% of the energy liberated from phosphagen (i.e., $46 \times .40$,

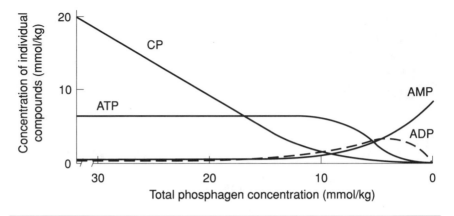

Figure 2.1   Depletion of phosphagen stores in human muscle during a burst of high intensity exercise. *Note*. Adapted from McGilvery (1975) by permission.

or 18.4 kJ/mole; 18.4 × .030, or 552 J/kg of wet muscle) can be applied to the bonding of actin and myosin. Depending on the mass of active muscle (5-20 kg), the phosphagen reserves are thus sufficient to allow the performance of a total of 3 to 12 kJ of external work. An all-out staircase sprint (with an external power output of up to 1.2 kW, or 1.2 kJ/s) can exhaust phosphagen reserves within a few seconds, and even when a person is cycling at a moderate power output of 100 W (0.1 kJ/s), the initial muscle store of ATP and CP would provide energy for no more than 2 min of exercise.

Sustained physical activity thus requires the repeated regeneration of the high energy phosphate bonds. In the presence of oxygen (aerobic metabolism), the chemical energy necessary for such a resynthesis is made available through the breakdown of foodstuffs in the Krebs (citric acid) cycle. Metabolic fuels include intramuscular glycogen and fat, plus free fatty acids and glucose from the bloodstream. The end products that must be eliminated are carbon dioxide and heat, the latter reflecting inefficiencies in the translation of chemical energy to mechanical work (see Figure 2.3). If oxygen is not available, the body relies on anaerobic metabolism. Energy is then derived only from carbohydrate, and metabolism halts at the lactate-pyruvate stage; lactate, the end product of the reaction, accumulates in the muscle cytoplasm.

In theory, any one of the processes involved in the sustained delivery of chemical energy or the removal of the waste products of metabolism could limit phosphagen regeneration, but in practice oxygen delivery seems the preeminent constraint.

Sustained Delivery of Chemical Energy

Some 75% of the energy needed to sustain vigorous aerobic exercise is derived from the breakdown of carbohydrate, mainly glycogen (Shephard, 1982b). Under

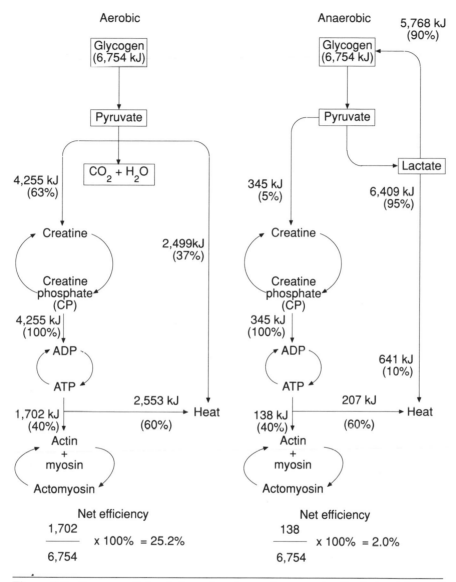

Figure 2.2 Sequence of chemical reactions in muscle contraction for the breakdown of 1 glucosyl equivalent to yield 37 moles ATP, with a total heat liberation of 6,754 kJ. Under aerobic conditions, 63% of this energy drives the phosphagen system; 40% of phosphagen energy is used in actin-myosin bonding. The overall thermodynamic efficiency is approximately 25% (i.e., 40% × 63/100). Under anaerobic conditions, the immediate yield of ATP is 3 moles per glucosyl equivalent, a thermodynamic efficiency of about 2% (i.e., 25 × 3/37). Much of the accumulated lactate is later metabolized elsewhere in the body. With a recycling efficiency of 90%, lactate is in effect reused 10 times, so that the ultimate efficiency of anaerobic metabolism can be as high as 20%.

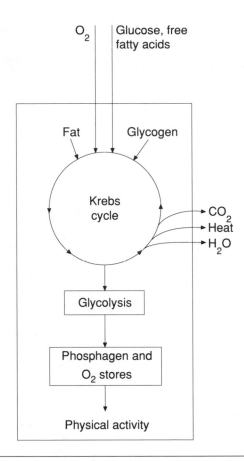

Figure 2.3   Sequence of processes involved in muscle contraction. In theory, endurance performance could be limited by the input of oxygen and foodstuffs to the Krebs (citric acid) cycle or by the buildup of heat, carbon dioxide, lactic acid, and other waste products. *Note*. Adapted from Shephard (1977a) by permission.

normal resting conditions, the muscle sarcoplasm stores about 400 g of glycogen (2.5 moles of glucosyl equivalents), and the liver contains 100 g (0.6 moles; Hultman & Greenhaff, 1992).

If these glycogen reserves were to be utilized over 60 min, they would provide enough fuel to sustain a gross energy expenditure of some 2.2 kJ/s, or 2,200 W. Assuming a mechanical efficiency of 25%, this would produce an external power output of 555 watts. The total energy expended over the hour (3,600 s) would then be 2.2 × 3,600, or 7,920 kJ. Given that an energy expenditure of 1 kJ requires an oxygen consumption of some 48 ml (2.14 mmol), it appears that a person would need to develop an oxygen consumption of more than 6.3 L/min (4.7 mmol/s) throughout the entire hour of exercise in order for the glycogen stores to become the factor limiting performance. In fact, such an oxygen consumption is beyond the ability even of most endurance athletes.

Nevertheless, the performance of repeated sprints fades towards the end of a number of team games such as soccer and ice hockey. I. Jacobs (1981) has suggested that the rate of glycogen metabolism begins to slow if intramuscular reserves of carbohydrate drop below 175 mmol/kg of dry weight, reflecting a 45% rather than 100% depletion of the normal initial reserves of 320 mmol/kg. The peak oxygen consumption of an ordinary sedentary person is only about one third of that found in an endurance athlete, so that it is still unlikely that the steady aerobic performance of the average individual will be limited by depletion of intramuscular glycogen, except on rare occasions when near maximum effort is sustained for 2 hr or more.

Carbon Dioxide Transport

Carbon dioxide transport normally does not limit either the rate of phosphagen regeneration or the performance of aerobic exercise in a young adult, but it can become a significant constraint in certain circumstances, for instance, during underwater exploration or in chronic respiratory disease. When underwater, the subject's ventilation is hampered by the increased density of respired gas, and the circulatory transport of carbon dioxide is also impeded by the influence of the increased partial pressure of oxygen on the combination of carbon dioxide with the hemoglobin molecule (Shephard, 1982b). In chronic respiratory disease, narrowing or collapse of the airways increases the work of breathing and limits peak ventilatory effort.

Lactate Accumulation

Brief but very intense muscular efforts impede local blood flow. The resulting accumulation of lactate and hydrogen ions can create so acidic an environment within the active muscle fibers (Hultman & Sahlin, 1980) that there is an inhibition of key, rate-limiting enzymes involved in the metabolism of glycogen (Danforth, 1965; Hofer & Pette, 1968), particularly phosphorylase (Constable, Favier, & Holloszy, 1986) and phosphofructokinase (Stanley & Connett, 1991; also see Figure 2.4). Intramuscular concentrations of lactate also rise (although at a slower rate) during sustained, rhythmic activity at intensities greater than about 70% of maximal oxygen intake (McLellan, 1987; Shephard, 1992c).

The intramuscular accumulation of lactate during vigorous exercise is a complex phenomenon, influenced by all of the variables that affect the transport of lactate to and from the active tissues (Zouloumian & Freund, 1981). The rate of diffusion of this substance from the active muscle fibers into the bloodstream is relatively slow and is influenced by the concentrations of extracellular buffers (Mainwood & Renaud, 1985; Wilkes, Gledhill, & Smyth, 1983), a fact that has encouraged some athletes to seek an improvement of their endurance performance by deliberately ingesting sodium bicarbonate. A second potential cause of lactate

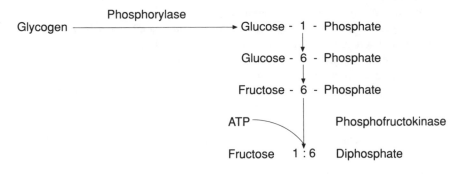

Figure 2.4   Rate-limiting steps in glycolysis. Phosphorylase and phosphofructokinase are adversely affected by a decrease of intramuscular pH. *Note.* Reprinted from Shephard (1977a) by permission.

accumulation is a deficiency of the enzymes needed to metabolize pyruvate to carbon dioxide and water (Connett, Gayeski, & Honig, 1984; Kaijser, 1970; Stainsby, 1986). However, in our present context, an important factor seems to be an inadequate delivery of oxygen to the active muscle fibers, with a consequent switching to alternative (i.e., anaerobic) pathways of energy release, a situation classically described as the anaerobic threshold.

Elimination of Heat

Body heat inevitably tends to accumulate during sustained exercise, because no more than 25% of the chemical energy released from body food stores is converted into useful, external mechanical work.

Even under temperate conditions, the rectal temperature of marathon runners may reach 40 to 41°C (Hubbard & Armstrong, 1989; Kavanagh & Shephard, 1977a; Pugh, Corbett, & Johnson, 1967; W.O. Roberts, 1989; Wyndham & Strydom, 1972). However, unless the climate is extreme, or the exerciser wears inappropriate clothing, neither the rise of body temperature nor the depletion of fluid and mineral reserves seems sufficient to become the critical factor limiting performance during the first hour of aerobic activity.

Oxygen Transport

By a simple process of elimination, we can see that in normal circumstances the main factor limiting dynamic physical activity over periods of 1 to 60 min is the steady transport of oxygen from the atmosphere to the working tissues.

However, the rate at which external work can be performed for any given oxygen-mediated rate of phosphagen regeneration depends on the individual's net mechanical efficiency, that is, the ratio of the external mechanical work that is performed to the additional energy cost of undertaking that activity. As we have seen, the nature of the chemical reactions that occur within the body imposes a ceiling of about 25% on the net efficiency of aerobic activity. The observed net efficiency in some commonly practiced, large-muscle tasks such as cycling and uphill walking or running approaches this figure. But in other activities such as swimming, the average mechanical efficiency is much lower and varies widely according to the skill of the performer. In tasks that involve displacement of the body mass, the energy cost of performing a given amount of external work is also greater for a heavier than for a lighter individual. Finally, there are certain special situations in which an accumulation of carbon dioxide or lactate can affect endurance performance.

The Role of Anaerobic Energy Release

When considering an individual's tolerance of fairly short periods of physical activity (1-10 min), we must consider not only the steady flow of oxygen to the working tissues but also the possible contribution of a locally accumulated *oxygen deficit*, the so-called oxygen debt (A.V. Hill, Long, & Lupton, 1924-1925).

An oxygen deficit develops during the first few minutes of exercise at a fixed power output and equals the cumulative difference between the actual and the steady-state oxygen consumption for the task. This reflects not only the work accomplished by the partial, anaerobic breakdown of glucose and glycogen to lactate, but also an alactate element, the latter corresponding to the depletion of body oxygen stores and the breakdown of high energy phosphates (diPrampero, 1971). The alactate component of the oxygen deficit must be made good after exercise has ceased, but a part of any accumulated lactate can be metabolized elsewhere in the body even as exercise proceeds. This is one reason why the oxygen deficit does not exactly match the excess postexercise oxygen consumption (as had been anticipated in early theories involving repayment of an oxygen debt). Hormonal and thermal stimuli may also sustain metabolism far into the recovery period, independently of anaerobic products that remain to be metabolized.

Quantification of Anaerobic Energy Release

Measurement of the oxygen deficit is technically quite difficult. If the subject is performing submaximal exercise at a steady rate, a plateau of oxygen consumption is reached where oxygen delivery equals oxygen usage. The observer can then estimate the deficit of oxygen consumption accumulated to this point (Bangsbø et al., 1990; Medbø et al., 1988). However, in order to determine the maximal anaerobic capacity, the exercise must be exhausting. A true steady-state is never reached under such conditions; a proportion of the work continues to be performed anaerobically until the intramuscular concentration of lactate and hydrogen ions becomes so high that the breakdown of glycogen is halted and the subject must stop exercising. There is then no observable final plateau of oxygen consumption that can be used to estimate the accumulated oxygen deficit. Medbø et al. (1988) have suggested that the equivalent steady oxygen cost of exhausting exercise can be estimated by extrapolating the linear relationship between treadmill speed and oxygen cost from submaximal activity to speeds of running that are exhausting within 2 to 3 min. Expressing the accumulated oxygen deficit in ml/kg, they claim a measurement precision of 3 ml/kg.

Another possibility is to continue measuring oxygen consumption from the end of exercise until the original resting readings have been regained. It is then assumed that the excess oxygen consumption observed during the recovery period corresponds reasonably closely with a repayment of the accumulated oxygen deficit. Classical calculations also assumed that a portion of the lactate (10% by diPrampero, 1971; 20% by A.V. Hill et al., 1924-1925) was metabolized to carbon dioxide and water, liberating sufficient energy to allow resynthesis of the remainder to glycogen. One fallacy in this reasoning is that some of the better oxygenated tissues metabolize lactate immediately, as exercise is proceeding. This reduces the apparent size of the oxygen deficit (Ahlborg & Felig, 1982), resulting in an underestimation of anaerobic capacity. Other factors operate in the opposite sense. Increases of ventilation, heart rate, tissue temperature, and catecholamine concentrations all lead to persistence of a high oxygen consumption during the recovery period. Also, because energy is needed to restore intracellular levels of sodium, potassium, and calcium ions and to replenish glycogen stores, oxygen consumption may show a small increase over initial resting values that, continuing for several hours after exercise (Gaesser & Brooks, 1984; Gore & Withers, 1990), makes estimates of the anaerobic component arbitrary and unsatisfactory (see Figure 2.5).

Another alternative is to determine lactate concentrations during the early part of the recovery period. It is not practical to make repeated determinations of intramuscular lactate concentrations (Costill, Sharp, Fink, & Katz, 1982), but blood lactate concentrations can be measured on specimens collected from the heated finger tip or the heated or vasodilated earlobe. Blood taken from the arm veins is less satisfactory because of circulatory time delays and the metabolism of lactate in other tissues (Robergs et al., 1990; Yoshida, Takeuchi, & Suda, 1982). Not all lactate comes from anaerobic metabolism. Further problems of interpretation arise due to the excretion of lactate in sweat and urine (Lamont, 1987), and to the nonuniform distribution of lactate in body water. Again, no allowance can be made for lactate that is metabolized during the exercise bout. Moreover, the alactate component of the oxygen deficit (sometimes as much as 40% of the total) is inevitably ignored if only lactate concentrations are measured.

Different authors have estimated the oxygen equivalence of anaerobic metabolism at volumes ranging from 5 to 20 L, with the excess postexercise oxygen consumption commonly exceeding the initial oxygen deficit. The present author favors the estimates proposed by diPrampero (1971), volumes ranging from 5 L (223 mmol) in a sedentary young man to 8 L (357 mmol) in a well-muscled male athlete (see Table 2.1). The maximal deficit can be accumulated in as little as 30 to 40 s, if one exerts an all-out effort; yet as soon as the intensity of exercise

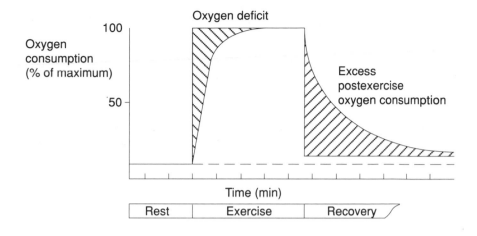

Figure 2.5   Oxygen deficit and postexercise oxygen consumption. Estimating the cumulative excess postexercise oxygen consumption is extremely difficult, because a small "tail" of increased consumption can persist for as long as 8 hr after exercise has ceased. *Note.* Adapted from Shephard (1977a) by permission.

falls appreciably below one's maximal aerobic power, restorative processes occur. Blood lactate concentrations fall most rapidly if the subject maintains muscle blood flow by continuing to exercise at 40% to 60% of maximal oxygen intake (Boileau, Misner, Dykstra, & Spitzer, 1983; Hermansen & Stensvold, 1972).

Contribution of Anaerobic Metabolism to Endurance Effort

The practical importance of anaerobic metabolism to the performance of an endurance task can be seen when its contribution is compared with that due to the steady transport of oxygen.

In the moderately athletic man of Table 2.1, the steady oxygen intake may be 5 L/min, or 3.7 mmol/s, so that over the first minute of all-out exercise, only 38% of energy needs are met aerobically (see Figure 2.6). If the activity is continued, the contribution of aerobic metabolism rises to 55% at 2 min, 75% at 5 min, and 86% at 10 min. By the end of the first hour, anaerobic metabolism has accounted for less than 3% of the total energy expenditure.

Irrespective of the duration of a bout of vigorous activity, there is an initial depletion of muscle phosphagen stores and an accumulation of lactate plus hydrogen ions, because a finite time is needed to adjust muscle blood flow, and thus the local delivery of oxygen, to the greater demands of exercise. In the early stages of an endurance competition, this inevitable oxygen deficit may be augmented by intense anaerobic efforts while athletes "jockey for position." The accumulation

Table 2.1
Potential Sources of "Anaerobic" Activity in a Moderately Athletic Young Man

Component	Tissue mass (kg)	Concentration decrease	Contribution (oxygen equivalent)
Depletion of oxygen stores			
Venous blood	4	100 ml/L	400ml (17.8 mmol)
Myoglobin	20	4-10 ml/L	80-200ml (3.6-8.9 mmol)
Body fluids	38	0.5 ml/L	19ml (0.8 mmol)
Phosphagen	20	25 mmol/kg (1.15kJ/kg)	1.65 L (73.6 mmol)
Lactate			
Muscle	20	44 mmol/kg	
Blood	5	11 mmol/L	
Total lactate production = 0.935 mole (combustion 10% = 0.0935 mole)			6.0 L (267.9 mmol)
Total			8.15 L (363.8 mmol)

Note. The calculation is based on the assumptions of a relatively complete depletion of phosphagen in 20 kg of active muscle, with 46 kJ of anaerobic effort equated to an oxygen intake of 1.1 L, a final blood lactate concentration of 11 mmol/L, and the resynthesis of 90% of the accumulated lactate, using energy derived from oxidation of the remaining 10%. Adapted from Shephard (1977a) by permission.

of lactate and the associated decrease of intramuscular pH lead to discomfort and weakness in the active muscles and an excessive ventilation relative to the oxygen that is delivered. The wise distance competitor thus learns to adjust his or her pace so that any early accumulation of lactate can be quickly metabolized as the race proceeds. Renewal of anaerobic effort is then deferred until a final 30-s sprint to the finishing line (A.V. Hill, 1925).

Plainly, a complete description of the endurance performer must consider the rate at which an oxygen deficit can be accumulated (the anaerobic power), the total capacity for anaerobic metabolism (the anaerobic capacity), and the percentage of maximal oxygen intake at which anaerobic activity first becomes a significant component of metabolism (sometimes termed the anaerobic threshold).

Margaria (1966) proposed a field test of anaerobic power, based on the timed ascent of a short flight of stairs. Caiozzo and Kyle (1980) suggested that if the subject carried a load such as a backpack, the pace could be slowed, allowing a more precise timing of the ascent. Measurement of the work performed over the first 5 s of an appropriately loaded, all-out cycle ergometer test has proven a popular alternative to staircase sprinting (Vandewalle, Pérès, & Monod, 1987). Scores on both types of procedure depend greatly on the subject's motivation and coordination.

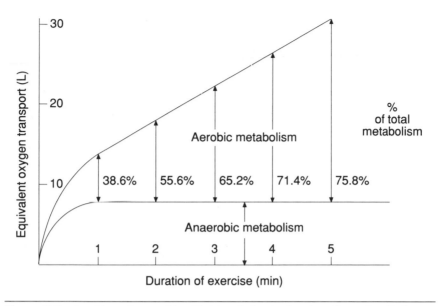

Figure 2.6   Aerobic and anaerobic effort in relation to duration of exercise. Peak anaerobic capacity is 8 L of oxygen and maximal oxygen consumption is 5 L/min.

The anaerobic capacity can be assessed from one's tolerance of an exhausting uphill treadmill run (Niinimaa, Wright, Shephard, & Clarke, 1977) or from the total amount of work performed during 30 to 45 s of all-out cycle ergometer exercise (Vandewalle et al., 1987).

The limitations of the anaerobic threshold have already been discussed. If a series of blood samples is collected during a progressive exercise test, note may be taken of the points when blood lactate readings exceed 2 and 4 mmol/L (McLellan, 1987; Shephard, 1992c). The first of the two blood lactate concentrations corresponds approximately with the accumulation of significant quantities of lactate in the active muscles (Systrom, Kanarck, Kohler, & Kazemi, 1990) and is often associated with a disproportionate increase of ventilation (assessed by an increase in the ventilatory equivalent for oxygen, $\dot{V}_E/\dot{V}_{0_2}$, and a rapid rise in the respiratory gas exchange ratio, $\dot{V}_{C0_2}/\dot{V}_{0_2}$). The second concentration signals a rapid efflux of lactate into the blood stream, commonly accompanied by an increase in the ventilatory equivalent for carbon dioxide, $\dot{V}_E/\dot{V}_{C0_2}$ (Ribeiro et al., 1985).

Though these anaerobic processes are important to the performance of an endurance athlete (Powers, Dodd, Deason, Byrd, & McKnight, 1983; Reybrouck, Ghesquiere, Cattaert, Fagard, & Amery, 1983; Schnabel & Kinderman, 1983), they are of much less importance to ordinary citizens, who rarely reach the threshold of anaerobic metabolism during their normal activities. It is indeed uncertain how much new information a determination of either anaerobic capacity or anaerobic threshold adds to a standard determination of maximal oxygen intake. However, in patients where it is judged hazardous to undertake a maximal test, an estimation of anaerobic threshold can provide some indication of aerobic function (Kavanagh, Mertens, Baigrie, Myers, & Shephard, 1991; Parkhouse, McKenzie, Rhodes, Dunwoody, & Wiley, 1982).

Individual Components of the Oxygen Transfer Process

The sequential arrangement of the various processes involved in the transport of oxygen from the atmosphere to the working tissues (ventilation, pulmonary gas exchange, blood transport, and tissue gas exchange) is illustrated in Figure 2.7. (This diagram first appeared in the February 1968 issue of the *Ontario Medical Review* and is reprinted with the permission of the Ontario Medical Association.)

Ventilation by the bellows action of the chest brings an almost continuous stream of ambient air close to the alveolar-capillary interface within the lungs. However, part of the respired gas is wasted in ventilating the dead space of the airways, where no gas exchange can occur, and only that fraction of the inspirate reaching the alveoli, the *alveolar ventilation*, contributes to oxygen exchange. Part of the measured intake of oxygen is consumed by the chest muscles and heart, and this fraction also is not available to the muscles engaged in performing the intended external work.

Pulmonary gas exchange occurs across the interface between the alveolar gas spaces and pulmonary capillary blood. The resistance to gas transfer offered by this interface is commonly called the *pulmonary diffusing capacity*, or in some European literature, the *transfer factor*.

Blood transport, the third stage in the process, transfers oxygen from the pulmonary capillaries to the capillaries of the active muscles. Here the peak rate of oxygen transport is determined by the individual's hemoglobin level and his or her maximal cardiac output. As with ventilation, a fraction of the available cardiac output is wasted; within the chest, there are small vascular shunts that bypass the ventilated regions of the lungs, and within the tissues, a substantial fraction of the cardiac output is directed to organs other than active skeletal muscle.

Tissue gas exchange comprises the final sequence of events that govern the movement of oxygen from the tissue capillaries to sites within the muscle mitochondria where aerobic metabolism proceeds. For convenience, these events can be considered jointly as the tissue diffusing capacity.

Limiting Processes—Evidence
From the Conductance Theory

In evaluating which processes impose a major limitation on oxygen intake, and thus endurance performance, it is helpful to develop a mathematical model of

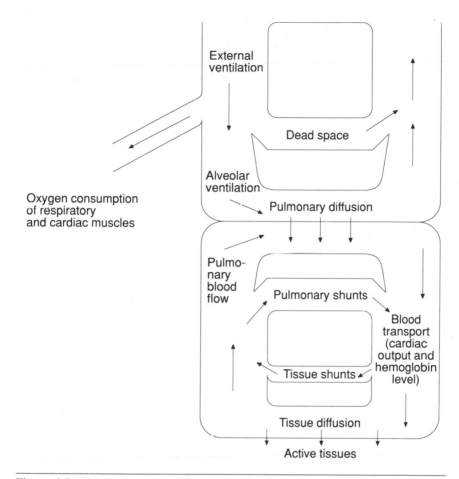

Figure 2.7   Transport of oxygen from atmosphere to working tissues. *Note*. Adapted from Shephard (1968a) by permission.

the oxygen transfer process corresponding to Figure 2.7. Hatch and Cook (1955) were the first to suggest that the individual elements of gas exchange could be treated as a sequence of metabolic conductances. In electrical terms, a conductance ($\dot{G}$) is the reciprocal of a resistance. It expresses the current flow (I) through an element per unit of potential difference (E):

$$\dot{G} = I/E$$

Let us suppose that we have four conductances arranged in series. If a current I is passed through such a circuit, an overall potential difference E is developed, and this distributes itself between the four elements in proportion to their respective resistances, or in other words to the reciprocal of their respective conductances.

In humans, the volume flow of substances such as oxygen can be regarded as the equivalent of an electrical current, and the concentration gradient for the substance under consideration becomes the analogue of potential difference. Note that for the purpose of this analysis, the concentration gradient is expressed as a dimensionless concentration (ml/L), rather than as a gradient of partial pressure, measured in kPa.

The individual's overall conductance for oxygen, $\dot{G}_{0_2}$, is thus a function of the maximal oxygen intake ($\dot{V}_{0_2max}$) and the oxygen concentration gradient from inspired air ($C_{I,0_2}$) to metabolic sites within the active muscle fibers ($C_{\bar{t},0_2}$):

$$\dot{G}_{0_2} = \dot{V}_{0_2max}/(C_{I,0_2} - C_{\bar{t},0_2})$$

The units for $\dot{G}$ are then the traditional L/min STPD, or mmol/s, depending on the units that have been chosen to represent $\dot{V}_{0_2max}$.

As discussed below, similar equations can be developed for the four individual stages of oxygen transfer (alveolar ventilatory conductance, pulmonary diffusion, bloodstream conductance, and tissue diffusion). The overall oxygen conductance ($\dot{G}_{0_2}$) can then be obtained by reciprocal summation of the four individual elements:

$$1/\dot{G} = 1/\dot{V}_A + [B/1-B)]/\lambda\dot{Q} + 1/\lambda Q + [K/(1-K)]/\lambda Q$$

Alveolar Ventilatory and Bloodstream Conductances

Alveolar ventilation ($\dot{V}_A$) can be regarded as a conductance, with a corresponding gradient of oxygen concentration from the atmosphere to alveolar gas ($C_{I,0_2} - C_{A,0_2}$):

$$\dot{V}_A = \dot{V}_{0_2max} / (C_{I,0_2} - C_{A,0_2})$$

For example, if $\dot{V}_A$ = 80 L/min,
$C_{I,0_2}$ = 209 ml/L, and
C_A = 160 ml/L,
then 80 = $\dot{V}_{0_2max}/(209 - 160)$ and
$\dot{V}_{0_2max}$ = 3,920 ml/min STPD, or 2.92 mmol/s.

In much the same way, blood transport can be regarded as the product of two conductance terms, $\dot{Q}_{max}$ (the peak cardiac output), and *lambda* (the solubility coefficient for oxygen, an expression of both the hemoglobin content of unit volume of blood and the manner in which the hemoglobin of a particular individual reacts with oxygen). Again, there is an appropriate gradient of oxygen concentration, in this case from arterial blood ($C_{a,0_2}$) to mixed venous blood ($C_{\bar{v},0_2}$):

$$\lambda\dot{Q} = \dot{V}_{0_2max}/(C_{a,0_2} - C_{\bar{v},0_2})$$

Pulmonary and Tissue Diffusion

The choice of conductance terms relating to pulmonary and tissue diffusion presents a little more difficulty. Indeed, at first sight, the remaining gradients, from alveolar gas to arterial blood ($C_{A,O_2} - C_{a,O_2}$) and from mixed venous blood to the active tissues ($C_{\bar{v},O_2} - C_{t,O_2}$) seem incorrect. Moreover, physiologists have traditionally expressed the two diffusing capacities, $\dot{D}_L$ and $\dot{D}_t$, as the rate of gas transfer (ml/min) per unit of partial pressure gradient, measured between alveolar gas and mean pulmonary capillary blood ($P_{A,O_2} - P_{\bar{pc},O_2}$) and between mean tissue capillary blood and the tissues ($P_{\bar{tc},O_2} - P_{t,O_2}$).

For the purpose of the conductance calculation, the two diffusional conductances must be converted from the traditional respiratory physiological units of ml/min per mm Hg to L/min per ml/L, using the appropriate conversion factor α (i.e., $\alpha\dot{D}_L$ and $\alpha\dot{D}_t$). Figure 2.7 suggests an explanation of the apparently anomalous concentration gradients associated with these two conductances. In reality, neither is a simple series arrangement. The transfer of gases across the pulmonary and the tissue capillary interfaces depends upon an interaction between the rate of blood flow in a given channel and the corresponding local diffusing capacity. It is thus necessary to create new conductances expressing the nature of these interactions (Shephard, 1972).

For the lungs, the conductance term becomes $(1 - B)/B\ \lambda\dot{Q}$, and for the tissues, the corresponding term is $(1 - K)/K\ \lambda\dot{Q}$. The derivation of the constants B and K is beyond the scope of this book, but we may note that both contain integrals related to the shape of the oxygen dissociation curve, with $B = e^{(-\dot{D}_L/\int \lambda\dot{Q})}$, and $K = e^{(-\dot{D}_t/\int \lambda\dot{Q})}$. We may thus write

$$(1 - B)/B\ \lambda\dot{Q} = \dot{V}_{O_2}/(C_{A,O_2} - C_{a,O_2})$$

and

$$(1 - K)/K\ \lambda\dot{Q} = \dot{V}_{O_2,max}\ (C_{\bar{v},O_2} - C_{t,O_2}).$$

Limitations of the Conductance Theorem

There are a number of obvious limitations to this simplified mathematical representation of the cardiorespiratory system (Shephard, 1971a), including certain external constraints, inhomogeneities of ventilation, the complex natures of diffusing capacities, cardiac conductance, and tissue solubilities, and time delays related to the capacity of the oxygen transport system. Situations can be envisaged where it is undesirable to maximize individual conductances, and it remains unclear whether oxygen, carbon dioxide, and lactate transport have equal importance in terms of continuing muscle function. If, for example, a lack of oxygen has a graver import than a buildup of lactate, then the simple comparison of overall conductances for these two substances may be misleading.

The conductance concept assumes an absence of external constraints; thus oxygen transport can increase progressively until all elements in the conducting sequence are maximally stressed. However, in practice other factors may halt exercise before such a limit is reached. For example, if the subject is poorly motivated, unpleasant sensations arising in the chest (dyspnea) or the working muscles (local fatigue) may stop an activity when the subject is far from peak heart rate or cardiac output.

Problems also arise from temporal and spatial inhomogeneities of ventilation. For the purpose of the conductance analysis, the lungs are represented as a simple chamber, uniformly and continuously ventilated, whereas we know that the chest bellows is a complex system, that the distribution of ventilation and perfusion is far from uniform, and that both ventilation and blood flow tend to be discontinuous, cyclic processes. The effective value of $\dot{V}_A$ applicable to the conductance equation is thus determined in part by the temporal and spatial matching of blood flow within the lungs.

Both pulmonary and tissue diffusing capacities are complex terms. The pulmonary diffusion term $\alpha\dot{D}_L$ reflects not only the ease with which oxygen diffuses across the alveolar and pulmonary capillary membranes in response to a given concentration gradient, but also the rate of reaction between oxygen and intracapillary hemoglobin (and thus the volume of blood in the pulmonary capillaries). Analogous considerations apply to the tissue diffusion term $\alpha\dot{D}_t$. Neither $\alpha\dot{D}_L$ nor $\alpha\dot{D}_t$ is completely independent of cardiac output, though the model implies such. An increase of cardiac output may distend existing capillaries, or it may open up new vessels. In either case, there will be an increase in both the effective surface available for diffusion and in the capillary blood volume, and this will be reflected in larger values for both $\alpha\dot{D}_L$ and $\alpha\dot{D}_t$.

Among the complexities of cardiac conductance, we may note that the peak cardiac output is not a fixed value determined by the strength of the cardiac musculature. Rather, it is influenced by venous return and thus preloading of the ventricles, by the response of the cardiac muscle to sympathetic nerve activity and catecholamines (both of which can modify the contractility of the myocardium), and by the impedance resisting expulsion of the ventricular contents (afterloading of the heart). Furthermore, the conductance model assumes that the tissues behave as a single, homogenous oxygen sink with an equivalent diffusing capacity $\alpha\dot{D}_t$ and terminal oxygen concentration $C_{\bar{t},O_2}$. But in fact, a substantial part of the peak blood flow observed during maximal exertion is directed to tissues other than muscle, particularly the skin, and the terminal oxygen concentrations are very different for the various components of the circulation.

Solubility factors for oxygen, carbon dioxide, and lactate all differ from one tissue to another, making it difficult to relate local pressure or concentration gradients to the corresponding conductances. Further, the properties of the red cell pigment are such that the average value of the blood solubility term λ increases with a decrease in the alveolar oxygen concentration (see Figure 2.8).

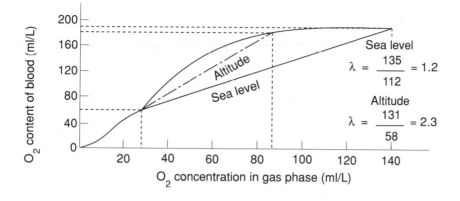

Figure 2.8   Illustration of the method of calculating the solubility of oxygen in unit volume of blood (λ). The average slope between arterial and mixed venous points is used in the calculation. Note that if the partial pressure of oxygen in the gas phase is reduced, the subject is brought to the steep part of the oxygen dissociation curve, and the effective value of λ is increased. However, at high altitude this advantage is partially offset, because a given oxygen pressure gradient is equivalent to a larger gradient in the dimensionless concentration units (ml/L) used in the conductance equation. *Note.* Adapted from Shephard (1977a) by permission.

In effect, there is an increase in λ as the blood passes from the arterial to the venous side of the circulation, and the calculation of pulmonary and tissue diffusion conductances must be based on an integral of λ, reflecting the changes occurring in the capillaries.

Time delays between the mouth and the active tissues are imposed by the capacities of the various conductances such as the lungs and the circulation, although these are not of major importance in bouts of exercise having a duration of 1 min or longer (Essfeld, Hoffmann, & Stegemann, 1991).

The overall objective of metabolic transport is to allow the skeletal muscles to perform external work, and this objective is not necessarily achieved by maximizing overall conductance. For instance, a large overall oxygen conductance may be realized by maximizing alveolar ventilation or cardiac output but at the expense of a gross increase in the work of the respiratory or cardiac muscles. In consequence, the oxygen available for the performance of useful external work may be less than would have been delivered by more modest respiratory or cardiac efforts (Morrison, Van Malsen, & Noakes, 1983). By way of practical example, one adaptation that favors the working ability of populations indigenous to high altitudes is a decrease in the sensitivity of the respiratory control mechanism and thus a lessening of the ventilatory response to a given amount of exercise (Lahiri & Milledge, 1968).

Despite these various important limitations, the conductance equation provides a convenient framework for summarizing interrelationships between the various determinants of oxygen transfer. Moreover, the overall oxygen conductance can be compared with the conductance of other metabolic transport systems such as those governing the transfer of carbon dioxide, lactate, and body heat, in order to assess which system is the most likely to limit endurance effort.

Effective Alveolar Ventilation

Early investigators suggested that the vital capacity of the lungs provided a useful measure of physical fitness (Dreyer, 1920), and more recently, correlations have been shown between vital capacity and performance in a number of types of endurance competition (Cordain, Tucker, Moon, & Stager, 1990; Cordain & Stager, 1988; Ishiko, 1967). However, much of the observed correlation reflects (1) the prevalence of chronic chest disease among participants in early studies, (2) a mutual dependence of vital capacity and performance on body size (G.R. Cumming, 1971), (3) a contribution of vital capacity to buoyancy in distance swimmers (Cordain & Stager, 1988), and (4) an influence of shoulder muscle strength on lung function in groups such as rowers and swimmers (Clanton, Dixon, Drake, & Gadek, 1987). Some types of endurance training (particularly distance running) even weaken muscles in the upper part of the body, which can reduce the power of the chest bellows and increase the residual lung volume (Cordain, Glissan, Latin, Tucker, & Stager, 1987).

Peak Pumping Ability of the Chest

During vigorous aerobic exercise, very deep inspirations are taken, bringing the chest to a volume where the ability of the thoracic muscles to generate pressure is compromised (de Troyer & Yernault, 1980). Likewise, very vigorous expirations could theoretically induce a collapse of the intrathoracic airways, so that added expiratory efforts merely narrow the air passages rather than augment expiratory airflow (Aaron, Johnson, Pegelow, & Dempsey, 1990; Shephard, 1982b). Airway collapse is not encountered in normal subjects when breathing at normal ambient pressures (Dempsey, 1986), but it can occasionally arise in such individuals if the pressure gradient along the airways is increased by exposure to high ambient pressures, as when exercising at great depths underwater (Mead, 1980; Shephard, 1982b). The likelihood of airway collapse is increased by the loss of elastic recoil and damage to airway cartilages that occurs with aging, and the problem is commonly encountered in individuals who have developed emphysema or chronic obstructive lung disease.

Nevertheless, the peak pumping ability of the thoracic bellows does not usually limit the endurance performance of a young, healthy adult. There is at least a small margin between the peak airflows reached during maximal exercise and those that can be developed voluntarily at comparable lung volumes (Denison, Waller, Turton, & Sopwith, 1982; Hesser, Linnarsson, & Fagreus, 1981). If the maximum voluntary ventilation (MVV) is measured at an optimum respiratory rate, using low-resistance apparatus that does not impede ventilation, figures of 160 to 200 and 120 to 160 L/min body temperature and pressure saturated (BTPS) are typical of ordinary young men and women, respectively, and scores may be at least 20% greater in endurance competitors (Shephard, 1982b). The ventilation observed during 15 min of all-out endurance exercise is usually only about two thirds of these figures.

Unfortunately, this does not prove conclusively that the larger respiratory minute volumes could be either developed acutely or sustained during prolonged bouts of exercise. The resting subject cannot realize a full MVV at respiratory rates of less than 90 breaths/min (Shephard, 1957), whereas the respiratory rate adopted during sustained aerobic exercise is typically only about 40 breaths/min (somewhat higher in trained than in untrained subjects, [Folinsbee, Wallace, Bedi, & Horvath, 1983] and increasing if the effort is prolonged [Hanson, Claremont, Dempsey, & Reddan, 1982]). The choice of respiratory rate while exercising sometimes reflects an entrainment of rhythms such as the running or pedalling pace (Bechbache, Chow, Duffin, & Orsini, 1979; Kirby, Nugent, Marlow, MacLeod, & Marble, 1989; Kohl, Koller, & Jager, 1981; Paterson, Cunningham, & Bumstead, 1986). A rate of 35 to 40 breaths/min was once held to minimize the work of the respiratory muscles, but this conclusion was based on tests using fixed respiratory minute volumes. In fact, the greater mechanical cost of choosing a somewhat slower respiratory rate may be more than offset because the subject then has a longer period for gas exchange and the ventilatory demand is reduced.

Sustained Pumping Ability of the Chest Bellows

A major limitation of the MVV test is that it is normally concluded within 15 s, a much shorter period than a typical bout of aerobic activity. It is thus arguable that although young adults have a substantial initial margin of ventilatory capacity, this is rapidly attenuated during sustained exercise, because subjects dislike the unpleasant sensations of vigorous breathing, the respiratory muscles become fatigued, or bronchospasm is provoked by oral inhalation of a combination of cold, dry air and air pollutants.

Although endurance athletes talk much about the sensation of "second wind" (Shephard, 1974, August), unpleasant breathlessness (dyspnea) does not usually limit their performance. In contrast, poorly motivated, sedentary people frequently stop exercising because they find the task unpleasant. This judgment is reached through a compounding of local muscular discomfort and general perceptions of exertion with the specific sensations of unaccustomed vigorous breathing. In a progressive maximal exercise test, the worst feelings of breathlessness are usually encountered 1 to 2 min after ceasing the activity as lactate and hydrogen ions diffuse from the working muscles to the bloodstream. Because time is required to transport these metabolites into the bloodstream and across the blood-brain barrier, breathlessness is particularly likely to limit attempts at prolonged and just submaximal effort (Shephard, 1987b). Perceptions of dyspnea or local muscular weakness may halt such exercise even though the mechanical ability of the respiratory apparatus is not fully taxed (see Table 2.2).

The intensity of respiratory sensations (S_R) reported by a given person depends on any external resistance to breathing (as assessed by pressures at the mouth, P_m), the duration of inspiration (t_i), and the frequency of respiration (f_R), according to an equation of the type (Killian, 1987; Killian, Summers, & Basalygo, 1985):

$$S_R = K \cdot P_m^{1.4} \cdot t_i^{0.52} \cdot f_R^{0.26}.$$

Another important variable is the tidal volume relative to the capacity of the chest bellows. It was once held that dyspnea arose if exercise demanded a respiratory minute volume that used more than 50% of the vital capacity each breath (e.g., a ventilation of more than 100 L/min with a vital capacity of 5 L and a respiratory rate of 40 breaths/min). However, careful ratings of respiratory sensations show that ventilation first becomes perceptible at greater than 20% of peak power output, equivalent to a much smaller fractional usage of vital capacity. As the work rate is further increased, the sensation grows, becoming severe at 70% to 80% of peak aerobic power (Killian, 1987). The quality of the sensation also seems to differ, and the ventilatory threshold for dyspnea is thus greater during aerobic exercise than when an equivalent hyperventilation is induced by a manipulation of inspired gas mixtures (L. Adams, Chronos, & Guz, 1982; Stark, Gambles, & Lewis, 1981; but not Swinburn, Wakefield, & Jones, 1984).

N.L. Jones (1984) put the average subjectively acceptable ceiling of tidal volume at 74% of the individual's vital capacity, less a constant of 1.11 L (in other words, 56% of a 6-L vital capacity, but only 46% of a 4-L vital capacity). However, depending on motivation, the level of aerobic fitness (L. Adams, Chronos, Lane, & Guz, 1986), and the extent of habituation to feelings of breathlessness (well developed both in athletes and those with chronic respiratory

Table 2.2
Factors Reported as Limiting a Progressive Cycle Ergometer Test

Limiting factor	Percent of sample		
	$FEV_{1.0} < 60\%$	$FEV_{1.0}$ 60-90%	$FEV_{1.0} > 90\%$
Breathlessness	39%	31%	22%
Leg effort	22%	39%	49%
Breathlessness + leg effort	39%	28%	28%
Chest pain	0	3%	1%

Note. Data is for 458 subjects, classified in relation to the individual's 1-s forced expiratory volume ($FEV_{1.0}$), expressed as a percentage of the normal value for a subject of the same age, sex, and height. Reprinted from Killian (1987) by permission.

disease), the threshold of unpleasant chest sensations during a bout of physical activity can vary widely from 33% to 75% of the individual's ventilatory reserve (Gilbert & Auchincloss, 1969). Factors tending to increase feelings of breathlessness in the sedentary exerciser include a large functional residual gas volume and thus an unfavorable muscle length for the generation of inspiratory pressures, a high internal flow resistance (Killian, 1987), rapid inspiration (P. LeBlanc, Bowie, Summers, Jones, & Killian, 1986), and inspiratory muscle weakness (N.L. Jones, 1984), and performance of exercise such as cycle ergometry, in which there is a rapid accumulation of lactate at relatively low intensities of effort (Cockcroft, Beaumont, Adams, & Guz, 1985). In contrast, the likelihood of exercise-induced dyspnea is reduced in the endurance athlete because the anaerobic threshold is a large fraction of the individual's maximal oxygen intake, the length of the inspiratory muscles is kept in a favorable range by beginning each inspiration within the expiratory reserve volume (Killian, 1987), and the relative consumption of fat is high even during vigorous exercise (fat demands a larger oxygen consumption per kJ of energy released, but produces a smaller quantity of ventilation-stimulating carbon dioxide).

The older individual with chronic obstructive lung disease is particularly vulnerable to dyspnea, and a vicious cycle may develop. Lack of fitness, muscle weakness, and a resultant accumulation of lactate cause dyspnea even during moderate exercise. Habitual activity is thus reduced, with a further loss of fitness and a worsening of dyspnea (Mertens et al., 1978).

The respiratory muscles can eventually become fatigued if a subject sustains a high rate of ventilation (B.J. Martin, Chen, & Kolka, 1984; B.J. Martin, 1987), although one's susceptibility to such fatigue depends on the type, intensity, and duration of exercise, with much interindividual variation. Potential contributing factors (Shephard, 1987b) include weakness of the thoracic muscles due to a lack of training or a specific pathology, a local accumulation of lactate (seen even in short-term hyperventilation; Cobley, Cooke, Freedman, & Moxham, 1981), local glycogen depletion due to prior use of the chest muscles (Gorski, Namiot, & Giedrojc, 1978; Moore & Gollnick, 1982; but not Fregosi & Dempsey, 1986), fatigue at the neuromuscular junction, an increase of airway resistance due to such causes as exercise-induced bronchospasm (McFadden, 1987; Shephard, 1977b), a secondary reaction to inhaled air-pollutants (Folinsbee, 1990), or a secondary effect from a deterioration of posture as an athlete approaches exhaustion (F. Haas, Simnowitz, Axen, Gaudino, & Haas, 1982). However, any fatigue-related decrease of MVV is minimal over the first 60 min of vigorous physical activity, at least in trained subjects (Bender & Martin, 1985). Indeed, Anholm, Stray-Gunderson, Ramanathan, & Johnson (1989) saw no decrease relative to a 4-min MVV score after 62 min of exercise at 77% of the subjects' maximal oxygen intake, and Loke, Mahler, & Virgulto (1982) found only a 10% decrease in MVV over the course of a marathon run. Furthermore, though training of the respiratory muscles increases both the local activity of aerobic enzymes (Moore & Gollnick, 1982) and ventilatory power (B.J. Martin & Chen, 1982), it does not seem to increase maximal oxygen transport (D.W. Morgan, Kohrt,

Bates, & Skinner, 1987). A ventilatory limitation of endurance performance is particularly likely to develop in individuals with exercise-induced bronchospasm (Shephard, 1977b). In such people, exposure to cold, dry air can quickly reduce the maximum voluntary ventilation by 20% to 30%, so that physical activity becomes halted by acute breathlessness.

Experimental observations show that healthy young adults can sustain some 70% to 75% of the MVV over 4 min of resting hyperventilation (Freedman, 1970). Likewise, if an exercising subject is persuaded to increase the respiratory rate to 100 breaths/min, some 75% to 80% of the resting MVV (still more than the usual peak exercise ventilation) can be sustained throughout a 15 min test. Moreover, the main factor limiting an even greater ventilatory effort seems psychological rather than physiological, a reaction to the unpleasant sensations associated with repeated, rapid chest movements (Shephard, 1974c). With strong encouragement, subjects can push themselves from 80% to 100% of MVV, even in the 15th min of exercise. Nevertheless, respiratory sensations are reduced and ventilation can be increased with a small improvement of exercise endurance, if turbulent airflow and thus the respiratory work rate is reduced by breathing gas mixtures that contain 80% helium (Aaron, Henke, Pegelow, & Dempsey, 1985; Ward, Poon, & Whipp, 1980).

The MVV falls with age, being 20% to 25% less in the sixth decade of life than in young adults. But it seems that the maximum exercise ventilation is reduced proportionately, so that the normal margin between the MVV and exercise ventilation is usually maintained throughout the span of working life. One exception to this generalization is if the normal age-related loss of respiratory function has been exacerbated by a combination of chronic respiratory disease and exposure to air pollutants, including cigarette smoke. In such individuals, attempts at aerobic exercise may be limited by a distressing breathlessness (Shephard, 1976), and a parallel is seen between poor dynamic lung volumes and a low maximal oxygen intake (Babb, Viggiano, Hurley, Staats, & Rodarte, 1991).

Influence of Dead Space

The major component of the total dead space (a volume of 100-130 ml and 130-160 ml in young women and young men, respectively) is attributable to the anatomical dead space of the conducting airways. A sizeable minor component (30-40 ml), termed the *alveolar dead space*, reflects an inhomogeneity of gas in the terminal airways plus a temporal or a spatial mismatching of ventilation and blood flow within the lungs.

The size of the anatomical dead space increases with expansion of the lungs. Thus, if exercise leads to an increase in the mean alveolar gas volume, there is some augmentation of the anatomical dead space. On the other hand, the matching of alveolar ventilation and blood flow is improved by moderate exercise (Bake, Bjure, & Widimsky, 1968; Bryan et al., 1964). The increase of tidal volume leads to a more uniform distribution of inspired gas, and a rise of pulmonary arterial pressures increases the perfusion of alveoli in the upper parts of the lungs. Inequalities of ventilation and perfusion persist in the horizontal plane, but, nevertheless, the alveolar dead space may become smaller than when the person is sitting at rest.

Most of the dead space (a volume of up to 500 ml observed during vigorous exercise) is due, not to unmixed gas in the large conducting airways of the anatomical dead space, but to the very brief time available for a mixing of gas between the terminal air passages and the alveolar spaces (Beeckmans & Shephard, 1971). The extent of such stratified inhomogeneity within the smaller airways (Fredberg, 1980; Hlastala, 1982), although important from the viewpoint of gas exchange, is less than would be predicted from computer models of the respiratory tract (L.G. Baker, Ultman, & Rhoades, 1974; Beeckmans & Shephard, 1971). It thus seems that alveolar gas mixing is aided by a combination of local turbulence at airway bifurcations, convection, and axial streaming of inspired air (Engel, Wood, Utz, Macklem, 1973; L.R. Johnson & Van Liew, 1974). Final equilibration is also helped by physical movements of the bronchi and possibly the massaging action of the heart beat. Nevertheless, little of the inspirate is transported directly to the alveoli. Gas traverses the final few millimeters of the airway by molecular diffusion (E.A. Harris, Buchanan, & Whitlock, 1987). The interface between mixed and inspired gas progressively retreats up the bronchial tree, leaving a diminished volume of dead gas in the conducting airways (see Figure 2.9), the extent of this mixing process depending on the length of the postinspiratory pause.

At rest, some 30% of external ventilation is wasted in the dead space. The influence of exercise on this wastage is controversial. Some authors have reported that the ratio of alveolar to external ventilation ($\dot{V}_A/\dot{V}_E$) remains at about 0.7, but others have suggested that $\dot{V}_A$ approximates $\dot{V}_E$ more closely as the respiratory minute volume is increased. Most observations have been made at respiratory rates selected by the subjects themselves, typically in the range 25 to 50 breaths/min. The optimum respiratory frequency from the viewpoint of minimizing dead space seems a rate of about 32 breaths/min (Shephard & Bar-Or, 1970), but these authors found that even at the highest rates likely during exercise, the ratio $\dot{V}_A/\dot{V}_E$ is no smaller than 0.70 to 0.75 in an adult and 0.80 in a child.

Given that the dead space is a smaller fraction of ventilation during exercise than when at rest, it is unlikely that it imposes a major limitation on aerobic performance. S.E. Brown et al. (1984) found that the deliberate addition of 250 to 500 ml of dead space to the airway had no influence on the maximal oxygen intake of normal adults, although it did reduce the peak oxygen transport in patients with chronic chest disease. The dead space is particularly likely to assume importance if ventilation is already marginal or if dyspnea is the primary factor restricting a subject's performance. In such situations, a 10% decrease of alveolar ventilation due to either a slowing of respiratory rate or a shift in chemosensitivity could reduce the oxygen cost of breathing sufficiently to yield a matching 10% gain in endurance performance (Dicker, Lofthus, Thornton, & Brooks, 1980; Hsieh & Hermiston, 1983) at the expense of some upward drift of P_{a,CO_2}.

Ventilatory Conductance

From the viewpoint of the conductance equation, we may accept that young, healthy persons can develop 75% to 80% of their maximal voluntary ventilation

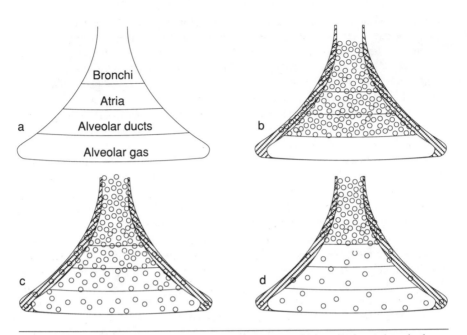

Figure 2.9 Stratified inhomogeneity: (a) situation at end of expiration, when the bronchial system is uniformly filled with expired gas; (b) situation at end of inspiration, when expansion of lungs and terminal airways has admitted inspired gas to conducting airway. As this gas is held in the lungs, it exchanges progressively with the alveolar space, (c) and (d), and the interface with unmixed, dead-space gas progressively retreats up the conducting airways. *Note.* Reprinted from Shephard (1977a) by permission.

during a sustained bout of aerobic exercise and that 75% of this respired volume will mix with alveolar gas. The maximal alveolar ventilation is thus likely to be in the range 85 to 120 L/min BTPS, or 65 to 100 L/min in STPD units. (Note that all conductances are expressed under standard conditions of temperature and pressure, dry gas, or STPD, rather than at body temperature and pressure saturated, or BTPS, which is the air movement sensed by the individual.)

The Oxygen Cost of Breathing

One assumption implicit in the oxygen conductance analysis is that if overall oxygen transport is increased, this will benefit muscles performing useful aerobic activities. However, an appreciable fraction of the observed total oxygen intake is consumed by the conducting system itself to sustain metabolism in the heart and respiratory muscles. Could the oxygen needs of the transport mechanism become large enough to limit peak aerobic performance?

Hypothesis of a Critical Limit to Ventilation

If a healthy young person remains at rest, the oxygen used by the respiratory muscles is quite small, probably less than 10 ml/min, or 7.4 μmol/s (Otis, 1964). However, such costs increase disproportionately with an increase of respiratory minute volume (Aaron et al., 1990). Turbulent airflow replaces the more economical, viscous flow through a growing fraction of the bronchial tree; a larger part of the respiratory energy consumption is diverted to mechanical displacement of the liver and other heavy abdominal viscera; the efficiency of the respiratory pump decreases as accessory muscles with poorer mechanical efficiency begin to contribute to ventilation; and finally, chest movements may become so rapid that the optimum speed of muscle shortening is exceeded.

If the added oxygen cost of a further increase in respiratory effort $(\Delta \dot{V}_{O_2 R}/\Delta \dot{V}_E)$ is plotted against the resulting augmentation of oxygen transport $(\Delta \dot{V}_{O_2}/\Delta \dot{V}_E)$, it is possible to envisage a subject reaching a critical point (see Figure 2.10) at which the extra respiratory oxygen consumption equals or exceeds the total additional oxygen intake resulting from the added ventilation. Any further increase of ventilation is then not only uneconomical, but actually reduces the delivery of oxygen to the muscles that are performing useful external work.

Experimental Values

It is technically quite difficult to measure the oxygen consumption of the heart and respiratory muscles during exercise, in part because the figure of interest is overshadowed by the oxygen consumption of the limb muscles, and in part because the techniques usually adopted (such as voluntary hyperventilation or the addition of carbon dioxide to the inspirate) in themselves modify many of the determinants of respiratory work such as mean thoracic volume, airway dimensions, and the pattern of the breathing cycle.

Shephard (1966a) indicated that the oxygen cost of breathing in near-maximal aerobic exercise was about 4 to 5 ml of oxygen per liter of airflow, four to five times the resting figure. Aaron et al. (1990) recently attempted to mimic the respiratory patterns of vigorous aerobic exercise in resting subjects; using this approach, they found somewhat lower values, rising from 1.8 ml/L at the ventilations corresponding to 70% of maximal oxygen intake to 2.9 ml/L at those ventilations expected at 100% of maximal oxygen intake. Because subjects were resting, their technique inevitably minimized the cardiac component of oxygen cost, although hyperventilation in itself increases cardiac output to some extent. The two data sets thus seem at least of a comparable order.

Perhaps more importantly, deliberate hyperventilation during near-maximal exercise quickly leads to a decline in the ratio $\Delta \dot{V}_{O_2}/\Delta \dot{V}_E$, from a normal figure of 30 to 40 ml of oxygen per liter of ventilation to less than 5 ml for each liter increment of ventilation. Any increase of the peak respiratory minute volume would thus contribute little to oxygen transport unless there were a matching increase of maximal cardiac output.

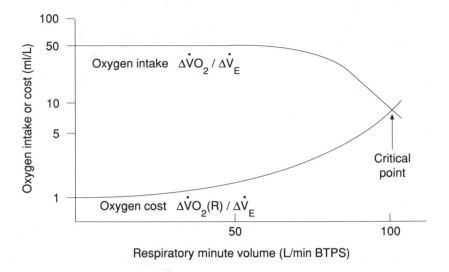

Figure 2.10 Influence of initial respiratory minute volume on oxygen cost of added respiratory effort ($\Delta\dot{V}_{0_2R}/\Delta\dot{V}_E$), and added oxygen intake resulting from increased respiratory effort ($\Delta\dot{V}_{0_2}/\Delta\dot{V}_E$). Note that for the subject illustrated (a sedentary young woman), the critical point at which the oxygen consumed exceeds the extra oxygen delivered is at approximately 100 L/min BTPS. *Note.* Adapted from Shephard (1977a) by permission.

Location of Critical Point

The critical point which $\Delta\dot{V}_{0_2R}/\Delta\dot{V}_E$ exceeds $\Delta\dot{V}_{0_2}/\Delta\dot{V}_E$ apparently exceeds the ventilation normally attained during endurance exercise, corresponding to a respired volume of about 100 L/min and 130 L/min in sedentary young women and men, respectively.

If the crossover point occurred at a similar respiratory minute volume in endurance athletes, then the increase of oxygen intake achieved by a given increase of ventilation might be an important factor limiting performance for the sportsperson. However, the maximal cardiac output in an endurance athlete of either sex is substantially greater than that of a sedentary person, and for this reason the crossover point is not reached until a correspondingly larger respiratory minute volume has been developed. Indeed, in maximal aerobic exercise, the endurance athlete has a lower ventilatory equivalent ($\dot{V}_E/\dot{V}_{0_2}$) and thus a higher reciprocal ($\dot{V}_{0_2}/\dot{V}_E$, oxygen delivered per unit of ventilation) than a sedentary subject.

On the other hand, the crossover value is readily exceeded in older subjects if airflow resistance (and thus the oxygen cost of breathing) is increased by chronic obstructive lung disease (Levison & Cherniak, 1968). Such individuals may well be forced to cease exercising at a relatively low heart rate, before their cardiac function has been fully taxed.

Modifications of Critical Point

During prolonged aerobic exercise, a combination of such factors as an accumulation of lactate and hydrogen ions (metabolic acidosis), a rising core temperature, pulmonary congestion, and respiratory muscle fatigue give rise to a ventilatory drift (Dempsey & Manohar, 1992). Ventilation becomes mechanically inefficient, and even a younger person is carried closer to the crossover point.

It might also be anticipated that imposition of an external resistance to breathing would increase the likelihood of exceeding the critical point during exercise. However, in practice, even a substantial external resistance (e.g., breathing through a gas mask) has little effect on either the oxygen cost of a given type of aerobic exercise or the rate at which it can be performed by a healthy young adult (Demedts & Anthonisen, 1973; Deroanne, Juchmes, Hausman, Pirnay, & Petit, 1968; Flook & Kelman, 1973; Shephard, 1962). This reflects human adaptability rather than a lack of oxygen cost from the added respiratory loading.

Adaptive mechanisms open to a healthy young person faced by an external respiratory load include (1) the adoption of a slower, deeper, and mechanically more efficient pattern of breathing, (2) some increase in the partial pressure of carbon dioxide in the alveoli, with a resultant dilatation of the bronchi and a reduction of internal airflow resistance, and (3) an increase of the mean thoracic gas volume, leading to mechanical expansion of the airways and a decrease of internal airflow resistance.

Pulmonary Diffusing Capacity

Because the body normally contains very little carbon monoxide, respiratory physiologists find it easier to measure the pulmonary diffusing capacity as a transfer of carbon monoxide than as the corresponding oxygen intake. Oxygen crosses the alveolar membrane somewhat more easily than carbon monoxide for any given partial pressure gradient, so that the maximum value of $\dot{D}_{L,O_2}$ is 1.23 times the maximum value of $\dot{D}_{L,CO}$.

The respiratory physiologist usually expresses the rate of gas transfer per unit of partial pressure (kPa or Torr), but for the purpose of the conductance equation, the oxygen diffusing capacity must be expressed as the volume of gas transferred per unit of concentration gradient (ml/L). Accordingly, a correction factor α is applied, such that $\alpha = (\pi - 47)/1,000$, where π is the barometric pressure, measured in Torr, and 47 is the corresponding partial pressure of water vapor within the body.

Cross-sectional comparisons show a larger resting pulmonary diffusing capacity in endurance athletes than in sedentary individuals (Anderson & Shephard, 1968b), although this may reflect an association between a large pulmonary diffusing capacity and a large maximal cardiac output (Andersen & Magel, 1970) rather than an important contribution of pulmonary diffusion to endurance performance. Certainly, there is no good evidence that the carbon monoxide diffusing capacity reaches a plateau value in either sedentary or athletic individuals, even at heart rates corresponding to peak oxygen intake (Anderson & Shephard, 1968a).

Experimental Values

If a moderately athletic young man undertakes maximal aerobic exercise, the carbon monoxide diffusing capacity ranges from 375 to 525 ml/min per kPa of driving pressure, or 50 to 70 ml/min per Torr. The corresponding value of $\alpha \dot{D}_{L,O_2}$ is between 45 and 60 L/min.

This last figure is much less than the hypothetical conductance of 450 to 500 L/min, predicted from the anatomical dimensions of the alveolar-capillary barrier (a surface area of 80 m^2, a harmonic mean thickness of 0.55 μm), the water solubility, and the diffusion coefficient for oxygen (Weibel, 1973). A part of the difference between the hypothetical and the experimental values is due to the time required for oxygen to react with the hemoglobin in the red cells. The delay creates a back-pressure of oxygen within the plasma, equivalent to the introduction of an additional series resistance between alveolar gas and the bloodstream. The imposed resistance varies inversely with the product of the rate of reaction (θ) and the volume of blood in the pulmonary capillaries (Q_c). Thus, if $\dot{D}_M$ is the conductance of the alveolar membrane proper, we may write

$$1/\dot{D}_L = 1/\dot{D}_M + 1/(\theta Q_c).$$

A true value for the membrane diffusing capacity can be obtained from the uptake of isotopically marked respiratory gases (Schuster, 1987), but more usually $\dot{D}_M$ is estimated from the observed values of $\dot{D}_L$ and θQ_c. The reaction constant (θ) for oxygen is close to unity. The anatomical value of Q_c is in the range 100 to 200 ml (Weibel, 1973), but physiological estimates based on the rate of gas transfer in resting subjects are substantially smaller. Given the limited distensibility of the pulmonary vascular bed, it seems unlikely that the functional value of Q_c exceeds 200 ml even in maximal aerobic exercise.

Thus, we may set an upper limit of 200 ml/min per Torr, or 143 L/min, to the conductance θQ_c. Taking $\dot{D}_L$ as 50 L/min, $\dot{D}_M$ would then be 77 L/min, still only about a sixth of the anatomical estimate. The probable reason for the remaining discrepancy is that the pulmonary capillaries cover only a small part of the available alveolar surface. Coverage increases during exercise, and there is an associated increase of $\dot{D}_M$ (Anderson & Shephard, 1968a). We may conclude that while the alveolar and capillary membranes would pose a negligible barrier to oxygen transfer if they were coextensive, a measurable resistance is normally found because parts of the alveolar surface are unrelated to perfused capillaries, and vice versa.

Alternative Evidence on Alveolar-Capillary Gas Exchange

Given technical difficulties in measuring the peak pulmonary diffusing capacity accurately (Anderson & Shephard, 1968a, 1968b), it is useful to consider other evidence concerning the equilibration of oxygen between alveolar gas and pulmonary capillary blood, based on transit times, alveolar-capillary oxygen concentration gradients, and arterial oxygen saturation.

CAPILLARY TRANSIT TIME. Under resting conditions, the transit time required for red cells to pass through the pulmonary capillaries ranges from 0.35 to 1.7 s, with an average of 0.8 s (Staub & Schultz, 1968). Calculations by these authors suggested that such times were adequate to allow both diffusion across the pulmonary membrane and the subsequent reaction of oxygen with intracorpuscular hemoglobin. Miyamoto and Moll (1971) estimated a similar average capillary path length, but argued that a minimum of 0.5 s was required for complete equilibration. However, their calculations neglected the facilitation of oxygen transfer by rotation of the red cells, their occasional displacement from the axial stream within the capillaries, and a possible movement of hemoglobin and cytochrome molecules within individual erythrocytes (E.P. Hill, Power, & Longo, 1973).

We may thus conclude that if the subject is at rest, there is adequate time for alveolar-capillary equilibration in even the shortest capillaries. Nevertheless, the margin is not large, and problems could arise if exercise induced a large increase of perfusion rates.

OXYGEN CONCENTRATION GRADIENTS. The small size of the oxygen concentration gradient from alveolar gas to pulmonary capillary or arterial blood provides further evidence that there is only a limited overall resistance to oxygen uptake at the alveolar-capillary interface. From a technical point of view, the most conveniently measured oxygen pressure gradient is that most appropriate to the conductance equation—from alveolar gas to arterial blood ($C_{A,O_2} - C_{a,O_2}$). The size of this gradient reflects not only incomplete equilibration of oxygen at the pulmonary interface, but also a mismatching of ventilation and perfusion within the lungs, and a fraction of the total cardiac output that bypasses the lungs in frank venous-arterial shunts.

The cross section of the pulmonary vessels shows about a threefold expansion in maximal aerobic exercise. Because cardiac output increases five- to sevenfold, the velocity of pulmonary blood flow must increase during maximal effort, and the average time available for gas transfer across the pulmonary membrane shortens from 0.75 or 0.80 s to 0.33 s. Moreover, the oxygen content of venous blood entering the lungs is much reduced in vigorous aerobic exercise; this increases the quantity of oxygen that must be transferred per unit of blood flow in order to realize 100% oxygen saturation of pulmonary venous blood. It also pushes the subject to the steep part of her or his oxygen dissociation curve (see Figure 2.8) where an increase in the effective solubility of oxygen in the blood reduces the ratio $\dot{D}_L / \lambda \dot{Q}$, further hampering equilibration at the alveolar interface.

Offsetting these handicaps, the increase of pulmonary capillary blood volume increases both the capillary surface area (a determinant of $\dot{D}_M$) and the product θQ_c, a rise of pulmonary arterial pressure facilitates perfusion of the upper part of the lungs (improving the match between $\dot{V}_A$ and $\dot{Q}$; West, 1977), and an increase of ventilation may push the $\dot{V}_A/\dot{Q}$ ratio from a resting figure of about 1 to 5 or 6 in maximal exercise. Thus, there is commonly a small increase of $P_{a_{O_2}}$ and a decrease of $P_{a_{CO_2}}$ during vigorous aerobic exercise (Asmussen & Nielsen, 1960).

Despite the composite nature of the alveolar-arterial gradient, it is quite small in young adults, typical values being 0.67 to 1.33 kPa (5-10 Torr) at rest, but 2.7 to 3.3 kPa (20-25 Torr) in near-maximal exercise. It has thus been argued that under resting conditions equilibration across the pulmonary membrane is virtually complete and that a relatively full equilibration is achieved even during vigorous aerobic effort (Shephard, 1987b), one occasional exception being the fit endurance athlete with a very large maximal cardiac output (Dempsey, 1986; Dempsey & Manohar, 1992).

ARTERIAL OXYGEN SATURATION.   The blood leaving the lungs in the pulmonary veins is normally almost fully saturated with oxygen, both at rest and during exercise. Nevertheless, a small decrease of arterial oxygen saturation can sometimes develop in well-trained athletes as they approach maximal aerobic effort (Gledhill, Spriet, Froese, Wilkes, & Meyers, 1980; Holmgren & Linderholm, 1958; Linderholm, 1959).

Changes in the temperature and pH of the blood induced by vigorous exercise complicate accurate measurements of arterial oxygen saturation, but recent evidence (Dempsey & Manohar, 1992; Powers, Dodd, Woodyard, Beadle, & Church, 1984; Powers et al., 1988; Williams, Powers, & Stuart, 1986) confirms the view that in some subjects with large maximal oxygen intakes, the arterial oxygen saturation may drop below 90% during brief bouts of very vigorous effort.

Although this probably reflects a diffusional limitation of gas exchange, there are some other potential explanations. For example, well-oxygenated pulmonary venous blood could have been diluted by poorly oxygenated blood that has bypassed the lungs (due to a poor matching of ventilation and perfusion or to frank venous-arterial shunts). The vertical matching of ventilation and perfusion improves during vigorous exercise (West, 1977), especially in endurance athletes (Todero, Pigorini, Rossi, & Venerando, 1979), but horizontal inequalities of ventilation and perfusion persist and may even increase (Hammond, Gale, Kapiton, Ries, & Wagner, 1986). Moreover, exercise reduces the oxygen content of venous blood, increasing the impact of poor ventilation-perfusion matching or a given venous-arterial shunt on arterial oxygen pressures (Dempsey & Manohar, 1992).

The practical importance of the arterial unsaturation can be assessed from the effects of a deliberate increase of alveolar oxygen pressure, using such tactics as voluntary hyperventilation, anaerobic exercise (Cockcroft et al., 1985), oxygen inspiration (Torre-Buono, Wagner, Saltzman, Gale, & Moon, 1985), or the breathing of an oxygen-helium mixture. Such maneuvers lead to small increases in both arterial oxygen saturation and peak oxygen intake (Dempsey & Manohar, 1992; P.W. Jones & Wakefield, 1984). On the other hand, significant arterial unsaturation seems unlikely to develop in the average person who is exercising at a moderate intensity that can be sustained for a few minutes to an hour.

Factors Modifying Pulmonary Diffusing Capacity

Are there any adverse changes in pulmonary diffusing capacity with prolonged exercise?

The rate of lymphatic drainage from the lungs increases during heavy physical activity (Coates, O'Brodovich, Jefferies, & Gray, 1984; Younes & Bshoutzy, 1989), and indirect evidence, such as an increase of residual gas volume and a decrease of $\dot{D}_L$, has suggested the possibility that subclinical edema may develop during prolonged bouts of vigorous exercise such as participation in a triathlon competition (Buono, Wilmore, & Roby, 1983; Maron, Hamilton, & Maksud, 1979; Miles, Enoch, & Grevey, 1986). But unless the subject is overhydrated, there is no radiographic evidence that edema develops (Gallagher, Huda, Rigby, Greenberg, & Younes, 1988), and any accumulation of extravascular fluid seems insufficient to hamper gas exchange (O'Brodovich, 1992). The main difficulty in gas exchange at the alveolar-capillary interface arises from a shortening of the equilibration time induced by exercise. During peak aerobic effort, the average red cell remains in the pulmonary capillary bed for only 0.33 s; in some capillary channels the transit time is much shorter than this. From the conductance equations, the key factor in equilibration across the alveolar interface is the ratio of peak diffusing capacity to peak cardiac output, or $\dot{D}_L / \lambda \dot{Q}$ (Haab, 1982; Shephard, 1971a). Maximal exercise increases $\lambda \dot{Q}$ more than $\dot{D}_L$, and the endurance athlete, having a large maximal cardiac output, is further handicapped relative to a sedentary person unless the athlete also has an above average exercise-induced increase of peak $\dot{D}_L$.

The normal shape of the oxygen dissociation curve nevertheless protects most subjects against the development of substantial arterial unsaturation during maximal aerobic exercise. The effective oxygen solubility factor *lambda* increases from around 1.2 to about 2.3 as the saturation of arterial blood falls from 97% to 90%. A decrease of P_{a,O_2} thus leads to only a small deterioration of oxygen transport unless the partial pressure gradient from alveolar gas to arterial blood widens to 50 Torr or more (Linderholm, 1959).

If the partial pressure gradient does exceed 50 Torr, then the subject is brought onto the steep part of her or his oxygen dissociation curve, the arterial oxygen saturation decreases rapidly, and there is a corresponding decrease in the oxygen transported per unit of cardiac output. Shepard (1958) calculated that in order to keep the arterial oxygen saturation above 90% at a maximal oxygen intake of 4 L/min (3.0 mmol/s), $\dot{D}_L$ should exceed 43 L/min, and if the maximal oxygen intake was 6 L/min (4.5 mmol/s), a figure of 71 L/min was required. Such figures are of the same order as the measured maximal diffusing capacity, emphasizing that although little physiological advantage would be gained from an increase of $\dot{D}_L$, a diminution of diffusing capacity would have serious repercussions on oxygen transport.

Effective Cardiac Output

The maximal cardiac output $\dot{Q}$ that can be attained during aerobic exercise is the product of maximal heart rate and maximal stroke volume. The heart rate is modulated by the balance of parasympathetic and sympathetic tone, and as the intensity of exercise is increased, by the stimulating (chronotropic) action of circulating catecholamines on the cardiac pacemaker (Shephard, 1982b). The stroke volume is influenced by the blood volume and thus the venous return to the heart (the preloading of the ventricles), the inherent pumping ability of the cardiac muscle or myocardial contractility at any given preload (as modified by the inotropic effects of catecholamines and sympathetic nerve activity), and the external impedance to systolic ejection imposed by systemic blood pressure and the compliance of the arterial tree (the afterloading of the heart).

The effectiveness of a given cardiac output in meeting the oxygen needs of the active tissues is influenced by the fraction of the total pulmonary blood flow that perfuses well-ventilated alveoli, the oxygen-carrying capacity of unit volume of blood, and the proportion of this oxygen content extracted by the active tissues (the arteriovenous oxygen difference). Account must also be taken of the distribution of the systemic blood flow between active muscles, inactive muscles, skin, and viscera. Finally, similar to ventilation, there is a theoretical upper limit of cardiac output, beyond which increases in the consumption of oxygen by the heart muscle itself outweigh any additional increases of peak oxygen intake.

Maximal Heart Rate

If a progressive exercise test is undertaken, the heart rate increases almost as a linear function of power output and oxygen consumption between 50% and 90% of maximal oxygen intake (I. Åstrand, 1960; Shephard, 1982b); but as maximal aerobic effort is approached, there is a tendency for the heart rate to plateau. However, it remains unclear why the heart rate peaks.

One factor is that further increases of sympathetic discharge induce progressively smaller increments of heart rate as maximal values are approached (Ribeiro, Ibanez, & Stein, 1991). The limitations of peak heart rate associated with breath-holding (Ahn et al., 1989) and exposure to very high altitudes (Pugh, 1962) both suggest that a deficient oxygen supply to the cardiac pacemaker may place a ceiling on heart rate. This certainly seems to be the case in occasional patients with atherosclerosis of the blood vessels supplying the pacemaker region (the sick sinus syndrome). However, the maximal heart rate also declines inevitably with age, yet the peak readings of an elderly person cannot be restored to their youthful values simply by administering oxygen during an exercise stress test.

Problems of venous filling may also be implicated. Certainly, venous return limits function during artificial pacing of the heart (Kissling & Jacob, 1973). Moreover, the rate of diastolic lengthening of the ventricle is faster in young than in elderly subjects (Shephard, 1987a). On the other hand, though the speed of diastolic lengthening is usually high in well-trained endurance athletes (Matsuda et al., 1983), they often have somewhat lower peak heart rates than sedentary individuals. Furthermore, there is no obvious relationship between the peaking of heart rate and the work rate at which stroke volume begins to decrease, making it unlikely that inadequate ventricular filling is an important limiting factor even at heart rates as high as 200 beats/min.

EXPERIMENTAL VALUES.   Heart rates as high as 250 to 300 beats/min may be developed for a few seconds during such heavily resisted activities as an awkward ski-turn; but in sustained rhythmic exercise, the heart rates of young men and women plateau at values a little under 200 beats/min. The term *maximal* will subsequently be applied to these plateau readings.

Maximal values are sometimes 5 to 10 beats/min lower in endurance athletes than in sedentary subjects, particularly if tests are made using sport-specific apparatus (Dal Monte, Faina, & Menchinelli, 1992). Vigorous aerobic training sometimes reduces the peak heart rate by a similar margin. On the other hand, endurance athletes tend to develop maximal values similar to sedentary subjects if they are asked to perform an activity that is unrelated to their selected sport (Shephard, 1982b).

The maximal heart rate decreases steadily throughout adult life (see Figure 2.11; also Fox & Haskell, 1968; Londeree & Moeschberger, 1982, 1984). There is much interindividual variability, and at least in sedentary subjects the maxima at any given age (Shephard, 1987b) are somewhat greater than suggested by the classical formula of 220 – age in years (P.O. Åstrand & Rodahl, 1986). Maximal values are also reduced at very high altitudes, although untrained subjects show no effect at altitudes below 2,000 m and athletes can sustain sea level maxima to 4,000 m (Kollias & Buskirk, 1974).

INFLUENCE OF MYOCARDIAL ISCHEMIA.   Healthy young subjects do not usually show signs of myocardial oxygen lack, even during maximal aerobic effort. In contrast, as many as a third of subjects 60 years and older develop clinical or electrocardiographic evidence of myocardial ischemia during a progressive exercise test as they approach exhaustion (Sidney & Shephard, 1977a; see chapter 3). Ischemia may present as angina, the onset of abnormal cardiac rhythms (particularly runs of premature ventricular contractions early in the cycle of cardiac repolarization; Cullen, Wearne, Stenhouse, & Cumpston, 1983), a depression of the ST segment of the electrocardiogram (Hollenberg, Go, Massie, Wisneski, & Gertz, 1985; Okin, Kligfield, Ameisen, Goldberg, & Borer, 1988; Staniloff, Diamond, & Pollock, 1984; Wohlfart, Pahlm, Sörnmo, Albrechtsson, & Lárusdottir, 1990), a failure of ventricular pumping, or upon cardiac catheterization, a transition from lactate uptake to lactate excretion in the coronary circulation (Blomqvist, 1974).

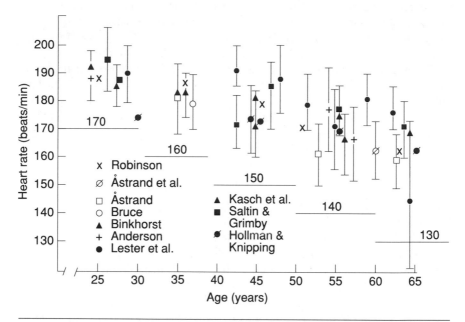

Figure 2.11   Effect of age on maximal heart rate. The horizontal bars represent approximately 85% of the maximal heart rate. *Note.* Reprinted from Fox and Haskell (1969) by permission.

Myocardial ischemia may limit both peak heart rate and cardiac stroke volume. In a small number of older subjects, the heart rate fails to increase to the anticipated maximal value during aerobic exercise because of a deficiency in the oxygen supply to the sinuatrial node (i.e., the sick sinus syndrome; Powles, Sutton, & Jones, 1974; Wohlfart et al., 1990). In other individuals, the onset of angina, alarming electrocardiographic changes, and such evidence of failing left ventricular function as a gallop rhythm or a falling systemic blood pressure lead to a symptom-limitation of maximal effort or a halting of the test by the supervising physician (American College of Sports Medicine, 1991; Sheffield, 1974).

Maximal Stroke Volume

The stroke volume of the heart is influenced by preloading of the ventricles, myocardial contractility, and afterloading. All of these variables change during exercise. The end result is that when a bout of aerobic exercise is performed sitting or standing, the normal heart shows a substantial increase of stroke volume to a maximal value, sustained from 50% to near 100% of maximal oxygen intake.

BLOOD VOLUME AND PRELOADING OF THE VENTRICLES.   Preloading of the ventricles influences the stroke volume markedly through the classical Frank-Starling mechanism (Shephard, 1982b). Provided there is not also a large increase of ventricular afterloading, the stroke volume rises progressively as diastolic filling increases. Filling of the ventricles depends directly on the venous return and thus the central blood volume (Asmussen & Christensen, 1939), but these variables are influenced in turn by the total blood volume.

One important consideration is the effectiveness of neural mechanisms regulating the tone of the venous reservoirs. Failure of venous regulation impairs physical working capacity; examples of such failure include the syndrome of vasoregulatory asthenia (a condition that affects some sedentary young adults) and the administration of an excessive dose of antihypertensive medication (a problem that all too commonly leads to hypotensive episodes among elderly individuals). During aerobic exercise, the tone of the cutaneous veins normally increases roughly in proportion to the severity of effort (Rowell, 1974, 1986), and such exercise can also enhance central blood volume through a 35% reduction in splanchnic blood volume (Wade & Bishop, 1962).

There is usually a 5% to 10% reduction of total blood volume during the first few minutes of vigorous physical activity (Rowell, 1974, 1985, 1986), due mainly to exudation of fluid into the active tissues. If the weather is warm, a rapid rise of core temperature leads to early sweating, a reversal of the normal increase in venous tone, and an increased exudation of fluid, further reducing the central blood volume and restricting the subject's ability to sustain a high work rate (Rowell, 1985; Saltin, 1964). However, there is no immediate decrease of maximal oxygen intake (Saltin, Gagge, Bergh, & Stolwijk, 1972) because the regulation of body temperature is not a limiting factor in the usual 10- to 15-min exercise bout associated with the measurement of aerobic power. On the other hand, the maximal oxygen intake is reduced if the body has been preheated before the test of aerobic power is begun (Pirnay, Deroanne, & Petit, 1970).

Aerobic training is commonly associated with an increase in total blood volume. In the early stages of such training, any potential gains of performance are commonly offset by an associated hemodilution and thus a decrease of hemoglobin concentration (H.J. Green, Jones, Hughson, Painter, & Farrance, 1987). But once adaptation is complete, there is a close (although not necessarily a causal) correlation between blood volume and maximal oxygen intake (Holmgren, 1967a).

The effects of artificially induced manipulations of blood volume have been studied in connection with wrestling and blood doping (autotransfusion). Wrestlers who deprive themselves of fluid in an attempt to enter an unnaturally low weight category suffer a decrease of physical working capacity that persists for at least 5 hr after rehydration (Herbert & Ribisl, 1972). Early investigators found inconsistent changes of working capacity following autotransfusion (M.H. Williams, 1974), but the variability of response was traced to a deterioration of blood specimens during storage (Gledhill, 1992). Well-controlled experiments have now shown an almost proportionate decrease of oxygen transport following bloodletting and a correspondingly supranormal endurance performance if appropriately preserved blood is reinfused after the subject has had time to regenerate a normal red cell count (Gledhill, 1992). Although there may be transient changes in circulating blood volume and thus in cardiac stroke volume with blood loss and subsequent reinfusion, the main effect of such maneuvers can be traced to changes in the hemoglobin content of unit volume of blood and thus the solubility factor lambda in the conductance equation.

In summary, there are some circumstances in which an acute decrease of blood volume can impair stroke volume, decreasing both endurance performance and oxygen transport. Such a development is particularly likely if the capacity of the system is strained by a combination of heat relaxation of the venous reservoirs, loss of fluid from the circulation, and sustained exercise. Conversely, a moderate increase of total blood volume and circulating hemoglobin gives a substantial advantage to an endurance performer.

MYOCARDIAL CONTRACTILITY.   The contractility of the myocardium is increased by a combination of intrinsic mechanisms related to heart rate, sympathetic nerve activity, and circulating catecholamine concentrations. During moderate aerobic exercise, an increase of venous return and thus of ventricular preloading accounts for most of the increase in stroke volume; but as maximal aerobic effort is approached, the influence of enhanced myocardial contractility becomes increasingly important.

Both sympathetic stimuli and catecholamine concentrations are likely to be greater during athletic competition than when a person is tested in the laboratory (Blimkie, Cunningham, & Leung, 1977). On the other hand, contractility may be impaired by a poor oxygen supply to the ventricles (e.g., in coronary vascular disease) or by excessive diastolic filling (in decompensated congestive heart failure). Cardiac denervation, such as occurs in heterotopic cardiac transplantation, also results in a less than normal increase of myocardial contractility during exercise (Shephard, 1991d).

AFTERLOADING OF THE VENTRICLES.   The myocardium has a finite working capacity, and thus the cardiac ejection fraction is influenced by the impedance resisting emptying of the ventricles, roughly equivalent to the systolic blood pressure.

Rhythmic exercise of the large skeletal muscles generally gives rise to some increase of systolic pressure, with little change of diastolic readings. A large increase of pressure is a harbinger of future resting hypertension (Jackson, Squires, Grimes, & Beard, 1983; Jetté, Landry, Sidney, & Blümchen, 1988). Increases of systolic pressure are also greater in older subjects (Montoye, 1984), in part because a given task requires use of a larger fraction of total aerobic power output. Higher pressures are seen when there is difficulty in perfusing the active muscles (e.g., in tasks that use small or weak muscles), or when making movements of the arms above the head (I. Åstrand, 1971; Lewis et al., 1983). Flow restriction seems greatest deep within the muscle belly, where the local pressure is highest, and occlusion is particularly marked in short, bulging muscles (Segersted et al., 1984). Bezucha, Lenser, Hanson, and Nagle (1982) noted a similar rise of blood pressure in one- and two-leg cycle ergometry if the two tests were arranged to demand a comparable relative effort. However, at high work rates, seated exercise seems to induce a greater cardiac work rate than supine activity (Moldover & Downey, 1983).

Resisted contractions that demand more than 15% to 25% of the maximal voluntary force for the muscle concerned (Byström & Kilböm, 1990; Järvholm, Styf, Suurkula, & Herberts, 1988) quickly restrict blood flow (Royce, 1958) and lead to major increases in both systolic and diastolic pressures, with corresponding augmentation in the work of the heart (Bull, Davies, Lind, & White, 1989; Gandevia & Hobbs, 1990; Lind & McNicol, 1967; Misner et al., 1990). The response seems proportional to the fraction of maximal voluntary force that is exerted (C.T.M. Davies & Starkie, 1985) and to the proportion of fast-twitch fibers that are activated (Frisk-Holmberg, Essén, Fredrickson, Ström, & Witell, 1983), but it is also influenced by the muscle mass that is involved in the exercise (Nagle, Seals, & Hanson, 1989).

The extent of ventricular afterloading in any given subject depends in part on the condition of the large arteries (peripheral vascular disease reduces arterial compliance, so that a given stroke volume gives rise to a larger rise of systolic pressure), in part on the tone of vasoregulatory mechanisms, and in part on the adequacy of perfusion of the active muscles (strong muscles and a large capillary-fiber ratio favor perfusion, whereas peripheral vascular disease may restrict it).

EXPERIMENTAL FINDINGS.   The effect of aerobic exercise on the stroke volume of a normal young adult varies with body posture. In the supine or semirecumbent position typical of much clinical testing, there is little increase of stroke volume over the range from rest to moderate effort (Magder, Daughters, Hung, Alderman, & Ingels, 1987). However, when subjects begin exercise sitting on a cycle ergometer, or standing on a treadmill, the leg veins are initially well filled. Exercise then tends to empty the dependent venous reservoirs, through direct compression of the large veins, an increase of thoracic suction, and (as the intensity of effort increases) an increase of venous tone (Holmgren, 1967a, 1967b). The resultant increase in preloading of the heart, coupled with an increase of myocardial contractility, increases stroke volume. Typically, maximal values are reached at about 30% to 50% of aerobic power (Simmons & Shephard, 1971b). Thereafter, stroke volume usually remains constant or may even decline, and any further increases of cardiac output depend on an increase of heart rate.

The maximal stroke volume varies somewhat with the aerobic fitness of the individual and with the mode of exercise that is being performed. Endurance athletes show a faster ventricular relaxation than sedentary individuals; they are thus able to develop a larger end-diastolic volume and a larger stroke volume (Dickuth, Horstman, Staiger, Reindell, & Keul, 1989; Fagard, Van den Broeke, & Amery, 1989; Rubal, Moody, Damore, Bunker, & Diaz, 1986). Treadmill exercise also yields a larger peak value (100-160 ml in young women, 120-180 ml in young men) than standard cycle ergometry (85-145 and 105-165 ml in women and men, respectively; Shephard et al., 1968b). The figures observed when using a standard cycle ergometer are in turn larger than the values observed when operating an arm ergometer (Simmons & Shephard, 1971b), although the deficit of stroke volume in aerobic arm exercise can be made good if moderate leg exercise is undertaken simultaneously (Toner, Glickman, & McArdle, 1990).

There have been suggestions that well-trained, older individuals who are free of ischemic heart disease attempt to compensate for the age-related limitation of maximal heart rate (Weisfeldt, Gerstenblith, & Lakatta, 1985) by increasing their peak stroke volume at the expense of an increased maximal end-diastolic volume. However, many older subjects show a decrease rather than an increase of stroke volume as maximal effort is approached (Niinimaa & Shephard, 1978), presumably because poor myocardial oxygen delivery weakens the force of ventricular contraction.

PROLONGED EXERCISE AND CARDIOVASCULAR DRIFT.   At any age, a bout of prolonged but submaximal aerobic exercise leads to a progressive diminution of stroke volume, with an offsetting increase of heart rate (R.B. Armstrong, 1987; J.M. Johnson, 1977, 1987; Rowell, 1974, 1985, 1986; Savard, Kiens, & Saltin, 1987).

Possible explanations of this cardiovascular drift include a mechanical slowing of ventricular systole (Ekelund & Holmgren, 1967; Seals et al., 1988), the development of heterogenous motion in the left ventricular wall (Douglas, O'Toole, & Woolard, 1990), a reduction of vagal discharge (Hartley et al., 1970), a heat-induced increase of heart rate (7 beats/min for a 1°C rise of rectal temperature; José, Stitt, & Collison, 1970) with an associated reduction of stroke volume (J.M. Johnson, 1987), a progressive increase of both cutaneous and muscle blood flow (R.B. Armstrong, 1987), a relaxation of venous tone (Zitnik et al., 1971), and an exudation of fluid into the tissues (Miles, Sawka, Glaser, & Petrofsky, 1983) related to both the increased osmolality of the tissue fluids and to capillary vasodilatation (Stick, Heinemann, & Witzleb, 1990).

Saltin (1973) argued that peripheral pooling was a relatively unimportant cause of cardiovascular drift, because stroke volume decreased almost equally in a prolonged bout of supine exercise. Further, in his experience, the decrease of stroke volume associated with prolonged heavy, submaximal effort could be corrected by a brief period of maximal exercise. However, others have argued that the main responsibility for the decline of stroke volume lies with peripheral pooling and a resultant decrease of ventricular filling (Molé & Coulson, 1985; Tibbits, 1985).

Maximal Cardiac Output

The maximal cardiac output is the product of the peak heart rate and the corresponding stroke volume. The peak cardiac output per unit of body mass is generally much lower in humans than in animal species (Rowell, 1988), amounting to perhaps 20 to 25 L/min in normal young women and men, and 25 to 35 L/min in endurance athletes, but falling to 15 to 20 L/min at an age of 65 years (Niinimaa & Shephard, 1978).

Over much of the range from rest to maximal aerobic effort, there is a linear relationship between cardiac output and oxygen intake (I. Åstrand, 1960; Pirnay, Lamy, Dujardin, Deroanne, & Petit, 1972), although the tendency to a fall of blood pressure and failure of cerebral perfusion during a sustained maximal effort suggests that there may be some decline of cardiac output as exhaustion is approached (Shephard et al., 1968b).

The value of $\dot{Q}$ appropriate to the conductance equation is a little less than the peak cardiac output, because perfusion of the lungs is never 100% efficient. The level of arterial unsaturation observed during maximal effort allows us to set an upper limit. If arterial blood has an oxygen saturation of 90% (Dempsey & Manohar, 1992) and mixed venous blood has a saturation of 15%, then the inefficiency of perfusion amounts to about 12% of the observed maximal cardiac output.

DISTRIBUTION OF CARDIAC OUTPUT.   Under resting conditions, muscle and skin blood flow together account for about a quarter of the cardiac output (about 1.5 L/min), while the remainder (about 4.6 L/min) is distributed to other parts of the body. Most tissues are relatively well perfused, and on average less than a quarter of the available oxygen is extracted from the blood as it passes around the circulation (an arteriovenous oxygen concentration difference of 40-50 ml/L).

During maximal aerobic exercise, the situation is very different. Almost all of the available oxygen is extracted from blood perfusing the active muscles (see Table 2.3). Blood flow is also diverted to the active muscles from other parts of the body (Musch, 1988; Musch, Haidet, Ordway, Longhurst, & Mitchell, 1987; Rowell, 1974, 1985, 1986; Wade & Bishop, 1962). Visceral perfusion is most affected, but there is some reduction of blood flow to inactive muscles (Bevegard & Shepherd, 1967; Ozolin, 1986), and as peak effort is approached, there may be a cutaneous vasoconstriction. The greatest redistribution of blood flow is induced by a combination of exercise and heat exposure. In such circumstances, the blood flow to the liver and kidneys may be less than 50% of normal, and the fractional extraction of oxygen from the visceral bloodstream is greatly increased (Poortmans, 1984; Rowell, 1985).

A limit to such circulatory adaptations is set by the susceptibility of the viscera to oxygen lack. If heavy aerobic exercise is performed under adverse environmental conditions, the delivery of oxygen to the liver and kidneys may drop to the point where a mild tissue protest is registered. Impaired liver function may reduce the activity of key enzymes such as serum cholinesterase (Gorski, Oscai, & Palmer, 1990; Nagel, Seiler, Franz, & Kung, 1990), and disturbances of renal function may cause protein and red cells to escape into the urine (Gilli, DePaoli-Vitali, Tataranni, & Farinelli, 1984; Poortmans, Rampaer, & Wolfs, 1989). But at most, a blood flow of 2.0 to 2.5 L/min (some 10% of the peak cardiac output) can be redirected to the working muscles by economies in perfusion of the viscera and inactive muscles.

A reduction in skin blood flow offers a more important potential mechanism of sustaining muscle blood flow during exhausting exercise. Skin blood flows

Table 2.3
Arteriovenous O₂ Differences in Various Tissues in a Moderately
Athletic Young Man During Maximal Aerobic Exercise

Tissue	Volume (L)	Oxygen consumption (ml/min)	Blood flow (L/min)	Arteriovenous O_2 difference (ml/L)
Muscle	28	4,550	24.5	186
Skin	10	12	6.0	2
Other organs	32	138	1.5	92
All tissues	70	4,700	32.0	147

Note. Reprinted from Shephard (1977a) by permission.

as large as 7 to 10 L/min have been observed during sustained heat stress (Detry, Brengelmann, Rowell, & Wyss, 1972; Rowell, 1974, 1985, 1986). Likewise, during near-maximal effort, the blood flow to the skin can account for about a quarter of the total cardiac output, although a sudden blanching of the skin suggests that there is an intense vasoconstriction as maximal effort is approached (Shephard et al., 1968a). The blood flow demands of the skin when exercising in a hot environment are reduced by an upright posture (J.M. Johnson, Rowell, & Brengelmann, 1974), by heat acclimatization (Eichna, Park, Nelson, Horvath, & Palmes, 1950), and by training (Simmons & Shephard, 1971a). There is thus some interaction between heat acclimatization and endurance training (P. Marcus, 1972).

During vigorous aerobic exercise, both the skin blood flow and the total cardiac output vary with the duration of the activity. Saltin (1973) found a peak cardiac output of 23.8 L/min in a 3- to 4-min maximal effort, rising to 26.7 L/min with more protracted exercise. Because of the greater cutaneous vasodilatation in the protracted experiment, systemic pressures were much lower than in brief exercise (respective mean values of 14.6 and 19.8 kPa). Presumably, the reduced afterloading of the heart allowed a larger cardiac output and thus a greater skin blood flow to be achieved without either an increase of overall cardiac work rate or a reduction in blood flow to the muscles and viscera.

THE SOLUBILITY COEFFICIENT λ. The overall cardiovascular conductance for a soluble gas, such as oxygen, depends on the product of peak cardiac output and the corresponding solubility coefficient λ. The normal value of the oxygen solubility coefficient increases from 1.2 to 2.4 with the fall in oxygen saturation of the blood on passing from the flat arterial to the steeper venous portion of the oxygen dissociation curve (see Figure 2.8). Note that the integrated value of λ, relevant to the interaction between pulmonary diffusion and blood transport of oxygen at the alveolar interface, is much smaller (in the range 0.3-0.4) because the blood is almost fully saturated with oxygen during most of its time in the pulmonary capillaries.

HEMOGLOBIN LEVEL.   The most important factor influencing λ is the blood hemoglobin concentration. The average woman has a hemoglobin level that is 10% to 18% lower than that of a man, due in part to menstrual losses of iron and in part to lower concentrations of androgens. Women thus have lower values of λ than men, which explains a part of the observed gender difference in aerobic power (Drinkwater, 1984).

Some well-trained endurance athletes also have a tendency to anemia (Clement, Asmundson, & Medhurst, 1977). This has been blamed on such factors as fads of diet (Mahlamarki & Mahlamarki, 1988), poor iron absorption due to a high-fat diet (Ehn, Carlmark, & Höglund, 1980), losses of iron in the sweat (Fredrickson, Puhl, & Runyan, 1980; Verde, Shephard, Corey, & Moore, 1984), a decreased formation or an increased destruction of red cells (Puhl, Runyan, & Kruse, 1981; Reinhart, Stäubli, & Straub, 1983), and hemorrhage from the intestines or the bladder (Eichner, 1989; D.E. Martin et al., 1986; J.G. Stewart et al., 1984). However, the main cause of athletic anemia is probably a hemodilution associated with an expansion of the plasma volume (H.J. Green et al., 1984; Kanstrup & Ekblöm, 1984), and if the total hemoglobin content of the body is estimated, a supposedly anemic athlete usually shows very normal values (J.H. Ross & Attwood, 1984).

In animals, either exercise or fear can cause a contraction of the spleen, increasing both the total blood volume and also the oxygen-carrying capacity of unit volume of blood (Manohar, 1987); but this type of response does not seem to occur in humans. Although sustained exercise leads to a temporary 5% to 10% increase in red cell count per unit volume of blood, this is due rather to various forms of water loss such as sweating and exudation of fluid from the blood into the tissues.

Prolonged arterial oxygen unsaturation (for example, congenital cyanotic heart disease or life at altitudes greater than 3,000 m) stimulates the bone marrow, increasing the formation of red cells, and boosting hemoglobin concentrations by up to 50%. Unfortunately, large increases of the red cell count can cause other less advantageous changes, including a rise of blood viscosity, an increased resistance to blood flow (but see Celsing, Svedenhag, Philstedt, & Ekblöm, 1986), and a greater vulnerability to intravascular clotting. It was once suggested that endurance athletes might enhance their competitive performance by a period of training at an altitude of 2,000 to 3,000 m. In theory, a small and temporary advantage is gained in this fashion (Dick, 1992; Shephard, 1974a, 1992d). However, training schedules are usually interrupted by the combination of altitude sojourn and unfamiliar surroundings, and unless the subjects are initially poorly trained, the net result is often a deterioration rather than an improvement of aerobic performance (Shephard, 1974a; 1992d). The red cell count and the hemoglobin level may be increased for the first few days after return to sea level, but normal values are quickly restored by a combination of hemolysis and reduced red cell formation once the stimulus of a low arterial oxygen content has been removed (Shephard, 1992d).

OTHER MODIFYING FACTORS. If the oxygen saturation of arterial blood falls, the affected person operates on the steepest portion of his or her oxygen dissociation curve, increasing the effective value of λ. This characteristic of blood oxygen transport makes an important contribution to the ability of the body to exercise, both at high altitudes (Houston & Riley, 1947) and in the presence of right-to-left intracardiac shunts (i.e., cyanotic heart disease; Ernsting & Shephard, 1951).

Changes in the 2, 3-diphosphoglycerate content of the red corpuscles can also modify the shape of the oxygen dissociation curve and thus change the value of λ. For instance, either a single bout of endurance exercise (Meen, Holter, & Refsum, 1981) or a more prolonged period of endurance training can increase the slope of the oxygen dissociation curve and thus augment the value of λ (Böning, Schweigart, Tibes, Hammer, & Meier, 1974; Veicsteinas, Ferretti, Margonato, Rosa, & Tagliabue, 1984). However, it is less clear whether such changes modify overall oxygen transport in the manner that the oxygen conductance equation would suggest (Cade et al., 1984; Flenley, Fairweather, Cooke, & Kirby, 1973).

FUNCTIONAL SIGNIFICANCE. The practical importance of the oxygen-carrying capacity of the blood and thus the solubility factor λ is most evident in experimental studies of carbon monoxide poisoning. In such circumstances, the decrease of maximal oxygen intake is almost directly proportional to the percentage of red cell pigment that has been converted to carboxyhemoglobin (Horvath, Raven, Dahms, & Gray, 1975).

Studies of autotransfusion also demonstrate the important influence of changes in hemoglobin level on both maximal oxygen intake (Gledhill, 1992) and endurance performance (Berglund & Hemmingson, 1987; Brien & Simon, 1987).

In acute bloodletting or severe anemia (at hemoglobin concentrations of 50-80 g/L, or 0.8-1.3 mmol/L), the maximal oxygen intake is greatly reduced, but oxygen transport is restored to more normal values after correction of the anemia (C.T.M. Davies & Van Haaren, 1973a, 1973b; Kanstrup & Ekblöm, 1984). On the other hand, in chronic mild anemia (110-120 g of hemoglobin per liter of blood, or 1.7-1.9 mmol/L), responses to submaximal exercise remain normal, and no reduction of maximal oxygen intake is seen (Vellar & Hermansen, 1971). One possible explanation of this paradox is that the lowering of blood viscosity associated with a mild anemia permits the subject to develop a larger maximal cardiac output; nevertheless, the adverse effects of a high red cell count on blood viscosity are less marked in vivo than in vitro (Celsing et al., 1986), because of the vasodilatation and warming of the blood that are induced by exercise.

The Oxygen Expenditure of the Heart

As with the respiratory muscles, there is at least a theoretical possibility that an increase in the oxygen expenditure of the ventricular muscle could outweigh the additional oxygen transported by an increase of cardiac output.

Under resting conditions, some 20% of myocardial oxygen consumption is attributable to the basal metabolism of the heart, and a further 1% is due to the energy cost of activating cardiac tissue. The energy cost of pumping blood around the arterial system accounts for no more than 3% of the total myocardial oxygen consumption. The main sources of metabolic expense are the development and maintenance of tension within the ventricular walls (Shephard, 1982b).

The work rate of the resting heart thus depends largely on the determinants of ventricular wall tension (that is, the intraventricular pressure, the square of the ventricular radius, and the inverse of wall thickness), on the number of times such tension is developed each minute (the heart rate), and the efficiency of conversion of chemical energy into mechanical work, which is an inverse function of myocardial contractility.

During exercise, the contractility of the heart is increased, in part by the rise of heart rate itself, but to a larger extent by an augmentation of beta-adrenergic discharge. The stroke volume increases with physical activity, but even in maximal aerobic effort, the external work associated with the pumping of blood around the circulation (the product of pressure and stroke volume) accounts for no more than 10% to 15% of cardiac metabolism (Burton, 1965; Shephard, 1982b). The major component of the myocardial oxygen consumption thus remains the development of intraventricular tension, and the energy expenditure of the heart continues to depend heavily on the systemic blood pressure.

EXPERIMENTAL VALUES. The resting dog heart consumes oxygen at a rate of about 75 nmol/s or 100 μl/min per gram of tissue, increasing to a figure of 0.45 μmol/s or 600 μl/min per gram in vigorous aerobic effort (Van Citters & Franklin, 1969). Figures for the pony (Manohar, 1988) and the human heart (Jorgensen, 1972) are of a similar order. Thus, with a heart weighing 300 g, the resting oxygen consumption would be 22 μmol/s, or 30 ml/min, and a maximal oxygen consumption of 134 μmol/s, or 180 ml/min, might be reached during vigorous aerobic exercise.

The oxygen expended per liter of cardiac output (5-6 ml/L) is similar during rest and exercise and is small relative to the oxygen that is transported (50 ml/L at rest; 150 ml/L during maximal exercise). It is thus unlikely that the average person ever reaches the point where the increase of oxygen expenditure associated with a further increase of cardiac output exceeds the resulting gain in overall oxygen intake. Nevertheless, the oxygen needs of the heart make an appreciable charge on the overall oxygen transport account and can add to the problems caused by the increasing oxygen cost of respiration during vigorous aerobic activity.

Tissue Diffusing Capacity

The effective tissue diffusing capacity can be estimated empirically from the known maximal oxygen intake and the probable gradient of oxygen tension from the tissue capillaries to the ultimate site of oxygen consumption within the active muscle cells.

Determination of intracellular $NAD^+/NADH$ ratios suggests that resting cellular metabolism drops by about 50% if the local oxygen pressure falls to 1 Torr (0.13 kPa; Chance, 1957; Granger, Goodman, & Cook, 1975), although in the mitochondria (where the majority of oxidative reactions occur), the critical oxygen pressure is as much as 1 to 2 orders smaller than this (Chance, 1957, 1977; Chance & Pring, 1968; Granger et al., 1975). Such findings may be compared with in vivo estimates of intramuscular oxygen pressures, based on the behavior of myoglobin during tetanic stimulation of the soleus muscle (Millikan, 1937). The saturation of the pigment suggested that the oxygen pressure within the cytoplasm of the active muscle remained between 3 Torr (0.4 kPa) and 5 Torr (0.66 kPa).

Alternative estimates of tissue oxygen pressures have been derived from femoral venous blood samples. This approach has sometimes yielded pressures as high as 22 Torr (2.9 kPa, corresponding to an oxygen content of 60 ml/L; Doll, Keul, & Maiwald, 1968), but such data are hard to reconcile with mixed venous oxygen contents of 30 to 40 ml/L, and one must suppose that the femoral venous specimens were heavily contaminated with blood draining from the superficial cutaneous veins.

A third option has been to examine the venous effluent from isolated muscle preparations. The results obtained by this technique have sometimes been complicated by an inadequate perfusion of the working muscle, but Stainsby (1986) observed a pressure of 6 to 10 Torr (0.8-1.3 kPa) in the blood flowing from muscle that was consuming oxygen at a rate equivalent to 3 L/min in a human subject.

A final alternative is to use the graphic method suggested by Bohr (1909) to estimate the oxygen tension within the tissue capillaries. To the extent that the tissue oxygen pressure is nonuniform, this method underestimates tissue diffusing capacity, but nevertheless it remains a useful model (Stainsby, Snyder, & Welch, 1988). Given a pulmonary venous oxygen tension of 115 Torr (15.4 kPa), an oxygen tension of 5 Torr (0.66 kPa) in the muscle veins, and an average oxygen tension of 4.5 Torr (0.6 kPa) in the surrounding tissues, the Bohr integration indicates a mean tension of 17.5 Torr (2.3 kPa) in the tissue capillaries, with a gradient of some 17.5 Torr (2.3 kPa) from the capillaries to the cytoplasm. Given a maximal oxygen intake of 4 L/min, the tissue diffusing capacity would then amount to 308 ml/min per Torr, or 219 L/min in the units of our conductance equation.

Evidence for a Peripheral Limitation of Function

Argument over the possible contribution of peripheral factors to endurance performance has continued for several decades. The peak muscle blood flow seems much larger in vivo than in isolated muscle preparations, with figures as large as 200 to 500 ml/min per 100 g of tissue being cited (Andersen & Saltin, 1985; Laughlin & Armstrong, 1985; Musch, Haidet, Ordway, Longhurst, & Mitchell, 1987; Reading et al., 1992; Rowell, 1988). Thus, if the bulk of the active muscle is large (e.g., the 20 kg anticipated in treadmill running), the potential blood flow through the active muscle (40-100 L/min) would far exceed the pumping ability of the average heart.

Although there are strong arguments favoring a central flow limitation when the bulk of active muscle is large, peripheral impedance becomes of growing importance as the volume of active muscle is decreased (e.g., single leg or arm exercise; LeJemtal, Maskin, Lucido, & Chadwicj, 1986; Shephard et al., 1988a). Indeed, even in two-leg ergometry, complaints of muscular weakness and fatigue with an early accumulation of lactate suggest that peripheral factors impose some limitations on aerobic effort (Shephard et al., 1968b). Clausen (1973) found that the blood flow to the vastus lateralis muscle (as indicated by the somewhat fallible technique of ^{133}Xenon clearance; Sejersen & Tonnesen, 1972) reached a plateau at some 70% of maximal oxygen intake. It may be that at higher intensities of effort, blood flow is directed to other intramuscular pathways. But if Clausen's data are taken at face value, the simplest explanation would be that the tension developed within an actively contracting muscle can rise to a sufficient level to restrict local perfusion. During isometric exercise, such a restriction first appears at about 15% of maximal voluntary force, and occlusion becomes complete at about 70% of maximal effort (Kilbom, 1976; Royce, 1958). During cycle ergometry, measurements of peak pedal torque suggest that exertion demands up to 25% of peak quadriceps force (Hoes, Binkhorst, Smeekes-Kuyl, & Vissurs, 1968).

The discussion of central versus peripheral factors is to some extent semantic, because the performance of the heart can be impaired by a failure of peripheral venous return (causing inadequate preloading of the ventricles), by an excessive rise of systemic blood pressure associated with weak skeletal muscles that are contracting at a large fraction of their maximal voluntary force or an inadequate vasodilatation in the active tissues (causing excessive afterloading of the heart), or by a peripheral symptom such as muscle pain that halts exercise before any aspect of central cardiorespiratory function has been fully stressed (Hartling et al., 1989). Nevertheless, it is useful to conclude our analysis of oxygen conductances by reviewing the main arguments that have been advanced by peripheralists, such as Kaijser (1970).

VARIATION OF PEAK OXYGEN INTAKE WITH MODE OF EXERCISE. If aerobic power were entirely centrally limited, it would be independent of the mode of exercise. However, even in young adults, step-test and cycle-ergometer values are, respectively, 3% to 4% and 6% to 7% smaller than the values obtained during uphill treadmill running (P.O. Åstrand & Saltin, 1961a; Shephard et al., 1968a). In older subjects with weak quadriceps muscles, the cycle ergometer may yield proportionately even lower results relative to step or treadmill tests (Bailey, Shephard, & Mirwald, 1976).

Arm ergometer exercise normally shows an oxygen consumption plateau that is only 70% of the treadmill maximum (Shephard et al., 1988a); part of the oxygen consumption during arm exercise is attributable to maintenance of body posture, and the peak external power output is an even smaller fraction of that seen in leg exercise. Thus, if the trunk is immobilized by strapping, the peak oxygen intake observed on the arm ergometer is only about a third of that for two-leg ergometry (C.T.M. Davies & Sargeant, 1974). On the other hand, the peak effort developed on an arm ergometer comes much closer to the treadmill figure in athletes such as canoeists and whitewater paddlers who have well-developed arm and shoulder muscles (Shephard, 1987c; Tesch, 1983; Vaccaro, Clarke, A.F. Morris, & Gray, 1984).

During cycle ergometer exercise, the cardiac output falls substantially short of the figures attained during uphill treadmill running (Simmons & Shephard, 1971b), providing further evidence that there is some peripheral limitation of the cycle ergometer task. During arm ergometry, the active muscle mass is probably only about 4 kg, compared to 20 kg in leg ergometry (Shephard et al., 1988a). Nevertheless, if 70% of treadmill maximal oxygen intake can be developed in such a situation, then application of the conductance equation suggests that the peripheral muscles must be adding no more than 43% to the centrally based impedance of oxygen transport encountered during treadmill running.

EFFECT OF VARIATIONS IN AMBIENT PRESSURE.   If circulatory transport is limiting an individual's maximal oxygen intake, then differences in arterial oxygen content induced by increases or decreases of ambient pressure should cause parallel changes in peak oxygen transport. Kaijser (1970) failed to find any increase in the somewhat subjective criterion of endurance time when his subjects were operating a cycle ergometer at an ambient pressure of 3 atmospheres. However, he made no measurements of maximal oxygen intake. Moreover, it seems likely that because of the very high ambient pressures that he used, the performance of his subjects was limited by an accumulation of carbon dioxide rather than by problems of oxygen transport.

The effect of variations in ambient pressure on oxygen transport is complicated by the nonlinearity of the oxygen dissociation curve. Nevertheless, most authors other than Kaijser (1970) have found an increment of oxygen transport with an increase in the oxygen pressure gradient (Forgraeus, 1973; Shephard, 1982b) and a decrease of oxygen transport as the inspired oxygen pressure is reduced (Kollias & Buskirk, 1974; Shephard, 1974a, 1992d). Shephard et al. (1988a) further noted that as the volume of active muscle was reduced, the task became increasingly limited by peripheral factors, and the handicap imposed by a low partial pressure of inspired oxygen was correspondingly diminished.

The distribution of pressure gradients emphasizes the dominance of central factors in two-leg cycle ergometry. Even in the experiments of Kaijser (1970), the venous oxygen pressure was only 65 Torr (8.6 kPa) when working at an ambient pressure of 3 atmospheres. Thus, the major part of the pressure drop from inspired air (oxygen pressure 1,800 Torr, or 240 kPa) must have occurred in the lungs and circulation rather than in the active tissues.

SPECIFICITY OF TRAINING.   If aerobic training is based on a program of arm exercise, relatively little of the improvement in oxygen transport that is observed during a subsequent arm ergometer test generalizes to the performance of leg exercise (Clausen, 1977; Sinoway et al., 1987). On the other hand, if the subject is trained on a normal, two-leg cycle ergometer, 57% of the increase in oxygen transport is transferred to the subsequent performance of all-out exercise on the arm ergometer (Clausen, 1977). Likewise, a program of treadmill training produces equal gains of aerobic performance on the treadmill *and* the cycle ergometer, although cycle ergometer training has a much smaller impact on subsequent treadmill performance (Pechar, McArdle, Katch, Magel, & deLucca, 1974).

Such observations support the view that there is some peripheral limitation of arm exercise, and possibly also of cycle ergometry, but that the large-muscle leg exercise performed on a treadmill is centrally limited. The 57% transfer of gains from the leg to the arm task agrees quite well with the conclusion that during arm work, peripheral factors add 43% to the impedance associated with central limitations of oxygen transport.

EFFECTS OF CHANGES IN CARDIAC OUTPUT.   If cardiac output limits oxygen transport, then an increase of maximal cardiac output should augment maximal oxygen intake. This is not always the case. P.O. Åstrand and Saltin (1961b) found that peak cardiac output increased as the duration of maximal effort was extended from 3 to 5 min to 6 to 10 min, but the peak oxygen transport remained unchanged. Likewise, beta-blocking agents such as propranolol decrease peak cardiac output without affecting maximal oxygen intake (P.O. Åstrand, Ekblöm, & A.N. Goldberg, 1971).

At first inspection, such observations might seem to argue against a central cardiac limitation of oxygen transport. The probable explanation is that both prolonged exercise and beta-blocking drugs (Gordon, van Rensburg, Russell, Kielblock, & Myburgh, 1987) alter the distribution of the available cardiac output between the active muscles and other channels such as the cutaneous circulation; the central flow to the muscles remains limiting, but is obscured by changes in skin blood flow. The nature of the response to beta-blocking drugs also depends on protocol (particularly the rate of increase of work rate; Hughson, 1989), and if a sufficient dose is administered, a 5% to 15% reduction of maximal oxygen intake occurs, although this still does not match the 30% to 35% decrease of peak heart rate (Gordon et al., 1987; Tesch, 1985).

EFFECT OF CHANGES IN MUSCLE TEMPERATURE.   If the limbs are warmed before testing, the maximal oxygen consumption increases, and if they are cooled, it decreases (Kaijser, 1970). Nevertheless, the magnitude of these changes in oxygen consumption (1 L/min for a 10°C-change in tissue temperature) is smaller than the effect predicted by the law of Arrhenius (i.e., a doubling of metabolic rate for a 10°C-change of tissue temperature). Cooling also reduces both maximal heart rate and the maximal arteriovenous oxygen difference.

Kaijser (1970) interpreted the narrowing of the overall arteriovenous oxygen difference with cooling as proof that the associated decrease of maximal oxygen intake was due to a thermally induced reduction in the activity of tissue enzyme systems that normally limit oxygen transport. However, there are other tenable explanations: (1) In a cold environment, the volume of blood perfusing the active muscles is reduced, and it thus undergoes a greater relative dilution by blood from other sources, such as the viscera; and (2) because cooling causes peripheral vasoconstriction, increasing the diffusion pathway from the tissue capillaries to the active sites within the muscle fibers, there may be an adaptive augmentation of oxygen pressure in the muscle capillaries. This last explanation implies that the muscle capillary system rather than tissue enzymes is a factor potentially limiting endurance performance.

BIOCHEMICAL RESPONSES TO TRAINING.   The activity of rate-limiting enzymes such as phosphofructokinase and succinic dehydrogenase increases in response to aerobic training (Henriksson, 1992a, 1992b; Holloszy, 1973; Saltin, 1973), and the trained subject also shows some widening of the maximal arterio-venous oxygen difference.

Some authors have inferred from these changes that the enzymes concerned normally limit endurance performance. However, anaerobic training can induce much larger increases of activity in many tissue enzymes (Gollnick & Hermansen, 1973). Further, the time course of the changes in oxygen transport induced by aerobic training and the cessation of such training does not seem to parallel gains of enzyme activity (Henriksson, 1992a, 1992b; also see chapter 4). Finally, the oxygen content of venous blood leaving the active muscles is such that there is little scope for a development of tissue enzymes to increase extraction; Saltin (1973) found only 6 ml of oxygen per liter of femoral venous blood.

It seems more likely that the training-induced widening of the arteriovenous oxygen difference reflects the direction of a larger fraction of the total cardiac output to the active muscles, with less dilution of the mixed venous blood by flow from low-extraction regions such as the skin (Simmons & Shephard, 1971a). Not only is the endurance-trained subject's need for skin blood flow reduced by earlier sweating and a reduction of subcutaneous fat, but the increase of total cardiac output reduces the impact of a given skin flow on the oxygen saturation of mixed venous blood.

What alternative explanation can be advanced for the doubling of tissue enzyme activity that develops during the course of aerobic training? One possible reason might be that the tissues are compensating for a lengthening of the oxygen diffusion path. Saltin (1973) observed that a 15% gain of maximal oxygen intake was associated with a 37% increase of muscle fiber area. Often, such muscle hypertrophy is accompanied by an increase in the number of capillaries per muscle fiber (Shephard & Plyley, 1992), but in the absence of such an adjustment of blood supply, an increase of enzyme activities might serve a similar purpose. Another advantage of an increased enzyme activity is that less phosphagen depletion is needed to activate mechanisms of oxygen transport at the beginning of exercise (Saltin & Karlsson, 1971). Lastly, and probably most importantly, if enzyme activity is increased, then the steady-state combustion of carbohydrate tends to be replaced by the metabolism of fat (Holloszy, 1973), thus conserving glycogen for periods when the muscles contract too strongly—or too long each cycle—to permit their unrestricted perfusion.

Although there is some truth in a number of the arguments advanced for a peripheral limitation of oxygen transport, particularly when the active muscle mass is small, calculations of tissue diffusing capacity and application of the conductance equation support the thesis that the tissues do not normally offer a major impedance to oxygen delivery during large-muscle tasks.

Overall Conductance Equation

In summary, it is useful to incorporate the various constants that we have determined into the conductance equation for oxygen. Tissue diffusing capacity is so large that the fourth term in the equation may be neglected, except when performing a small-muscle task or when the local circulation is restricted by a condition such as Burger's disease.

In a healthy but sedentary young woman, we might find $\dot{V}_A = 60$ L/min, and $\lambda\dot{Q} = 20$ L/min. Using a nomogram to integrate λ for the alveolar interface (Shephard, 1971a), we find that the cumbersome term $B/(1-B)$ is about 0.006, so that the overall conductance equation reads:

$$1/\dot{G}_{O_2} = 1/60 + 0.006/20 + 1/20.$$

The overall conductance is 14.9 L/min, and (with an oxygen concentration gradient of 209 ml/L from the atmosphere to the mitochondrion) a peak oxygen intake of 3.12 L/min would be expected. In a moderately athletic young man, $\dot{V}_A = 90$ L/min, $B/(1-B) = 0.010$, and $\lambda\dot{Q}$ is perhaps 35 L/min. The overall conductance for such an individual is 25.0 L/min, and with an oxygen concentration gradient of 209 ml/L, a maximal oxygen intake of 5.23 L/min can be anticipated. Both of these estimates are somewhat higher than commonly observed figures, emphasizing, that at least in the adult, oxygen transport does not normally behave as a perfectly matched system (Shephard, 1971a).

If the equations are taken at their face value, the third term of the equation (effectively, the product of maximal cardiac output and the oxygen-carrying capacity of the blood) is dominant. However, the situation is complicated by the normal shape of the oxygen dissociation curve, which limits the increase of oxygen transport that can be accomplished by a given increase of alveolar ventilation. The equation also takes no account of the possible adverse effect of an increase of blood viscosity with an increase of red cell count, a response that could limit $\dot{Q}$ and thus hold $\lambda\dot{Q}$ constant despite an increase of λ. Finally, it leaves largely unanswered such questions as the relative importance of central factors (e.g., cardiac power, depressor reflexes) and peripheral variables (the nipping of major vessels in the fascia of contracting muscles, the adequacy of the intramuscular capillary bed, and a pooling of blood in inactive muscles) as determinants of the maximal cardiac output. The dominant role of blood transport seems clearly established for the child and the young adult, but other determinants of oxygen transport may become important in older men and women. It must also be remembered that disease can cause sufficient deterioration in any link in the oxygen conductance chain for this to become the main limiting factor.

Parallel conductance equations can be developed for the transfer of carbon dioxide, lactate, and heat (Shephard, 1992b). Carbon dioxide transport can limit performance in the presence of chronic respiratory disease, and the elimination of heat may become critical in a very warm environment. But in normal circumstances, oxygen conductance is the dominant determinant of endurance performance.

3
Chapter

Current Levels of Physical Activity and Health-Related Fitness

The nature of the relationships between physical activity, the health-related elements of the fitness spectrum, and health itself was discussed in chapter 1. Many population studies have concentrated on various measurements of fitness rather than physical activity. However, there are important limitations to such an approach, particularly when advising the individual, because inheritance accounts for a substantial part of the variation in both the basic elements of health-related fitness and the response of these elements to a regular program of physical activity (Bouchard, 1992).

Unfortunately, the assessment of physical activity also presents major problems (Powell, Stephens, Marti, Heineman, & Kreuter, 1991; Shephard, 1990d). The improvement of any one aspect of health-related fitness such as aerobic power represents the summated response to weeks, if not months, of physical activity. On any one specific day, physical activity patterns may differ widely from the norm for that individual, and it is difficult to provide representative measurements without studying a subject closely over a very long period. The expense of the investigation can then become prohibitive. Problems may also arise from invasion of personal privacy. Furthermore, the type of activity that is important to the development of health-related fitness and thus the health of the individual has yet to be resolved. Do we want to know the average level of physical activity for a typical day, or are we interested in that period of the day during which the energy expenditure exceeds a certain threshold? If we believe in a threshold, is this the same for all subjects, or does it vary with the person's age and initial level of aerobic fitness? And is it enough to measure the physiological response to physical activity (such as an increase of heart rate), or must the mode of exercise also be considered?

Despite these unanswered questions, the direct study of physical activity patterns holds substantial promise in future analyses of community health. Not only may it hold the key to new procedures for the assessment of personal health-related fitness, but it may find important practical applications as social scientists seek objective methods of testing both current community attitudes toward participation in physical activity, and the changes in those attitudes that can be induced by various motivational tactics.

Methodological Considerations in Population Studies

The collection of world-wide data on population levels of physical activity and health-related fitness was greatly stimulated by the Human Adaptability Project of the International Biological Programme, or IBP (Shephard, 1978). The basic objectives of the project were to evaluate how far particular physiological characteristics such as a high level of physical work capacity had helped indigenous groups in colonizing specific habitats and to trace the extent of potential adaptation to adverse habitats. It was hypothesized that low levels of health-related fitness would be endemic in developed nations, because such societies had abandoned the physically demanding cultures of neolithic hunter-gatherers and subsistence farmers, lifestyles to which the human body had become adapted over many centuries of evolution (G.A. Harrison, 1979; Weiner, 1964; Worthington, 1978). Tests were performed on athletes to provide evidence of the upper limit of human adaptability, and information was also collected on the manner in which various chronic diseases had restricted physical activity patterns and resultant levels of aerobic fitness.

An important cornerstone of the IBP project was the development of standardized methods for the measurement of both physical activity and health-related fitness (Weiner & Lourie, 1969; 1981). Additional information on the methodology appropriate to large-scale population surveys, on current patterns of physical activity in various communities, and on resulting levels of fitness has been presented by K.L. Andersen, Masironi, Rutenfranz, and Seliger (1978), Collins and Roberts (1988), Shephard (1986c), and Shephard and Parizkova (1991). Nevertheless, many of the original IBP investigations and more recent community studies leave key questions of experimental design unanswered. Were the samples that were tested representative of the populations under evaluation? Was the test environment adequately controlled? How were the results distorted by problems of cross-sectional or longitudinal methodology? What constraints on the reliability and validity of data were imposed by the use of simple measurement techniques appropriate to large-scale surveys? And were the surveys in themselves reactive, modifying physical activity patterns or health-related fitness?

Methods of Population Sampling

The IBP manuals of methodology (Weiner & Lourie, 1969, 1981) stressed the number of subjects that was needed to test whether apparent differences between populations were statistically significant, but they gave no further guidance on how to sample a given population, other than the very general recommendation that selection be at random.

Unfortunately, most physiologists have had little training in epidemiological methods, and many have thus based their conclusions on the testing of small convenience samples. Scores obtained on such groups often bear little relationship to true average values for the target population. Acceptable approaches test all members of a representative community, a cohort of a larger community, or a representative and appropriately stratified sample of an entire population. Nevertheless, problems may still arise if volunteer rates fall substantially short of 100%.

BIAS IN CONVENIENCE SAMPLES.   Convenience samples of "healthy young men" are typically drawn from laboratory staff or university students, and the latter are often enrolled in physical education courses or participating in athletic programs.

Exercise scientists have often inferred that the findings from such samples are relevant to all or at least to a substantial fraction of North Americans or Europeans (for instance, "white" males). Such an assumption is dubious for any of the reported physiological responses, but it is particularly suspect with regard to data on physical activity and health-related fitness, because convenience samples selectively recruit the "worried well" (Criqui, 1985). Volunteer samples commonly underrepresent the number of cigarette smokers in the general population. Typically, those tested are well-educated, single young men of above-average socioeconomic status. Both habitual physical activity and other manifestations of a healthy lifestyle are especially prevalent in such a group (Ferland, 1980; Fitness Canada, 1983; Health and Welfare Canada, 1988; Stephens & Craig, 1990; also see Table 3.1).

Because convenience sampling has been used, both the prevalence of physical activity and resultant levels of health-related fitness have been substantially overestimated in many developed societies. In contrast, when indigenous populations have been tested, the least active or the most acculturated members of a community have usually been the most accessible for evaluation, so that convenience sampling has underestimated fitness levels. Regular hunters are frequently absent from a settlement, and if a representative sample of the community is to be tested, the investigating scientist may need to live in a village for many months.

BIAS IN TESTING INDIGENOUS POPULATIONS.   Much of the available data on indigenous populations has been based on small, nonrepresentative samples of 8 to 12 people (Shephard, 1978). In consequence, quite erroneous impressions have been formed about such populations. For example, an earlier generation of Canadian scientists believed that the circumpolar Inuit had poor levels of both respiratory function (Beaudry, 1968; Hildes, Schaefer, Sayed, Fitzgerald, & Koch, 1976) and aerobic fitness (K.L. Andersen & Hart, 1963).

One of the larger IBP studies examined the Canadian Inuit community of Igloolik, which by the year 1990 had attained a population of about 1,000 people

Table 3.1
Influence of Educational Level and Occupation on Habitual Physical Activity

	High energy usage[a]		High time commitment[b]	
	1981	1988	1981	1988
Educational level				
Less than high school	17	31	50	74
High school	24	29	54	77
Some post-high school	26	31	62	81
University degree	27	33	64	89
Occupation				
Manager/professional	23	28	64	85
Sales/clerical	20	25	51	73
Blue-collar	19	30	52	76
Homemaker	13	22	51	77

Note. Numbers indicate percent of respondents. Data from (a) Stephens and Craig (1988); (b) Canada Fitness Survey (1983).
[a]>12.6 kJ/kg body mass/day.
[b]>3 hr/wk at least 9 months/yr.

(Shephard, 1978, 1980). Here, the epidemiologically acceptable decision was made to request the test participation of everyone over the age of 10 years. After a year of residence in the community, exercise scientists had secured informed consent from some 72% of the inhabitants. Nevertheless, the population averages for forced vital capacity and 1-s forced expiratory volume initially reported by the exercise scientists differed substantially from the values reported by a team of physicians who had visited the same settlement during the same year (see Table 3.2). The discrepancy was quickly traced to incomplete sampling of the population by *both* groups of investigators. The 28% of residents who had not volunteered for testing by the exercise scientists tended to be the sick members of the population, who were recruited selectively by the medical investigators. In contrast, the fittest members of the settlement (well represented in the sample tested by the exercise scientists) were not interested in an evaluation by the visiting physicians.

AGE AND SAMPLE BIAS.   Most investigators have found that a substantial fraction of older potential subjects either refuse to participate in testing or are excluded from physically demanding exercise assessments on medical grounds. This source of bias seems common to both indigenous and industrial or postindustrial societies (see Tables 3.3, 3.4; also S.N. Blair et al., 1989; Shephard, 1978, 1986c). The residual sample available for evaluation thus tends to include an

Table 3.2
Pulmonary Function Data for the Inuit of Igloolik

Subjects	One second forced expiratory volume (L, BTPS)		Forced vital capacity (L, BTPS)	
	Men	Women	Men	Women
Seen by both teams				
Medical team	3.64	1.98	4.94	2.80
Exercise scientists	3.69	1.99	4.87	2.82
Seen by medical team	3.14	1.88	4.41	2.66
Seen by exercise scientists	3.86	2.83	4.92	3.59
Population averages				
Medical team	3.39	1.90	4.68	2.68
Exercise scientists	3.76	2.74	4.89	3.25

Note. Adapted from Shephard (1978) by permission.

Table 3.3
Influence of Age on Percentage of Population Undertaking
Health-Related Fitness Testing

Age (yr)	Male participants (%)		Female participants (%)	
	Igloolik	CFS	Igloolik	CFS
10-19	77	80	65	74
20-39	67	68	56	57
40-59	41	48	48	40
>60	—	21	—	18

Note. Data from Shephard, 1978 (Inuit participating in the Igloolik survey); Canada Fitness Survey, 1983 (Canadians participating in the 1981 Canada Fitness Survey).

excessive proportion of those who are fit and have adopted a healthy, active lifestyle. There is no good method of determining the impact of this problem on health-related fitness scores for the population, although the bias in simple descriptive variables such as body mass index, resting heart rate, and resting blood pressure seems to be quite small (Stephens, 1989; also see Table 3.5).

One way of reducing sampling bias would be to make pretest screening procedures more disease specific. There is a need for simple tools that can be applied by paramedical personnel to large populations—methods having sufficient sensitivity to screen out people with serious disease and thus assure the safety of

Table 3.4
Recruitment of Middle-Aged and Older Men
to Various Studies of Health-Related Fitness

Study	Age (yr)	Recruitment (%)	Author
NHANES	25-74	70	Blair et al. (1989)
L.A. civil servants	40-59	75	Chapman (1964)*
Framingham residents	40-60+	66	Dawber et al. (1983)*
Albany civil servants	40-59	89	Doyle et al. (1957)*
Honolulu Japanese	45-59	81	Gordon et al. (1974)*
Puerto Rico residents	45-59	81	Gordon et al. (1974)*
Canadian Lipid Clinics	20-69	73	Hewitt et al. (1977)
Göteborg workers	40-67	84	Höglund & Gustafson (1975)
Minnesota businessmen	45-55	92	Keys et al. (1963)*
Yugoslavians	35-62	93	Kovaric et al. (1976)*
Evans Co., Georgia	45-64	92	McDonough et al. (1965)*
Israeli civil servants	40-59	86	Medalie et al. (1968)*
Tecumseh residents	40-59	83-88	Montoye (1975)
Chicago (W. Electric)	40-59	67	Paul et al. (1963)*
Lipid Research Clinics	20-69	85	Rifkind & Segal (1983)
California workers	40-59	66	Rosenmann et al. (1975)*
Chicago (Peoples' Gas)	40-59	92	Stamler (1973)*
Canada Fitness Survey	40-59	44	Stephens (1989)
Göthenburg men of 1913	50	88	Tibblin et al. (1975)*

For references marked by *, see Keys (1980).

Table 3.5
Response Bias in the Canada Fitness Survey of 1981

Age (yr)	Body mass index (kg/m²)		Resting heart rate (beats/min)		Blood pressure* (mm Hg)	
	Male	Female	Male	Female	Male	Female
7-19	100.0	99.5	99.3	99.5	99.8/100.0	99.8/99.7
20-39	100.0	98.7	99.3	99.3	99.3/99.5	99.6/99.6
40-54	98.9	97.2	98.2	98.6	97.3/97.6	97.3/97.5
55-69	98.1	96.2	97.7	98.0	94.4/95.8	93.4/94.8

Note. Data is based on a comparison of physical measurements for subjects participating in all tests with those completing the questionnaire, but excluded from the active tests of health-related fitness. Results for those excluded are expressed as percentages of the corresponding average results for the entire sample of a given age and sex.
*Systolic and diastolic readings

exercise tests, yet specific enough to exclude only a small proportion of healthy, older test volunteers. In Canada, the usual approach has been to use the Physical Activity Readiness Questionnaire (PAR-Q; Chisholm, Collis, Kulak, Davenport, & Gruber, 1975). The original version of the PAR-Q rejected about 20% of apparently healthy exercise test candidates (Shephard, Thomas, & Weller, 1991), but a recent revision of this screening device seems a useful advance (see Figure 3.1), excluding only about two thirds of the subjects who would have been rejected by use of the original PAR-Q instrument. Unfortunately, a proportion of subjects still give false positive responses to the revised PAR-Q, and it seems likely that some older volunteers will continue to be excluded unnecessarily from exercise testing by any simple paramedical screening process.

Post hoc attempts are sometimes made to adjust mean fitness scores for incomplete sampling of the population. Typically, survey participants are matched with nonparticipants in terms of such readily ascertainable, noninvasive characteristics as age, body mass index, and smoking habits. The most appropriate basis of adjustment would be in terms of habitual activity patterns, but unfortunately there are no simple yet valid methods of obtaining such information from uncooperative subjects.

SAMPLING BY COMMUNITY.   Despite potential sources of bias, one of the more satisfactory approaches to testing either a developed society or a discreet, indigenous population is to include in the sample all willing members of a community who meet certain minimal selection criteria.

Publicity regarding a health and fitness survey generally has a much greater impact when the investigation is concentrated in a small community than when the same volume of testing is distributed across an entire nation. The participation rate may be quite high when surveying a small community. For instance, Montoye (1975) reported an 83% overall response to a study of activity patterns and health-related fitness in the small city of Tecumseh, Michigan. Other investigations of discrete populations have recruited 62% to 93% of older men (see Table 3.4), compared to a disappointing 44% recruitment of 40- to 59-year-old men in the nationwide Canada Fitness Survey (Stephens, 1989). Nevertheless, much depends on what the subjects are expected to do. Montoye (1975) reported that participation in the physically demanding component of his test protocol decreased steeply with age, and only 50% of those aged 50 to 69 years completed a simple, submaximal step test. Because of such low participation rates, there is a substantial risk that average scores for the aerobic component of a fitness and activity survey will be biased by incomplete sampling of a community.

If relatively complete sampling is achieved, doubt may still remain about the generality of results, particularly if only a single community has been evaluated. The problem has been most obvious when tests have been conducted in isolated indigenous settlements. For example, the Inuit from different parts of the Arctic differ widely in their nutritional status and the extent of their acculturation to white society, with corresponding differences in reported levels of aerobic fitness and body fat (K.L. Andersen et al., 1978; Rode & Shephard, 1992; Shephard,

Yes   No

_____   _____   1. Has your doctor ever said that you have a heart condition and recommended only medically approved physical activity?

_____   _____   2. Do you have chest pain brought on by physical activity?

_____   _____   3. Have you developed chest pain at rest in the past month?

_____   _____   4. Do you lose consciousness or lose your balance as a result of dizziness?

_____   _____   5. Do you have a bone or joint problem that could be aggravated by the proposed physical activity?

_____   _____   6. Is your doctor currently prescribing medication for your blood pressure or heart condition (e.g., diuretics or water pills)?

_____   _____   7. Are you aware, through your own experience or a doctor's advice, of any other reason against your exercising without medical approval?

Note: 1. This questionnaire applies only to those 15 to 69 years of age.

2. If you have temporary illness, such as a fever, or are not feeling well at this time, you may wish to postpone the proposed activity.

3. If you are pregnant, you are advised to discuss the "PAR-X for Pregnancy" form with your physician before exercising.

4. If there are any changes in your status relative to the above questions, please bring this information to the immediate attention of your fitness professional.

I have read, understood, and completed this questionnaire.

Signature _____   Date _____

Signature of parent _____
or guardian (for participants under the age of majority)

Witness _____   Date_____

Figure 3.1   The Revised Physical Activity Readiness Questionnaire (PAR-Q).
Note. Reprinted from Shephard, Thomas, and Weller (1991) by permission.

1978; see Table 3.6). But even in developed societies, if a survey is restricted to one small city, this locale may attract a particular ethnic group, or job opportunities may be concentrated in a few specific industries that employ a preponderance of people from particular socioeconomic categories.

SAMPLING BY COHORT.   In larger cities, a study may grow to unmanageable size unless the recruitment of subjects is restricted to those born in a specific year (e.g., the Göteborg men-born-in-1913 survey; Wilhelmsen, Tibblin, & Werkö, 1972). The weakness of the cohort approach is that the experience of the group that is studied may differ from that of other cohorts living in the same region with respect to such factors as nutritional history, cumulative patterns of habitual activity, exposure to programs of health education, or encounters with the various stresses imposed by global warfare.

REPRESENTATIVE, STRATIFIED SAMPLING.   Another tactic is to recruit a representative or a stratified representative sample of a given city or nation. Bailey, Shephard, and Mirwald (1976) attempted to enlist the participation of a representative sample of the adults living in the medium-sized, prairie city of Saskatoon. People identified by drawing names in a specified sequence from the local telephone directory were invited to attend the university for a free assessment of health-related fitness (Bailey et al., 1976). Adoption of this tactic necessarily excluded certain categories of people from the survey: those living in various types of institution, those too poor to own a telephone, and those who had unlisted telephone numbers. But a much greater problem arose from subsequent attrition of the potential sample. Of 2,648 telephone respondents, 118 were immediately

Table 3.6
Average Skinfold Thickness and Maximal Oxygen Intake of
Various Circumpolar Populations

Settlement	Average skinfold thickness (mm)	Maximal oxygen intake	
		(μmol/[kg·s])	(ml/[kg·min])
Athabaskan Indians		36	49
Baffin Inuit		33	44
Finnish Skolts		35	47
Hokkaido Ainu		33	44
Igloolik Inuit	6.5	40	54
Nomadic Lapps		40	54
Point Hope Inuit		31	42
Upernavik Inuit		30	41
Wainwright Inuit	11.0	34	46

Note. Data from Shephard (1978); Andersen, Masironi, Rutenfranz, and Seliger (1978).

judged unsuitable for the aerobic component of the test battery (e.g., too old), 982 immediately refused to visit the test laboratories, and another 649 were unable to agree on a convenient time for testing. An additional 49 failed to keep their appointments, and 72 were excluded by the physician who was supervising the aerobic fitness test. Thus, only 29.4% of those who answered the initial telephone call completed the evaluation. This seems fairly typical of the success rate when an urban population is asked to attend a central location to participate in a substantial battery of health and fitness tests. Landry et al. (1980) also persuaded only 23.6% of 1,000 randomly selected Québecois to visit their laboratory for free fitness testing.

Howell and MacNab (1968) and R. Gauthier, Massicotte, Hermiston, and MacNab (1983) carried their health-related fitness tests to representative Canadian schools identified by Statistics Canada. The nth pupil in selected classes from the targeted schools was invited to participate in the fitness testing session, and if a refusal was encountered, the investigators proceeded to test the $n + 1$th pupil in the same class. The number of refusals was not stated in their published reports, but it is believed to have been quite low. Unfortunately, the data still had an important potential bias, because physical education was taught in the classes that were selected for testing.

Fitness Canada used the techniques and expertise of Statistics Canada to recruit a nationally representative sample of some 20,000 individuals aged 10 to 69 years for home-based assessments of activity patterns and health-related fitness (Fitness Canada, 1983). Their sample was cluster-stratified by province (the numbers tested were proportional to the square root of the population of a given province) and by place of residence (representatives were sought from rural areas, medium-sized towns, and large cities). Eighty teams of paramedical professionals telephoned selected households. The initial contact was followed by a household visit, during which subjects completed a physical activity questionnaire and performed a simple battery of health-related fitness tests (Shephard, 1986c; see Table 3.15, pages 126-127). Similar efforts to recruit representative national population samples have been made in the Canada Health Survey (1982), the Canada Health Promotion Survey (1988), the U.S. National Health and Nutrition Examination Surveys (S.N. Blair et al., 1989; McDowell, 1989), and the National Health Interview Survey (Pearce, 1989).

CONTROL OF TEST ENVIRONMENT AND EXPERIMENTAL CONDITIONS. The scores obtained on tests of aerobic fitness are influenced by a number of environmental factors, including the temperature of the testing location, its altitude, and its psychological ambience. However, many surveys have provided inadequate control of these variables.

There are wide cultural differences in concepts of a "comfortable" room temperature, ranging from 24° to 27°C in North America to as low as 13° to 16°C in the homes, schools, and offices of some hardy British. Many field tests are performed outdoors, and here an even wider range of temperatures may be encountered. Direct measurements of maximal oxygen intake tend to be a little below true peak values if the initial body temperature is low, but results are affected relatively little by warm conditions, unless the subject is dehydrated (Saltin, 1964). In contrast, there is a disproportionate increase of heart rate when a given submaximal work rate is attempted in a hot rather than a temperate environment. The high heart rate leads to an overestimate of the intensity of activity, and a corresponding underestimate of maximal oxygen intake by most simple prediction methods. A heat-induced increase of skin blood flow may also lead to an underestimation of the normal resting blood pressure. Finally, the speed on many field tests of performance-related fitness is slowed not only by hot weather, but also by adverse ground conditions and any opposing wind force (Shephard & Lavallée, 1978).

An increase of altitude leads to a decrease of both maximal heart rate and maximal oxygen intake (Shephard, 1992d). Tachycardia can influence estimates of the intensity of physical activity and the prediction of maximal oxygen intake from submaximal tests of aerobic fitness. The scores on some field tests of performance-related fitness are adversely affected by an altitude-induced decrease of oxygen transport, but this handicap may be partially offset by the performance-enhancing effects of a decreased air resistance and a slightly smaller gravitational acceleration at altitude. Both positive and negative effects on performance are minimal below 2,000 m, and such results are thus unlikely to be affected except in a few specific populations who live and are tested at medium and high altitudes.

Laboratory measurements of aerobic power and field tests of performance both rely on eliciting an all-out effort from the participants, and scores thus depend greatly on the success of the testing personnel in communicating with and overcoming the inhibitions of subjects. On the other hand, if the investigators are perceived to be overly tense, this can increase the subject's heart rate, causing overassessments of physical activity, underpredictions of maximal oxygen intake from submaximal test data, and overestimates of blood pressures both at rest and during exercise.

Finally, consistency in the response of subjects to a standard laboratory exercise test depends on the careful control of such extraneous behaviors as recent physical activity, heavy meals, cigarette smoking, and the use of alcohol and other drugs.

Problems of Cross-Sectional Surveys

Because of logistic difficulties in tracing populations with a high annual turnover rate, and the high costs of maintaining personnel and test equipment over the many years of a longitudinal survey, the majority of studies of physical activity and health-related fitness have been cross-sectional in type. Sometimes (AAHPERD, 1980; Canadian Assn. for Health, Physical Education and Recreation, 1980; R. Gauthier et al., 1983; Stephens & Craig, 1990) it has been possible to repeat surveys after the lapse of 5 to 15 years. In the case of the Canada Fitness Survey, the same individuals have been retested, allowing semilongitudinal comparisons between those participants whose physical activity increased and those whose activity remained constant or decreased over the intervening 7 years (Stephens & Craig, 1990). Still, interpopulation comparisons of cross-sectional data can be distorted by seasonal or climatic factors, selective migration, intercurrent pathologies, and cohort effects.

SEASONAL AND CLIMATIC FACTORS.   Sports and games show seasonal patterns in many countries. The trend to seasonal variations in outdoor work and leisure pursuits is particularly marked in regions of the world with a continental climate. Thus the observed patterns of habitual activity and resultant levels of health-related fitness depend on the time of year when data are collected.

Our study of French-Canadian schoolchildren continued over an entire year, individual children being tested within 2 weeks of their respective birthdays. Values for aerobic power were lowest during the summer, when school and community sports programs were not available to most students, with recovery in the late fall (see Table 3.7; also Shephard, Lavallée, Jéquier, 1978). Among blind children, a much larger loss of aerobic fitness was observed during the summer months when they no longer had access to specially adapted programs of physical education (diNatale, Lee, Ward, & Shephard, 1985). In Scandinavia, also, the physical condition of adolescent children deteriorates during the summer vacation months (P.O. Åstrand, 1961; Knuttgen & Steendahl, 1963).

Seasonal and climatic factors probably explain a substantial part of the apparent regional differences in the health-related fitness of adults who were tested in the Canada Fitness Survey (McPherson & Curtis, 1986). Aerobic fitness scores were substantially greater in the western provinces and were lowest in Québec. Observations of a representative sample of the Ontario population (Fitness Ontario, 1983) have shown that a substantially smaller proportion of the adult population is physically active in November than in June; for example, in June

Table 3.7
Seasonal Differences in Aerobic Fitness of
French-Canadian Children, Ages 6 to 11 Years

Months	Maximal oxygen intake	
	mmol/s	L/min
Jan-Feb	1.03	1.38
Mar-Apr	0.99	1.33
May-June	1.06	1.42
July-Aug	1.00	1.34
Sept-Oct	0.95	1.28
Nov-Dec	1.07	1.44

Note. Different groups of children of the same ages were tested in each 2-month period. Adapted from Shephard, Lavallée, et al. (1978) by permission.

1983, 44% of people were active three or more times a week, and 32% were inactive, but in November 1983, the values were 30% and 43%, respectively. Likewise, Stephens (1989) found that in June the hourly participation of a representative sample of Canadians in the 10 most popular recreational activities was almost twice that in November or December.

In contrast, we have seen little seasonal difference of health-related fitness among Inuit living in the Canadian arctic (Rode & Shephard, 1973; also see Table 3.8). Presumably, any decrease in the physical activity of the Inuit during the coldest winter months is offset by the extra energy cost of wearing heavy clothing and tramping over rough ice or through deep snow.

SELECTIVE MIGRATION.   Miall, Ashcroft, Lovell, and Moore (1967) noted a selective migration of tall individuals out of the mining valleys of South Wales. The normal age-related decrease of height was thus exaggerated in cross-sectional data from the affected communities. The impact of such migration-induced changes on the average body mass index of those remaining in the mining villages is obvious.

In recent years, the ethnic composition of the populations in central Canada and in the large urban centers of Australia has been greatly affected by migration. Successive waves of young adult immigrants have come from different parts of the world. Depending on the year in which a cross-sectional survey is conducted, one age-decade may thus include a predominance of people with British ancestry, another will be biased by economic migrants from southern Italy and Greece, and another by Hungarian refugees or Vietnamese boat people. The immigrants are initially the most healthy representatives of their parent country. Because of problems with their new language, many also tend to find heavy laboring jobs. Their cardiovascular mortality in the first few years after emigrating is thus lower than the average for either those still living in the country of their birth or for the native-born residents of their adopted home (Rose, 1970; also see Table 3.9). However, as the immigrants become more wealthy and adopt adverse lifestyle

Table 3.8
Seasonal Differences of Health-Related Fitness Among Inuit Males of Igloolik

	Aerobic power				Average skinfold thickness (mm)		Leg extension force (N)	
	[μmol/(kg·s)]		[ml/(kg·min)]					
Age (yr)	Summer	Winter	Summer	Winter	Summer	Winter	Summer	Winter
20-29	44.0	44.6	59.2	59.9	5.5	5.9	900	976
30-39	43.2	41.6	58.0	55.9	6.3	7.6	854	881
40-49	39.4	36.4	53.0	48.9	5.7	6.0	826	881

Note. Adapted from Rode and Shephard (1973) by permission.

Table 3.9
Early Mortality From Arteriosclerotic and
Degenerative Heart Disease in Selected Male Subjects

	Age-specific cardiac deaths per 100,000/year		
Group	40-49 yr	50-59 yr	60-69 yr
Italian immigrants to Australia			
(0-6 yr residence)	16	123	260
(7-19 yr residence)	51	170	376
(>20 yr residence)	130	344	680
Italians living in Italy	80	240	680
Australians, native-born	169	592	1,472

Note. Adapted from Rose (1970) by permission.

habits, their cardiovascular mortality moves progressively toward the average for native-born residents.

TOBACCO CONSUMPTION. Nicotine induces a temporary increase in the smoker's heart rate; typically, readings are augmented by 5 to 10 beats/min both at rest and in submaximal aerobic exercise (Rode, R. Ross, & Shephard, 1972). The specific effects of nicotine on the heart and airways are usually reversed within 1 hr. The hemoglobin of smokers also shows a 5% to 10% saturation with carbon monoxide, compared to values of 0.5% to 1.0% found in a typical urban nonsmoker. The affected hemoglobin is not available for oxygen carriage, and there is a corresponding reversible decrease of maximal oxygen intake (Apthorp, Bates, Marshall, & Mendel, 1958; Ekblom & Huof, 1972; Shephard, 1983b; Vogel & Gleser, 1972). About half of the carbon monoxide stored in the red cell pigment is lost from the body within 4 hr of cessation of smoking.

It is an appropriate question how long cigarettes should be withheld before testing aerobic fitness. If one is interested in the individual's work capacity under normal conditions, it is arguable that a smoker should be studied when the heart is nicotinized and the hemoglobin is contaminated with carbon monoxide, but in practice most data have been collected after at least 1 hr of abstinence from cigarettes.

In heavy smokers, a substantial fraction of the measured oxygen transport is consumed by the respiratory muscles (Rode & Shephard, 1971). Thus, a given level of aerobic power implies a lesser capacity for performing external work by a smoker than by a nonsmoker.

CHRONIC DISEASE. Remarkably few authors have discussed the medical conditions of their subjects. It is reasonable to assume that those with overt disease either did not volunteer or were excluded from most fitness surveys. On the other hand, subjects having chronic abnormalities compatible with normal life and employment may well have been tested, particularly in circumstances where investigators were not fluent in the language of the population under investigation. This is an important criticism, because a substantial proportion of older subjects are affected by one or more chronic diseases that limit some aspect of their health-related fitness.

J.R. Brown and Shephard (1967) noted that as many as a quarter of older Canadian women working in a large department store had some form of cardio-respiratory disease, and that the aerobic power of this subgroup was only 86% to 90% of the values seen in their healthy peers. The decision as to which subjects should be excluded from a population sample is quite difficult, because the dividing line between health and disease is fine. One possible criterion in those of working age is the ability to perform a full day's work. People with conditions such as mild anemia or postural hypotension should probably be regarded as lying at the poor end of a normal fitness distribution curve, rather than as being sick, because a vigorous aerobic conditioning program would likely restore both total hemoglobin reserves and venous tone in such individuals. On the other hand, those affected by conditions such as chronic bronchitis should probably be excluded from a normal sample, because a definite pathological process is involved.

The confounding of aging with the consequences of chronic disease is a particularly important source of difficulty in surveys of indigenous populations, because there is often a high prevalence of conditions such as tuberculosis or malaria among the older members of such communities (Shephard, 1978, 1980), and affected individuals have levels of aerobic fitness that are well below the average for their peers.

COHORT EFFECTS.   Cohort effects that have influenced health-related fitness and growth patterns in many countries include (1) wartime shortages of food (Schettler, 1977), (2) the more recent and deliberate trend toward decreased consumption of saturated animal fats (Florey, Melia, & Darby, 1978; U.S. Dept. of Health & Human Services, 1981), (3) the replacement of active recreation by television watching and other forms of passive entertainment (Alderson & Crutchley, 1990; Shephard et al., 1975; Sherif & Rattray, 1976; Tucker, 1990), (4) the growing use of motorized vehicles in both developed and developing societies (Rode & Shephard, 1992; Shephard, 1981), (5) the mechanization (Edholm, 1970) and subsequent automation of heavy industrial work, with a displacement of primary and secondary production to the developing world, and (6) an increase followed by a decline of cigarette consumption in developed societies (Jossa, 1985; Rosenbaum & Bursten, 1988; Shephard, 1981; U.S. Dept. of Health & Human Services, 1981), with an increase in the prevalence of cigarette addiction in the developing world.

Indigenous populations have commonly faced a superimposed process of acculturation to the lifestyle of developed societies (Rode & Shephard, 1992; Shephard & Rode, 1985), with such manifestations as a decrease in average family size, a shortening of the average period of lactation, a rapid decrease in traditional types of energy expenditure such as hunting and the cleaning of skins, the purchase of labor-saving domestic equipment, and a shift from game to store-purchased food. Moreover, these changes of lifestyle have been associated with a rapid decline of health-related fitness and an increase in the diseases of civilization such as diabetes and atherosclerosis (Reichley et al., 1987; Szathmary & Holt, 1983).

Problems of Longitudinal Surveys

Longitudinal surveys are widely assumed to indicate with irreproachable validity the course of growth and aging in any given community. But in practice, the interpretation of such results can be compromised by inconsistencies of methodology, test learning and habituation, secular trends, sample attenuation, and statistical artifacts.

METHODOLOGY.   Ideally, a longitudinal study of growth should follow the same group of children from their preschool years through to early adult life. Likewise, aging studies should follow the same individuals from early adult life to the retirement years. Methodology must then be held as constant as possible for many years. Laboratory personnel inevitably change over the course of such extended studies, and the customary approach of using laboratory staff for the biological calibration of equipment (N.L. Jones & Kane, 1979) thus needs reinforcement by physical methods of standardizing both equipment and procedures.

Measurements of health-related fitness such as skinfold thicknesses are particularly prone to interobserver and intraobserver variation (Edwards, Hammond, Healy, Tanner, & Whitehouse, 1955; Prahl-Andersen, Kowalski, & Heyendael, 1979; Womersley & Durnin, 1973, 1977). If the observer changes as a survey continues, it is vital that the readings obtained by the original investigator be calibrated against those reported by his or her replacement, and even if the observer remains unchanged, it is important to carry out periodic checks to ensure that the measuring technique has not evolved with frequent repetition of the test procedures.

Because of the need to retain a consistent test methodology, new technologies usually cannot be exploited in longitudinal research (D. Blair, Habicht, & Alekel, 1989). The procedures that are adopted for a survey may thus seem very dated by the time that a final report is prepared (Gilson & Hugh-Jones, 1955).

TEST LEARNING AND HABITUATION.   If measurements of aerobic fitness are repeated many times, the subject becomes progressively less anxious during successive tests (i.e., the process of habituation; Glaser, 1966; Shephard, 1969). In consequence, there is a decrease in cardiorespiratory and hormonal reactions to a standard bout of submaximal exercise, and this can be attributed mistakenly to a training response. Skill in test performance may also improve with repetition of the required procedures (the process of learning; Shephard, 1969). This further improves test scores, particularly in simple field measures of physical performance (Shephard, 1982a; Shephard et al., 1977). Finally, motivation may diminish if a subject becomes bored by the frequent repetition of assessments, and this can reduce scores on tests of cardiorespiratory function or muscle strength that require an all-out effort.

SECULAR TRENDS.   A longitudinal survey commonly confounds the effects of growth and aging with the consequences of secular changes in habitual physical activity, nutrition, and other aspects of personal lifestyle.

In the urban cultures of Europe and North America, studies of 30 to 40 years duration have been affected by industrial mechanization, which tended to increase productivity without any great reduction of energy expenditure (Edholm, 1970), and subsequent automation, which changed many heavy jobs into sedentary control operations. Over the same period, transportation has shifted from walking, cycling, and the use of buses to a widespread reliance on private cars, and a growing amount of free time has been devoted to passive recreation, particularly television watching. On the other hand, the upper echelons of society have participated in a fitness boom, statistics suggesting an increase followed by a plateauing of interest in active physical leisure over the past 2 decades. These various changes are documented both by self-reports of habitual activity patterns and by the less direct evidence of sports equipment purchases and investment in private sector recreational facilities such as health clubs (Shephard, 1986c, 1989a; Stephens, 1987; see Figure 3.2).

Dietary changes have been profound in recent years. Developed societies have progressively increased their consumption of refined sugars. Growing personal wealth has also allowed an increased consumption of meat, although in the

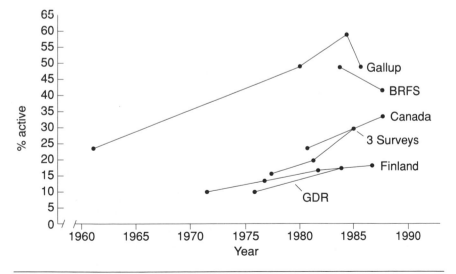

Figure 3.2   Percentage of population found to be active during various recent surveys. *Note.* Reprinted from Powell et al. (1991) by permission.

last 10 to 15 years health-conscious individuals have deliberately reduced their consumption of saturated animal fats.

Systematic alterations of lifestyle have been particularly rapid among indigenous communities, as these have become acculturated to western civilization (Greksa & Baker, 1982; Rode & Shephard, 1992; Shephard & Rode, 1985). Over 20 years or less, some populations have gone from a vigorous and independent nomadic existence to sedentary living that is dependent largely on governmental support. Food previously obtained by hunting and gathering, or subsistence agriculture has been replaced by store products, and the availability of cash has allowed increased purchases of cigarettes and alcohol. In consequence of these various behavioral changes, such groups have shown dramatic decreases in various indices of health-related fitness (see Figure 3.3).

SAMPLE ATTENUATION.   The size of a longitudinal sample inevitably undergoes progressive attenuation as an investigation progresses. Individuals move their placces of residence, change their hours of employment, sustain injuries, lose interest in a study, or are otherwise disqualified from participation in an experiment. For example, control subjects may elect to begin exercising (Shephard, 1989d), or school students may be moved for academic reasons from an experimental to a control class (Shephard et al., 1977).

The composition of a group that has been drawn from a geographically or linguistically isolated community may show a moderate and acceptable level of stability for a number of years, although in such a setting there is also a greater potential for the contamination of control subjects through accidental contact with members of the experimental group. The loss of schoolchildren from a 7-year prospective study conducted in the largely unilingual, francophone community of Trois Rivières, Québec, averaged only 4% a year (Shephard, 1982a). On the other hand, the population turnover in many large North American cities is 20% or higher a year, and a 4-year, multicenter, exercise-heart trial in southern Ontario suffered the very unsatisfactory cumulative dropout rate of over 60% (Shephard, 1981). Moreover, although there were no opportunities for direct contact between the experimental and the control subjects in that study, media publicity nevertheless encouraged many supposed control subjects to begin exercising (Shephard, 1989d).

Population displacement might seem less of a problem when a survey is organized on a national basis, as in the Canada Fitness Survey (1983). However, the high turnover rate of the North American population makes it extremely hard to trace the initial study participants if such a survey is repeated (Stephens & Craig, 1990).

Unfortunately, the loss of subjects from such an investigation is not a random process. Upwardly mobile, health-oriented, and healthy individuals have a greater propensity to migrate (see Table 3.9), and exercise programs also suffer a selective elimination of individuals who have adverse lifestyles, both by loss of interest and by death. Cigarette smokers, in particular, seem reluctant to remain in extended fitness studies (Massie & Shephard, 1971; Oldridge, 1979), perhaps because of peer pressure to abandon their addiction.

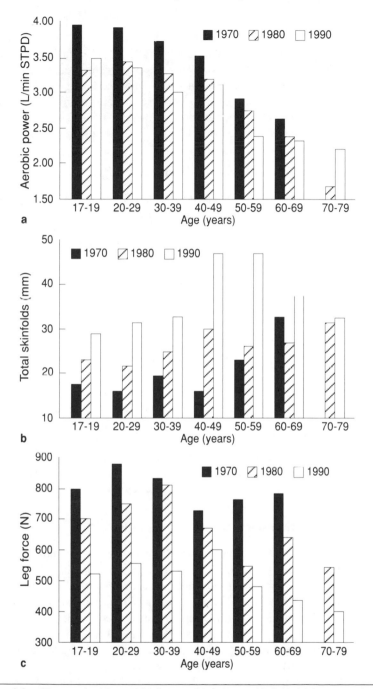

Figure 3.3   Changes in (a) aerobic fitness, (b) average skinfold thickness, and (c) maximal isometric quadriceps force in Inuit men of Igloolik over 20 years of accultura- tion. *Note.* Reprinted from Rode and Shephard (1992) by permission.

STATISTICAL ARTIFACTS.   The error of measurement of health-related variables (commonly, a coefficient of variation of 10%-15%) is such that population averages rather than individual test results are usually reported. However, problems of data smoothing then arise, particularly when analyzing results at the time of the pubertal growth spurt. Data for adolescent children must be aligned in terms of individual peak height velocities if the true course of growth is to be seen during the teenage years (Mirwald & Bailey, 1986; Preece & Baines, 1978).

Mixed Cross-Sectional and Longitudinal Designs

Some large-scale studies have retested the entire initial population periodically. If the same subjects have been tested, as for example, in the two Canada Fitness Surveys (Canada Fitness Survey, 1983; Stephens & Craig, 1990) and the three studies of the Igloolik population (Rode & Shephard, 1992), it becomes possible to compare the impact of secular trends on cross-sectional and longitudinal data. Mixed designs allow some of the advantages of a longitudinal approach without committing investigators and funding agencies to 30 to 40 years of data collection.

Measurement Techniques
Appropriate to Large-Scale Surveys

There is often disagreement on appropriate techniques of measurement, even when physical activity or health-related fitness is to be measured on a small, arbitrary sample of people in a well-equipped laboratory. Such disagreement is inevitably magnified by the compromises that are necessary when an attempt is made to collect data on a larger, representative sample of a community or a nation. Specific issues such as the interlaboratory standardization of methodology and the choice between a high- or low-technology approach must be resolved.

Interlaboratory Standardization of Methodology

An estimate of energy expenditure made from responses to a physical activity questionnaire or a determination of the chemical composition of a respiratory gas sample may be highly reproducible within a given laboratory, but such internal consistency may mask large, systematic interlaboratory differences in results (Cotes & Woolmer, 1962). There is thus a need for both interlaboratory agreement on basic procedures (Weiner & Lourie, 1969, 1981), and ongoing physicochemical and biological calibration of all techniques against common and valid external standards (N.L. Jones & Kane, 1979).

Unfortunately, more than two decades after conclusion of the IBP, we are still far from international agreement on a common set of procedures for measuring physical activity and health-related fitness. Apparently, the personal pride of individual investigators and the vested interests of rival national and international organizations have worked to conserve and even to multiply local variations of methodology.

Paradoxically, such problems are most prevalent among those undertaking high-technology surveys. Those using a low-technology approach have seemed more willing to accept and participate in preliminary orientation sessions, where observers have learned common techniques, cross-validating their individual observations against a common reference criterion.

High-Technology Approach to Measuring Physical Activity

If a single community is to be evaluated, a high-technology approach can usually be adopted. Some investigators have recommended extending a high-technology approach to nationwide surveys of physical activity and health-related fitness. Much of the necessary test equipment can be built into large, air-conditioned trailers to be driven from one city to another. One disadvantage is that a national survey then becomes a slow process. The months spent in a temporary accommodation are taxing for the observers who are involved, and difficulties can arise from seasonal differences in habitual activity patterns and resulting changes of fitness levels.

When studying remote locations, it may be possible to airlift the equipment of a modern laboratory into the region (Shephard, 1978). For example, we were able to fly a substantial amount of modern electronic equipment (and the necessary voltage stabilizers) 2,700 km north from Toronto to the arctic settlement of Igloolik for each of three community surveys of the Canadian Inuit (Rode & Shephard, 1992). However, the high costs of air transportation and the need to carry duplicate pieces of key apparatus makes such an approach very expensive.

High-technology equipment is inevitably costly to purchase, operate, and maintain. Typically, a single investigator can operate only a small number of recording units simultaneously. It is thus difficult to collect representative data by means of sophisticated monitors, and such apparatus is used mainly to validate and quantitate simpler methods of assessing habitual activity such as diary sheets and retrospective questionnaires that can be completed by the survey participants themselves. Available high-technology instruments include mechanical sensors of body movement such as pedometers and actometers, heart rate counters, respiration counters, oxygen consumption monitors, estimates of overall metabolism based on the ingestion of doubly-labeled water, and records of food intake. Details of these various methodologies are given by K.L. Andersen et al. (1978), Montoye (1985), Shephard (1978, 1986c; 1990d), and Verschuur (1987).

Because of cost factors, many high-technology measurements of physical activity patterns are limited to periods of 24 hr or less. It is thus important to ensure that the assessments are representative of a given subject's habits. Account must be taken of any differences of behavior between weekdays and weekends and between summer and winter conditions. Sampling is particularly critical when testing traditional, indigenous populations, because each month brings its own characteristic patterns of hunting or the cultivation of crops (see Figure 3.4).

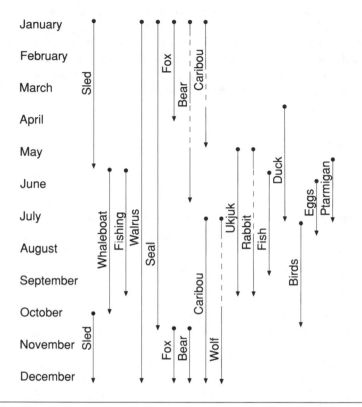

Figure 3.4   Hunting seasons reported by traditional Canadian Inuit living in the circumpolar community of Igloolik. *Note*. Reprinted from Godin and Shephard (1973a) by permission.

Some monitoring systems can operate for only a few minutes. There is then a considerable risk that recordings will be made when physical activity is at its most vigorous or that subjects will deliberately accelerate their pace of movement, because they know that measurements are being made.

If reliance is placed upon published tables of metabolic costs (see Table 3.10), it must be noted that energy expenditures vary widely with the pace of performance. The metabolic cost of many leisure pursuits has been estimated on top athletes; the average person is likely to engage in a given sport with much less vigor than an international competitor, and thus will have a lower energy demand. On the other hand, the average individual also moves much less efficiently than a superb athlete. Thus, the energy usage of an ordinary person may be substantially underestimated if the intensity of a leisure pursuit is gauged simply from the speed of its performance and the corresponding energy cost that has been observed in a well-trained athlete.

Finally, the validity of an earlier, seemingly accurate measurement of energy expenditure may quickly be erased by a change in technology. For example, the

Table 3.10
Average Gross Energy Cost of Selected Leisure Activities

Light activities	Energy cost (kJ/min)	Moderate activities	Energy cost (kJ/min)	Heavy activities	Energy cost (kJ/min)
Archery	13-24	Badminton	26	Basketball	38
Billiards	11	Canoeing	13-29	Boxing	38-60
Bowling	17	Cycling	17-84	Climbing	29-42
Cricket	21-33	Dancing	17-33	Cross-country	
Golf	20	Field hockey	36	running	42-46
Table tennis	15-22	Gardening	13-21	Rowing	17-47
Volleyball	15	Gymnastics	11-50	Soccer	21-50
		Horse-riding	13-42	Squash	42-76
		Skiing		Track	84
		cross-country	41-78		
		downhill	up to 32		
		Swimming	21-63		
		Tennis	24-36		

Note. Most figures refer to small samples of male subjects and have been standardized to a body mass of 65 kg. No account is taken of rest pauses. Data from Durnin and Passmore (1967).

introduction of new types of recreational equipment has changed the effort required in many common, leisure pursuits such as cycling. Likewise, mechanization and subsequent automation have greatly reduced the energy cost of many of the household and industrial tasks so painstakingly studied and summarized by Durnin and Passmore (1967).

MOTION SENSORS. Pedometers and actometers are usually attached to the subject's waist or thigh. They are intended to record a single impulse with each movement of the lower limbs (Kemper & Verschuur, 1977; Verschuur, 1987). The original design of pedometer used a watch mechanism to integrate impulses, but more modern motion sensors incorporate electronic counters. Devices of this type can assess activity patterns most effectively if the principal source of energy expenditure is a relatively stereotyped pattern of leg movement—for instance, when a subject is walking at a fixed pace. But a small modification of activity patterns can lead to a large distortion of results. For instance, if a person does no more than change from walking to jogging, the counter may record two impulses instead of one for each stride that is taken. Moreover, if the counter is fitted to the waist or the thigh, little or no account will be taken of any additional work that is performed by the arms. Kashiwazaki, Ianoka, Suzuki, and Kendo (1986) found that the correlation of pedometer data with direct measurements of energy expenditure ranged from 0.19 to 0.89, depending on the period of day and the types of activities that were being performed.

More accurate information can be obtained if a number of accelerometers are attached to different regions of the body (Montoye et al., 1983), particularly if the resulting signals are transmitted to a central receiver by telemetry. However, the essential simplicity of the pedometer approach is then lost, and a meaningful synthesis of the extensive movement records presents a major problem in data reduction.

HEART RATE RECORDERS.   There is a relatively linear relationship between heart rate and oxygen consumption, at least from 50% to 100% of maximal oxygen intake (I. Åstrand, 1960). Thus, if preliminary tests have established a heart rate-oxygen consumption line for a particular individual, subsequent measurements of heart rate can be used to estimate the oxygen consumption associated with a particular large-muscle activity.

Even when the subject is performing a standard laboratory task, such as treadmill running or cycle ergometry under ideal conditions, the coefficient of variation for the resultant estimate of oxygen consumption is about 10% (Shephard, 1968c). Under field conditions, variability is further increased, and the heart rate response to a given oxygen consumption is often substantially greater than that observed in the laboratory. Smaller muscle groups may be used, the task may incorporate resisted exercise or postural support, and there may be associated emotional excitement or exposure to high environmental temperatures (Shephard, 1968c).

Regardless of the method used to count the subject's heart rate, it is important to guard against instrumental artifacts. Poor contact of the ECG electrodes with the skin or incomplete removal of the surface layer of keratin can lead to electrical noise, with a gross undercounting or overcounting of heart beats. Integrating devices normally tally heart rates from the corresponding R-R intervals of the electrocardiogram, and miscounts can thus arise from large T waves or from premature ventricular contractions. Unfortunately, methods of eliminating such problems are very subjective; often, the primary tactic is merely to exclude very high and very low counts from consideration.

In industry, a cable can transmit the heart rate signal directly to a recording electrocardiograph, with on-line processing of heart rates. In many sports that are performed in a gymnasium or a stadium, the ECG signal can be transmitted telemetrically to an appropriate recording system (Niinimaa, Woch, & Shephard, 1978), although commercial apparatus has a poor frequency response (potentially distorting ECG waveforms), and the counts become unreliable if the subject moves further than a few hundred meters away from the recorder. The simplest devices for the study of free-living subjects use wrist watch mechanisms, electro-chemical cells, or solid-state circuits (Masironi & Mansourian, 1974) to accumulate heart beats over a specified period, such as 12 or 24 hr. The earliest prototypes of such equipment gave a single heart-beat total and thus only the possibility of calculating an average heart rate for the day. This information was not very helpful in assessing the number of minutes the subject had allocated to moderate or vigorous, health-related activity. Indeed, the score for a 24-hr period was often only a few beats above the value for complete rest, and the averaged figure was very vulnerable to distortion by artifactual signals.

More modern instruments indicate periods of the day when the heart rate falls within specified ranges (e.g., 80-100, 100-120, and > 120 beats/min). Health-related activity can then be distinguished from less intensive effort, and, given additional measuring cells, the lowest and the highest categories of heart rate can be automatically rejected as spurious data.

The most detailed information on heart rates is obtained by carrying a small cassette tape-recorder throughout a 24-hr period. Regrettably, commercial equipment of this type is expensive. It is also difficult to maintain a constant tape speed under field conditions, though the most sophisticated instruments superimpose a 60-Hz time base on the basic ECG recording, which allows heart rates to be corrected for any slowing of the tape that has been induced by body movements or exhaustion of the battery. Given much time and patience, the taped electrocardiographic complexes can be played back, displayed, and counted on a minute-by-minute basis. Heart rates can then be matched with the performance of specific activities recorded on the subject's diary sheet. Matching minimizes potential distortions of the heart rate-oxygen consumption relationship introduced by recent meals, cigarette smoking, excitement, anxiety, resisted exercise, changes of body posture, or high environmental temperatures.

VENTILATION AND OXYGEN CONSUMPTION METERS.   Most of the physical activities that contribute to maintenance of personal health are of a moderate rather than a high intensity. In theory, the respiratory minute volume, which is linearly related to oxygen consumption from 10% to 50% of maximal oxygen intake, should thus provide a better index of such activities than the heart rate, which is linearly related to oxygen consumption over the 50% to 90% range (I. Åstrand, 1960; Shephard, 1968c). However, in practice, the theoretical advantage of the respiratory measurements is offset by the need to wear a mouthpiece or a facemask, which substantially restricts the subject and modifies the oxygen cost of most types of physical activity. Moreover, unless the subject is watched very closely, there is a danger that expired gas will be lost by leakage, particularly if the investigator uses a simple facemask without a reflected seal.

If the wearing of an efficient gas-collecting mask or mouthpiece is compatible with the planned activities of the subject, most authors prefer to proceed with an analysis of expired gas, thus obtaining a more direct estimate of oxygen consumption. The earliest approach, still sometimes used in assessing the energy cost of sports activities (Niinimaa, Shephard, & Dyon, 1979), was to collect expired gas in a meteorological balloon or Douglas bag, which subjects carried on their backs. A tap was turned at a signal from the observer, and the expirate was collected for a known interval (e.g., 1 min). The resultant data were difficult to interpret unless the subject had been exercising at a consistent pace and had reached a steady level of oxygen consumption. A development of this technique, still used in sports such as swimming, is to push a modern, electronic metabolic cart alongside the exercising subject. Commercial forms of such apparatus give a print-out of ventilation, oxygen consumption, and gas exchange ratio at 20- to 30-s intervals throughout the period of gas collection.

Portable field equipment has also been devised to integrate a subject's oxygen consumption over periods of 5 to 60 min, though such devices are bulky enough to encumber the subject. They also have an appreciable mass (2-3 kg), and thus induce a 3% to 5% increase in the oxygen cost of most tasks. The equipment developed by Kofranyi and Michaelis (1949) included a mechanical flowmeter and a reciprocating sampling pump that diverted a 0.3% or 0.6% aliquot of expired gas to a small rubber or neoprene bag for subsequent chemical analysis at the base laboratory. The bag was quickly filled, and the apparatus could only be used for a few minutes at any one time. In consequence, many observers tended to collect data on the most vigorous portion of a movement sequence. Also, the capacity of the flowmeter (50-60 L/min) was exceeded by the ventilatory volumes attained in many types of athletic activity.

A rival system (the integrating motor pneumotachograph, or IMP) recorded the volume of airflow by the somewhat less rugged arrangement of displacing a sliding contact along an electrical potentiometer, thus varying the speed of a battery-driven integrating counter (Wolff, 1958). The system required rather more frequent and more sophisticated maintenance than the Kofranyi-Michaelis respirometer. The calibration of the IMP changed frequently and unpredictably. Indeed, if the subject took a deep breath, the potentiometer contact sometimes jammed at the end of its travel. One advantage of the IMP over the mechanical meter was that smaller aliquots (0.03% or 0.06%) of expired gas could be collected in small canisters for subsequent laboratory analysis; the volume of gas accumulated during a short burst of exercise was therefore small, but steady activities could be measured for up to 1 hr.

Further development of this equipment (the Oxylog recorder) now incorporates a turbine flowmeter, two electrochemical oxygen detectors, and a small tape-recorder, so that a continuous estimate of oxygen consumption can be recorded on tape or transmitted telemetrically (K.L. Andersen et al., 1988; Ikegami, Hiruta, Ikegami, & Miyamura, 1988). However, the precision remains disappointing; estimates of oxygen consumption have an accuracy no better than 10% to 20% relative to direct measurements when the equipment is used at high work rates (Ikegami et al., 1988).

DOUBLY LABELED WATER. The ingestion of water labeled with stable but nonradioactive isotopes of hydrogen (^2H) and oxygen (^{18}O) allows the estimation of carbon dioxide and water production. It is assumed that after equilibration, the ^2H is eliminated only as water, whereas the ^{18}O is eliminated both as water and as carbon dioxide. The carbon dioxide output can thus be calculated from the difference in elimination rates of the two isotopes. Because of the time required for equilibration with body pools of water, energy expenditures are usually averaged over 1 to 2 weeks.

Such measurements are therefore most suitable for correlating with 7- or 14-day records of food consumption. One recent report claimed that the double-labeling technique had about the same accuracy as that obtained from dietary records (Hoyt et al., 1991), although in the Tour de France (where the 24-hr energy expenditure averaged 3.4-3.9 times basal), Westerterp, Saris, van Es, and ten Hoor (1986) found that the energy consumption estimated by double labeling exceeded the recorded food intake by 12% to 35%. The doubly-labelled water is expensive (the current cost is up to $600 for a single analysis), imposing a major restriction on wider use of the technique.

RECORDS OF FOOD INTAKE.   Over short periods, records of food intake may differ substantially from other estimates of energy expenditure, but if observations made by a well-trained nutritionist are extended for 7 or 14 days, there is agreement to within 10% to 15% (Durnin & Passmore, 1967; Pollitt & Amante, 1984). The main disadvantage of the dietary approach is that it can estimate energy expenditures only over a long period, covering both work and recreation. It can give little indication of the shorter periods of more intensive activity, which are probably more important in the context of health.

High-Technology Approach to Measuring Health-Related Fitness

An ideal assessment of health-related fitness would provide accurate data on aerobic fitness, both absolute and relative, on the lactate threshold (and thus the subject's aerobic capacity, or ability to operate close to their aerobic power for a prolonged period), on blood pressure and electrocardiographic response to such effort, and on the total burden of body fat and its distribution. From the viewpoint of overall health, this information might usefully be supplemented by measurements of heart size, muscle strength, flexibility, bone health, and selected biochemical data, such as the glucose tolerance curve and the blood lipid profile.

AEROBIC FITNESS.   The aerobic fitness of an average person is best measured by the direct determination of maximal oxygen intake during uphill running or walking on a laboratory treadmill. After much discussion of protocol (Shephard, 1978; Shephard et al., 1968b), agreement is now emerging that the optimal approach begins with a warm-up of 2 to 3 min of running at 70% of the individual's estimated maximal oxygen intake. The treadmill speed that will demand 90% of the subject's maximal oxygen intake is estimated from this data. The definitive test then begins at 90% of maximal oxygen intake, with further small increases of treadmill slope or speed each minute in order to bring the subject to exhaustion within 9 to 11 min. Provided that the subject is well motivated, objective evidence of a central limitation of oxygen transport will be seen during the final minutes of such a test (Shephard, 1992b): Oxygen consumption increases by less than 1.5 μmol/(kg·s), or 2 ml/(kg·min), for a further increase of treadmill loading, the heart rate approximates the expected maximal value for the subject's age (Fox & Haskell, 1968; Londeree & Moeschberger, 1984; Shephard, 1987a), the respiratory gas exchange ratio exceeds 1.15, and the blood lactate concentration reaches values ranging from 10 to 11 mmol/L in a young adult to 8 mmol/L in a senior citizen (Shephard, 1987a). If a small number of such tests are performed under laboratory conditions, the data for any given individual have a test-retest reliability of about 4% (Wright, Sidney, & Shephard, 1978). It is less certain whether such precision can be sustained when a larger volume of data is collected under field conditions. Perhaps more seriously, a slight illness or minor variations in training schedule can alter the results for any given individual by as much as 10% of the average value for that person.

Some clinical laboratories do not measure oxygen consumption during treadmill testing, contenting themselves with reporting the final test stage that the subject reaches when following a fixed progressive protocol, such as the Bruce test (Shephard & Lavallée, 1978). The hope of the investigator is that the energy cost of walking or running at a given combination of treadmill speed and slope can be equated with a fixed oxygen demand expressed per kilogram of body mass. In practice, there is at least a 10% interindividual variation in the oxygen cost of treadmill walking, even in young adults (Shephard et al., 1968a). The error of assuming a constant energy cost is substantially widened if the test sample includes children or older adults (G.R. Cumming, 1978; Shephard, 1987a) or if the subject uses even light hand support.

In most field situations, a treadmill is not available. Alternative modes of exercise testing include the cycle ergometer, step test, and the sport-specific ergometers that are used when evaluating athletes (Dal Monte, Faina, & Menchinelli, 1992; Shephard, 1978). Relative to the treadmill criterion, the peak oxygen intake of the average person is about 4% lower when measured on a step test, 7% to 8% lower in seated cycle ergometry, and at least 12% lower in supine cycle ergometry (Shephard et al., 1968a). Particularly in unfit, older people, the peak effort on a cycle ergometer tends to be limited by peripheral muscle weakness and fatigue rather than by the peak oxygen delivery of the cardiorespiratory system (Kay & Shephard, 1969; Shephard, 1992b).

One attraction of the cycle ergometer is that the subject remains in a relatively fixed position, making it easier to measure blood pressures and to collect blood samples while the test is proceeding. The increments of work rate can also be graded rather precisely when determining the lactate threshold, and some investigators have claimed that the mechanical efficiency of effort shows little interindividual variability on this device. Certainly, a rough estimate of oxygen consumption can be made from the external mechanical work performed during either cycle ergometry or stepping (Shephard, 1978). A young adult operates a heavily loaded cycle ergometer with a net mechanical efficiency that averages about 23%. The oxygen consumption even of young subjects varies 4% to 5% around predictions based on this average value (Shephard et al., 1968b). Children and old people work less efficiently, for several reasons. The total power output of such individuals is lower than in a young adult, increasing the relative importance of unmeasured energy losses in the chain and bearings, and lack of experience in cycling may lead to flat-footed operation, reducing the exchange of energy between the pedals and the muscles of the calf. Also, in an older person, postural work and the energy lost through limb movements may be increased by an accumulation of body fat.

If the chosen form of work is a step test, it is quite possible both to measure oxygen consumption and to record the electrocardiogram, the necessary leads being supported by a firm post mounted at the side of the steps. The energy cost of stepping is determined by body mass, step height, and the stepping rhythm. The net mechanical efficiency for a complete, comfortably paced rhythm of ascent and descent (60-120 paces/min) is about 16%, and this figure varies surprisingly little with the leg length of the subject; a step 20.3 to 22.9 cm high can accomodate everyone from 10-year-old children to older adults. The oxygen consumption of individual subjects normally varies about 7% around predictions based on the 16% statistic (Shephard et al., 1968b), although the cost of ascent is modified further if the subject uses a hand support.

Predictions of maximal oxygen intake can be made from the responses to submaximal exercise. The systematic error of such predictions is fairly small, and the results may thus give an indication of the average level of aerobic fitness within a given community. However, the data are not sufficiently precise to indicate the physical condition of individual test candidates.

LACTATE THRESHOLD.   The intensity of activity when significant quantities of lactate accumulate in peripheral blood is often estimated from ventilatory measurements made during a progressive treadmill or cycle ergometer test (Shephard, 1992c). The determination is based most easily on the transition from a decreasing to an increasing ventilatory equivalent for oxygen ($\dot{V}_E/\dot{V}_{O_2}$). The respiratory gas exchange ratio ($\dot{V}_{CO_2}/\dot{V}_{O_2}$) also begins to increase rapidly at this stage in the test, although the ratio of ventilation to carbon dioxide output ($\dot{V}_E/\dot{V}_{CO_2}$). continues to fall. The most obvious break-point in the relationship of ($\dot{V}_E/\dot{V}_{O_2}$) to work rate is thought to correspond with the onset of acidosis in the active tissues; the blood lactate is about 2 mmol/L at this point.

Some authors have attempted to distinguish a second break-point in the curve (McLellan, 1987), when a rapid accumulation of lactate in the bloodstream begins (a blood lactate of about 4 mmol/L). At this stage in the test, there is a rapid increase in ventilation and carbon dioxide output relative to work rate. However, many authors argue that the typical curve is not consistent enough to warrant attempts at distinguishing the second break-point (Shephard, 1992c).

BLOOD PRESSURES.   Accurate measurement of blood pressures requires the introduction of a recording needle or catheter into a major artery. This is an accepted clinical procedure and is occasionally undertaken for research purposes, but it carries various risks that are not justified in most evaluations of health-related fitness.

Approximate values for resting and exercise blood pressures can be obtained by sphygmomanometry as part of a progressive exercise test. Unfortunately, international comparisons of the resulting data have been hampered by variations in measuring technique, such as differences in the speed of cuff deflation, and some observers have used the fifth rather than the fourth phase of the Korotkov sounds to indicate the diastolic pressure. Many observers tend to prefer the digits 0 and 5 when recording pressures, and results have also been influenced by the location where the data is collected (values are often higher when taken in a doctor's office than when recorded in the community; Shephard, Cox, & Simper, 1981; M.A. Young, Rowlands, Stallard, Watson, & Littler, 1983). During exercise, the cuff estimates of systolic pressure sometimes differ from intraarterial readings by 10 to 20 mm Hg, or 1.3 to 2.7 kPa (Kleinhauss & Franke, 1971; Rowell, Brengelmann, Blackmon, Bruce, & Murray, 1968), and there is often even greater difficulty in determining the diastolic pressure. Usually, there is no clear point at which the Korotkov sounds become muffled, and some authors have thus made the assumption (in general, supported by intraarterial measurements) that the diastolic pressure changes little during rhythmic, non-resisted exercise.

To a first approximation, the product of systolic blood pressure and heart rate gives an indication of cardiac work rate (the double product). Particularly if there is evidence of myocardial ischemia, such as anginal pain or electrocardiographic ST segmental depression, it is useful to note the double product at which such symptoms first appear and to note how this value changes in response to endurance training.

EXERCISE ELECTROCARDIOGRAM.   Whereas paramedical professionals use the electrocardiogram to obtain accurate heart rate data, the main purpose of examining the exercise electrocardiogram in a clinically supervised test is to detect silent myocardial ischemia. This is important to the safety of a test, and it also provides an indication of the subject's prognosis.

Early attempts to record the electrocardiogram of an exercising subject were often frustrated by a wandering electrical baseline, but this difficulty has been largely overcome. Investigators now appreciate the importance of reducing the input impedance of the recording electrodes by a preliminary abrasion of the skin, and any residual baseline shifts can be corrected by electronic signal averaging devices that are triggered by a normal QRS complex (Rautaharju, Friedrich, & Wolf, 1971).

If only a single-lead system is available, the exploring electrode is best placed in the CM_5 position (Blackburn et al., 1967; see Figure 3.5). It is preferable to use at least three unipolar electrode placements (CM_2, CM_4, and CM_6) in order to test for ischemia over a large area of the myocardium. There is some likelihood of a false negative stress test unless the subject can be persuaded to exercise to at least 85% of maximal oxygen intake. If the exercise electrocardiogram shows evidence of ST segmental depression (a horizontal or downsloping tracing, leading to more than 0.1 mV of depression 80 msec following the QRS complex), then the subject's risk of a future myocardial infarction or sudden death is increased at least twofold (Hollenberg et al., 1985; Okin et al., 1988; Shephard, 1981; Staniloff et al., 1984; Wohlfart et al., 1990; see Figure 3.6) and possibly as much as five- to sixfold (Giagnoni et al., 1983). Moreover, the increased risk seems to be independent of the subject's age, smoking habits, and blood pressure (Giagnoni et al., 1983). The assessment of ST depression becomes a little more precise if the record is calibrated for the overall electrocardiographic voltage,

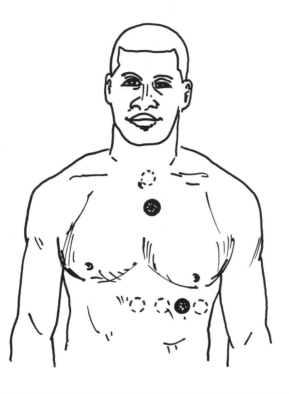

Figure 3.5   Recommended lead placements when recording the electrocardiogram during vigorous exercise. *Note*. Reprinted from Shephard (1977a) by permission.

which standardizes data in terms of the magnitude of the R wave (Berman, Wynne, Mallis, & Cohn, 1983; Ilsley et al., 1982).

Exercise may also induce premature ventricular contractions. Such abnormalities of heart rhythm are thought to carry an adverse prognosis if they are of polyfocal origin (as shown by variations in their waveform), if they occur early in the repolarization cycle (the R wave being superimposed on the T wave of the preceeding complex), and if they become more frequent or develop into runs of abnormal beats during exercise (Blackburn et al., 1973; Cullen et al., 1983; Jelinek, 1980; Kohn, Ibrahim, & Feldman, 1971). However, it is less clear whether abnormal rhythms give independent information relative to the warning provided by ST segmental depression (Yang, Wesley, & Froelicher, 1991).

It is finally important to emphasize that if there are no symptoms of myocardial ischemia, then electrocardiographic abnormalities of the ST segment and premature ventricular contractions give only a very fallible indication of the health of

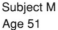

Subject M
Age 51

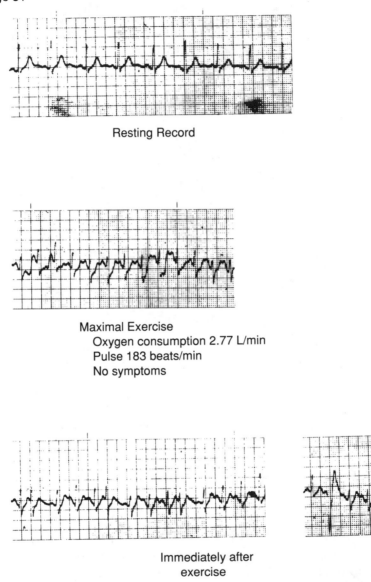

Resting Record

Maximal Exercise
Oxygen consumption 2.77 L/min
Pulse 183 beats/min
No symptoms

Immediately after
exercise

Figure 3.6 Abnormalities of the electrocardiogram during and immediately following vigorous exercise. The record shows ST segmental depression and polyphasic ventricular premature contractions. (The subject was a middle-aged man who was a heavy smoker. He worked as a janitor in an apartment building and, 4 weeks after testing, died suddenly while running up four flights of stairs to attend to a broken water main.) *Note.* Reprinted from Shephard (1977a) by permission.

the coronary vasculature in an individual. As many as two thirds of apparently positive exercise stress tests prove to be false positive results, with no adverse clinical consequences over a 5- or even a 10-year period (Shephard, 1981, 1987b).

HEMOGLOBIN LEVELS.   Procedures for the estimation of hemoglobin should follow the internationally agreed protocol (International Committee, 1967). Samples of capillary blood are treated with Drabkin's reagent, which converts the hemoglobin to cyanmethemoglobin, and the concentration of the latter is determined from the absorption of visible light at a wavelength of 540 nm. Disposable cuvettes are now available that are pretreated with an appropriate quantity of reagent. Readings are compared with those obtained using a standard cyanmethemoglobin preparation.

CARDIAC DIMENSIONS.   Early determinations of cardiac volume were based on linear measurements of the radiographic heart shadow in posteroanterior and lateral axes (Reindell, König, & Roskamm, 1966). A simple formula yielded a figure that was usually expressed in milliliters per kilogram body mass. Typical values were 10 to 11 ml/kg in an average person and 14 to 15 ml/kg in a well-trained endurance athlete.

Unfortunately, this approach did not distinguish clearly between an increase of wall thickness and an enlargement of the ventricular cavity, the latter being likely to develop with the increased stroke volume of a well-trained person. Recently, data on the thickness of various segments of the ventricular wall have been obtained by echocardiography, with a view to distinguishing a desirable training response from a pathological enlargement of the heart. Attention has focused on the relative thicknesses of the interventricular septum and the posterior ventricular wall; the maximal permitted ratio is 1.0 to 1.3 in healthy individuals (Rost & Hollmann, 1992). However, the interpretation of such findings remains unclear, particularly the possible relationship between hypertrophy of the interventricular septum and hypertrophic cardiomyopathy, which has been linked to the sudden death of endurance athletes.

OBESITY.   Hydrostatic weighing is commonly regarded as the method of choice in high-technology assessments of body fatness (Shephard, 1991b). However, there are a multiplicity of equations for converting density readings into percent body fat (see Table 3.11), reflecting interpopulation differences in the average density of lean tissues.

Measurements of skinfold thicknesses are quite susceptible to interobserver variation due to differences in such factors as caliper design, choice of measurement site, the method used to support the skinfold during measurements, and the period of skinfold compression that is allowed before a reading is taken (Shephard, 1991b). On the other hand, skinfold readings have an advantage over many alternative techniques in that fat is actually being measured, at least in the superficial tissues. Data can also be obtained on the central-versus-peripheral distribution of subcutaneous fat. Cardiovascular health is adversely affected by a masculine distribution of superficial fat (i.e., a high ratio of abdominal to limb

Table 3.11
Discrepancies in Body Density Predicted From Skinfold Readings
and in Percent Body Fat Predicted From Body Density

Estimates of body density for a common set of skinfold readings

Formula	Density (g/cc)	Age (yr)	Sex	Author
$1.1533 - 0.0643(\log_{10}\Sigma S)$	1.048	15	M	Durnin & Rahaman, 1967
$1.1610 - 0.0632(\log_{10}\Sigma S)$	1.057	22	M	Durnin & Rahaman, 1967
$1.1369 - 0.0598(\log_{10}\Sigma S)$	1.032	15	F	Durnin & Rahaman, 1967
$1.1581 - 0.0720(\log_{10}\Sigma S)$	1.032	22	F	Durnin & Rahaman, 1967
$1.1447 - 0.0612(\log_{10}\Sigma S)$	1.050		M	Durnin, personal commun.
$1.1309 - 0.0587(\log_{10}\Sigma S)$	1.036		F	Durnin, personal commun.
$1.130 - 0.055(\log_{10}S_t)$ $- 0.026(\log_{10}S_s)$	1.049	13-16	M	Pařízková, 1961
$1.114 - 0.031(\log_{10}S_t)$ $- 0.041(\log_{10}S_s)$	1.035	13-16	F	Pařízková, 1961
$1.0923 - 0.0202(S_t)$	1.074	22	M	Pascale et al., 1956
$1.0896 - 0.0179(S_s)$	1.068	22	M	Pascale et al., 1956
$1.0764 - 0.00088(S_t)$ $- 0.00081(S_s)$	1.051	20	F	Sloan et al., 1962

Estimates of body fat for a common set of body density readings

Formula	Body fat (%)	Author
$(5.548/D - 5.044)100$	19.0	Rathbun & Pace, 1945
$(4.971/D - 4.519)100$	17.1	Brozek et al., 1963a
$(4.570/D - 4.142)100$	16.9	Brozek et al., 1963a
$(4.0439/D - 3.6266)100$	18.8	Grande, 1961
$(1.10 - D)500$	20.0	MacMillan et al., 1965

Note. Where Σ is the sum of triceps, subscapular, and suprailiac skinfolds, S_t is the thickness of the triceps skinfold, S_s is the thickness of the subscapular skinfold, and D is the estimated body density. Reprinted from Shephard (1978) by permission.

skinfold readings; Lapidus et al., 1984; Reichley et al., 1987). One important criticism of skinfold data is that it provides no estimate of the quantity of internal, or visceral, fat. The proportion of internal to external fat generally increases as a person ages (Shephard, 1991b).

Circumference readings are more repeatable than skinfold determinations, particularly when observers have only limited anthropometric experience. Their disadvantage is that circumference reflects not only fat but also a much larger component of lean tissue and bone. Circumference data thus show a poor correlation with independent measures of obesity (Murray & Shephard, 1988).

Most methods of estimating lean tissue mass (e.g., determinations of the naturally occurring isotope ^{40}K or the dilution of ingested deuterated water) rely on past assessments of the body mineral or water content of very small numbers of cadavers (Shephard, 1991b). The overall lean mass or the local muscle volume of the active limbs may show a fairly close correlation with peak oxygen intake (C.T.M. Davies & Van Haaren, 1973b; Shephard et al., 1988a), but lean mass determinations do not provide a very satisfactory method of assessing obesity. The body fat (obtained by subtracting lean from total body mass) usually accounts for only a small proportion of the total body tissue, and a small error in the estimation of lean mass thus leads to a large error in the estimate of percent body fat.

Whole-body impedance is one method of estimating lean tissue, and thus body fat, that is currently quite popular with clinicians. A simple voltmeter records the electrical impedance to passage of a high-frequency electrical current between the wrists and the ankles (Chumlea & Baumgartner, 1990). In addition to the general objection to the estimation of body fat from lean tissue measurements, the impedance data depend substantially on both the form of the limbs and the trunk and on the distribution of electrical currents through and around fascial planes. Thus, impedance measurements are not well suited to interpopulation comparisons of body fat among subjects who differ in their average body build.

MUSCLE STRENGTH. Measurements of static and dynamic muscle strength and muscular endurance are often included as part of a battery of fitness tests. From the health perspective, muscle development influences the cardiovascular reactions to a given exercise task. If the muscles in one part of the body are weak, there may be an excessive rise of blood pressure when that body part is exercised. The preservation of muscle strength is also important to the quality of life for the very old.

The peak handgrip force is commonly measured in large-scale surveys, but such readings are not always well correlated with overall muscularity. Strength tends to be specific to the type of exercise, whether isotonic, isokinetic, or isometric, the direction of any movement that is permitted during testing, and the joint angle. Furthermore, a high peak strength does not always mean an outstanding muscular endurance.

An alternative overall assessment of muscularity is achieved by measuring the mass of lean muscle per unit of stature. This has the advantage that the observer does not have to obtain a maximal effort from the subject.

JOINT AND BONE HEALTH. Flexibility is difficult to determine in large-scale surveys, since in any one subject, the findings vary from one joint to another (Shephard, Berridge, & Montelpare, 1990), and again there are intraindividual differences between static and dynamic measurements. Further, the scores obtained on procedures such as the sit-and-reach test or its equivalent, the Kraus-Weber toe-touching test, depend substantially on the subject's leg length.

In young adults, a normal range of endurance exercise seems sufficient to maintain the range of motion of the major joints, and the determination of flexibility may not add much to a fitness assessment, unless there has been a local injury that is limiting activity. However, there is a progressive deterioration of joint function with aging (Shephard, 1987a). Thus, even if there has been no injury, the loss of flexibility in the frail elderly may be sufficient to limit their participation in aerobic exercise, causing a substantial deterioration in quality of life.

Bone health may be assessed for the skeleton as a whole or for specific regions of the body. A number of large hospital departments have facilities for measuring whole-body calcium, using neutron activation and a whole-body counter (Shephard, 1991c). More commonly, bone density is measured at local sites, such as the wrist or the lower part of the vertebral column, using the technique of dual-beam photon absorptiometry (E.L. Smith, Smith, & Gilligan, 1990).

METABOLIC VARIABLES.   A glucose tolerance curve provides a simple measure of the risk of developing diabetes and associated cardiovascular complications. Standard biochemical techniques are used to monitor blood glucose levels following the ingestion of a fixed dose of glucose. In general, aerobic training leads to a faster clearance of glucose from the bloodstream (see chapter 5).

A full, blood lipid profile currently requires the determination of total cholesterol, LDL- and HDL-cholesterol, and the subcomponents of HDL-cholesterol (particularly the protective HDL-2 component and the corresponding A-I apoprotein). It is important that these observations be validated against some well-standardized, external source. (Rifkind & Segal, 1983).

Low-Technology Approach to Measuring Physical Activity

Because of the high cost of equipment and the need for specialized personnel, most investigators have preferred to base large-scale surveys of physical activity and health-related fitness on simple procedures that use a minimum of equipment and do not require the presence of a supervising physician (Canada Fitness Survey, 1983; Shephard, 1986c). The only practical, large-scale approach to the assessment of physical activity is the use of a diary record or questionnaire (Edholm, 1970; Shephard, 1978).

DIARY RECORDS.   The subject is asked to keep a minute-by-minute record of his or her activities; notekeeping is facilitated by sheets that are ruled in minutes and hours and standard abbreviations for commonly encountered activities (e.g., S for sleeping, Si for sitting, St for standing, and W for walking). Appropriate abbreviations are entered in the diary each time that the activity of the subject changes, and succeeding minutes are marked by a horizontal line until the subject again changes activity.

The success of this type of record depends very much on the intelligence and enthusiastic cooperation of the subject. Commonly, the accuracy of reporting deteriorates after 1 or 2 days of record keeping. Further, the process of completing the diary sheets may be reactive. At work, the completion of records that are to be inspected by an independent observer may stimulate greater application to the paid task, even if confidentiality is assured. And in leisure hours, the thought of having to make additional diary entries may persuade a less motivated subject to continue reading or watching television, rather than taking up some other pursuit. On the other hand, data reduction can be a problem if a wide range of activities are reported.

Whereas representative, 24-hr records covering all activities are important when determining total daily energy expenditures, much simpler information may suffice from the viewpoint of health-related fitness. For example, weekly diary sheets can record brief details of the nature and duration of up to three vigorous aerobic activities a day (Shephard, 1982b). Kavanagh (1992) found that this type of record offered a valuable means of assessing the compliance of postcoronary patients enrolled in a progressive exercise program. Simple diaries have also been used quite successfully in large-scale, prospective studies of cardiovascular health in the Framingham community (Dawber, 1980) and among British executive civil servants (Morris, Clayton, Everitt, Semmence, & Burgess, 1990).

DIRECT OBSERVATION.   Technicians can be trained to keep minute-by-minute records of activity patterns analogous to the detailed, self-kept diaries. If the observer has a quiet, unobtrusive manner, the subject's activities are altered relatively little by either the investigator's note-taking or use of an electronic notepad. The accuracy of such data is generally greater than when the subjects themselves maintain the diaries. The main practical difficulty in implementing an observational approach is that often a technician can shadow only a single subject, so that surveying a large community becomes prohibitively expensive. Observation is best suited to the study of people living in close proximity to each other who are following a stereotyped daily regimen, for example, army recruits (Edholm et al., 1970; O'Hara et al., 1978), a company of submariners (Southgate & Shirling, 1970), or a group of postal carriers whose daily duties are closely constrained by union regulations (Shephard, 1983c). Sometimes, the observer's findings can be matched to direct measurements of oxygen consumption for the main daily activities. Such a combined methodology was applied successfully to the determination of total energy expenditures in various types of Inuit hunting expeditions on the arctic tundra (Godin & Shephard, 1973a).

RETROSPECTIVE QUESTIONNAIRES.   Retrospective physical activity assessments can range from answering a single, well-chosen question to completing a complex form, with or without the assistance of paramedical personnel. Some questionnaires run to 20 or more pages and cover behavior during the previous week, the previous month, or over an entire year. The quality of the information obtained becomes highly suspect if a complicated, self-administered procedure is applied to an entire population that presents a wide spectrum of intelligence and motivation. Also, subjects commonly exaggerate the extent of their involvement in physical activity when completing such instruments. The cause may be a limitation in the design of the questionnaire—the average tennis player, for example, may find no alternative but to classify the time occupied in changing, conversing, and searching for lost balls as playing tennis. The total time reported as spent in activities during a 24-hr day may also depart widely from the available 1,440 min, and an arbitrary scaling of either the entire day or the period purportedly occupied by physically active pursuits is then required. The completion of a detailed, retrospective questionnaire thus becomes a rather fallible method of obtaining information on habitual patterns of physical activity.

More accurate information can sometimes be obtained if a bulky form is replaced by a much simpler classification of physical activity. Shephard and McClure (1965) showed that in the stereotypic situation of an army unit, 36% of the interindividual variation in measures of aerobic fitness could be detected from the response of subjects to a single question regarding their involvement in sports or an aerobic training program. Likewise, a simple, five-level response was used to classify the habitual physical activity of Saskatoon residents (Bailey, Shephard, Mirwald, & McBride, 1974; Bailey, Shephard, & Mirwald, 1976); the choice of response ranged from *none* or *infrequent* through *regular* (i.e., 2-3 sessions a week of moderate aerobic activity such as jogging, tennis, squash, or swimming four lengths or more) to *very frequent* (i.e., 4-5 sessions a week) or *regular training* (i.e., 3-5 sessions a week of deliberate training for a specific sport). There were substantial differences of aerobic power between the five levels of response in both men and women. Respective values for the two sexes ranged from 22.2 and 19.4 μmol/(kg·s), 29.9 and 26.1 ml/(kg·min) in those reporting infrequent or no activity to 24.8 and 21.4 μmol/(kg·s), or 33.3 and 28.7 ml/(kg·min), for those with regular activity and 29.2 and 23.2 μmol/(kg·s), or 39.3 and 31.2 ml/(kg·min), for those with very frequent activity. Again, when a simple questionnaire was used to classify the activity patterns of subjects of an Inuit community, a substantial gradient of aerobic power was seen in terms of their reported involvement in traditional hunting pursuits (Shephard, 1978).

Godin and Shephard (1985) attempted a slightly more sophisticated, three-question rating of subjects' patterns of aerobic activity (see Figure 3.7). The 2-week test-retest reliability was 0.80 for reports of sweat-inducing activity, and 0.94 for reports of strenuous activity. The internal validity of the activity assessment was demonstrated relative to independent measurements of the individual's aerobic power (a 69% accuracy of classification relative to a simple step test) and body fat (a 66% accuracy of classification relative to skinfold measurements). Because the accuracy of reports was greater for strenuous than for more moderate activity, fit subjects were identified more consistently (80%) than those who were unfit, and thin subjects (89%) were classified more clearly than those who were fat.

The Canada Fitness Survey (1983) provides one example of a much more complicated test instrument. Separate sections of the questionnaire covered occupation, domestic chores, and leisure activity, and prompt cards were used to remind participants of activities that they might otherwise have overlooked.

Leisure Time Exercise Questionnaire

1. Considering a **7-day period** (a week), how many times on the average do you do the following kinds of exercise for **more than 15 minutes** during your **free time** (write the appropriate number in each circle).

Times per week

a) **Strenuous exercise**
   (heart beats rapidly)
   (i.e., running, jogging, hockey, football, soccer, squash, basketball, cross-country skiing, judo, roller skating, vigorous swimming, vigorous long-distance bicycling)

b) **Moderate exercise**
   (not exhausting)
   (i.e., fast walking, baseball, tennis, easy bicycling, volleyball, badminton, easy swimming, alpine skiing, popular and folk dancing)

c) **Mild exercise**
   (minimal effort)
   (i.e., yoga, archery, fishing from river bank, bowling, horseshoes, golf, snowmobiling, easy walking)

2. Considering a **7-day period** (a week), during your **leisure time**, how often do you engage in any regular activity long enough to **work up a sweat** (heart beats rapidly)?

Often	Sometimes	Never/rarely
❑	❑	❑

Figure 3.7   Questionnaire for the assessment of habitual activity. *Note.* Reprinted from Godin and Shephard (1985) by permission.

Apparently because of the complexity of the questions that were asked, little relationship was found between the estimates of either leisure energy expenditure or total daily energy expenditure and measures of health-related fitness (see Table 3.12). Indeed, those who reported low levels of leisure activity tended to achieve higher scores on many of the tests of health-related fitness. Arguably, the standard adopted in the original analysis for an *active* individual (i.e., having an estimated additional daily energy expenditure of 8.4 kJ/kg of body mass, or 0.5-0.6MJ) was too low, and it included a large segment of the population who were not active enough to anticipate any resultant gains of fitness. Moreover, Godin and Shephard (1985) pointed out that perceptions of participation become erroneous if attention is focused on low- and moderate-intensity exercise. An alternative classification, based on the much simpler criterion of the estimated intensity of reported activities (Shephard, 1986c), showed some gradient of aerobic power, skinfold readings, muscular endurance, and flexibility (see Table 3.12), although the proportion of the population classed as physically active dropped dramatically to only 5.1% of young men and 1.3% of young women.

The Campbell's survey of 1988 revised the definition of an active individual upwards to a person having a leisure expenditure of 12.6 kJ/kg/day (Stephens & Craig, 1990). When subjects were classified on the basis of this criterion, intercategory differences in the proportions of individuals with an excess body mass, an excessive average skinfold reading, and an adverse waist-hip ratio were still small but, particularly in the young adults, were in the expected direction (see Table 3.13).

The large amount of clerical work involved in analyzing a relatively complicated questionnaire, such as the Canada Fitness Survey document, may be justified in terms of the information it provides to those who design facilities and plan motivational tactics. But if the objective of a survey is simply to evaluate exercise habits as one aspect of community lifestyle, then a much simpler piece of information (such as the proportion of subjects who are performing the minimum physical activity needed to sustain cardiovascular condition) may be all that is required.

Low-Technology Approaches to Measuring Health-Related Fitness

In general, the search of those testing the health-related fitness of large populations has been for field procedures that use a minimum of equipment, and do not require the presence of a supervising physician (Canada Fitness Survey, 1983; Shephard, 1986c; see also Table 3.14). Simple assessments are made of aerobic power, body composition, muscle strength and flexibility, or tests of physical performance that can be equated with aerobic power, anaerobic power, and strength are measured on the track or in a gymnasium.

AEROBIC POWER.   Perhaps the most controversial issue has been the choice of a procedure for the field assessment of aerobic power. Candidate tests have included direct evaluation of the heart rate observed at a standard submaximal rate of working on a cycle ergometer or stepping bench, prediction of maximal

Table 3.12
Relationship Between Reported Amount of Daily Active
Physical Leisure and Selected Measures of Fitness

Variable	Men		Women	
	Active (>8.4 kkd*)	Moderately active/ sedentary (<8.4 kkd)	Active (>8.4 kkd)	Moderately active/ sedentary (<8.4 kJ/kg/d)
Body mass (kg/m)	.417	.423	.352	.354
Skinfold (mm)	10.8	10.4	12.8	12.4
Lean mass (g/cm)	.346	.354	.260	.264
$\dot{V}_{O_2max}$				
[μmol/(kg·s)]	33.9	34.7	25.5	26.3
[ml/(kg·min)]	45.6	46.7	34.3	35.2
Handgrip (N)	520	528	298	300
Sit-ups (n)	31.7	34.8	24.6	27.2
Sit-and-reach (cm)	29.8	30.4	31.7	33.4

Variable	Men			Women		
	Active (>8 METS)	Moderately active (>6 METS)	Sedentary (<6 METS)	Active (>8 METS)	Moderately active (>6 METS)	Sedentary (<6 METS)
Body mass (kg/m)	.422	.420	.420	.352	.347	.352
Skinfold (mm)	9.7	10.0	10.5	10.1	10.7	12.2
Lean mass (g/cm)	.354	.347	.348	.252	.258	.261
$\dot{V}_{O_2max}$						
[μmol/(kg·s)]	36.7	36.8	34.6	29.8	27.2	26.0
[ml/(kg·min)]	49.3	49.4	46.5	40.0	36.6	35.0
Handgrip (N)	521	523	525	324	300	304
Sit-ups (n)	39.6	37.4	34.1	35.8	35.6	27.2
Sit-and-reach (cm)	31.6	31.1	30.2	38.4	35.6	32.8

Note. Subjects aged 20 to 29 yrs. Data from Canada Fitness Survey (1983).
*kkd = kJ of energy expenditure per kg body mass per day.

Table 3.13
Relationship Between Reported Daily Leisure Activity
and Percentage of Subjects With Possible Health Risk

Group	Excess body mass[a]	Excess fat[b]	Waist-hip ratio[c]
Age 15-24 yrs			
>12.6 kJ/kg/day	16%	29%	<15%
> 4.2 kJ/kg/day	17%	38%	<15%
< 4.2 kJ/kg/day	20%	36%	<15%
Age 25-44 yrs			
>12.6 kJ/kg/day	35%	31%	15%
> 4.2 kJ/kg/day	35%	35%	20%
< 4.2 kJ/kg/day	39%	41%	29%
Age 45+ yrs			
>12.6 kJ/kg/day	51%	41%	52%
> 4.2 kJ/kg/day	50%	38%	52%
< 4.2 kJ/kg/day	54%	53%	52%

Note. Adapted from Stephens and Craig (1990) by permission.
[a]Body mass index > 25 kg/m^2.
[b]Average skinfold > 12 mm (males), > 15 mm (females).
[c]Ratio > 0.90 (males), > 0.80 (females).

oxygen intake based on the heart rate-power output relationship, or performance during an all-out walking or running test.

A cycle ergometer is relatively heavy, but it can be transported in a car to a central school or testing hall. The investigator may then decide to measure or to make a close linear interpolation of the physical working capacity at a fixed heart rate such as 170 beats/min (the so-called PWC$_{170}$ test; R. Gauthier et al., 1983; Howell & MacNab, 1968). An assessment of this type inevitably underestimates cardiorespiratory fitness when the heart rate is increased by anxiety or a hot environment (Shephard et al., 1968b). Further complications arise from a variable decline in maximal heart rate with age (Shephard, 1987a). Though the PWC$_{170}$ test demands only about 80% of maximal oxygen intake in a young adult, a heart rate of 170 beats/min may exceed peak aerobic effort for some 65-year-old subjects; therefore some authors measure a PWC$_{150}$ in older individuals. Others adjust the exercise loading so that the average person of any age is brought to 70% of maximal oxygen intake. Responses can then be compared in terms of deviations from the heart rate anticipated at 70% of peak aerobic effort (assuming this to decline linearly from 160 beats/min at age 25 to 120 beats/min at age 65).

The I. Åstrand (1960) prediction of maximal oxygen intake is based on the supposed linear relationship of heart rate to work rate or the corresponding oxygen consumption between 50% and 90% to 100% of maximal oxygen intake,

Table 3.14
Test Battery Used in Canada Fitness Survey of 1981

Variable	Comment
Questionnaire data	
Lifestyle	
Physical activity habits	
Anthropometric data	
Standing height	Gentle traction; estimated, if measurement not possible.
Body mass	Estimated, if necessary.
Skinfolds (biceps, triceps, sub-scapular, suprailiac, medial calf)	All measures repeated once, twice if difference exceeds 1 mm.
Girths (relaxed upper arm, chest, waist, hips, right thigh, right calf-maximum)	Steel tape used.
Bone diameters (biepicondylar humerus-elbow, biepicon-dylar femur-knee)	
Performance tests	
Blood pressure (for screening)	Systolic and diastolic (phase 4) after 5 min of rest before step test, also at 30-60 s and 2.5-3.0 min after completing the step test.
Step test (cardiovascular)	Canadian Home Fitness Test (advanced version—up to 3 bouts of 3-min exercise each); results as final heart rate or estimated $\dot{V}_{O_2max}$; also resting, intermediate, and 3-min post-test heart rates.
Grip strength (muscular strength)	Combined maximum, right and left hands, after two attempts each.
Push-ups (muscular endurance)	Males from toes, females from knees.
Sit-and-reach (trunk flexion)	Using a modified Wells and Dillon flexometer, after stretching.
Sit-ups (muscular endurance)	60 s maximum.

Note. Adapted from Canada Fitness Survey (1983) by permission.

as observed in healthy young adults. The subject performs one or more steady, 6-min bouts of exercise on a step or a cycle ergometer. If the researcher assumes the heart rates corresponding to 50% of aerobic power (128 beats/min in men; 135 beats/min in women) and 100% of aerobic power (195 beats/min in men, 198 beats/min in women), the prediction of maximal oxygen intake can then be based on a single, submaximal measurement of heart rate (f_h) and the corresponding power output or oxygen consumption ($\dot{V}_{O_2observed}$). A nomogram was originally developed to make the necessary calculations, but a small computer can now be programmed to carry out these operations:

For men,

$$\dot{V}_{O_2max} = 2\dot{V}_{O_2observed} \, (195 - 128)/(f_h - 61).$$

For women,

$$\dot{V}_{O_2max} = 2\dot{V}_{O_2observed} \, (198 - 135)/(f_h - 72).$$

The oxygen consumption is generally not measured in field testing, but it can be predicted from the corresponding work rate. A constant net mechanical efficiency is assumed, 23% when a subject is exercising on a cycle ergometer and 16% when he or she is making repeated ascents and descents of a double step. As with the PWC_{170}, the original version of the Åstrand test made no allowance for the decrease of maximal heart rate in older subjects. The more recent prediction procedure (I. Åstrand, 1960) incorporated an average age factor, which was used to reduce the predicted maximal oxygen intake; this can be simplified to 0.87 at age 35 years, 0.78 at 45 years, 0.71 at 55 years, and 0.65 at 65 years.

In Canada, predictions of aerobic power have been based extensively on use of the Canadian Home Fitness Test (CHFT) (Bailey et al., 1976; Shephard, Thomas, et al., 1991). When performing the CHFT, the subject repeatedly ascends and descends a 20.3-cm double step at an age- and gender-specific rhythm set by tape-recorded music. For a person of average aerobic fitness, the three test stages correspond to approximately 60%, 70%, and 80% of maximal oxygen intake. At the end of each 3-min test stage, exercise is halted briefly (a standard 25-s recovery interval), and the investigator counts the pulse rate from 5 to 15 s after each bout of exercise. If the heart rate is not too high, the subject proceeds to the next test stage. The aerobic fitness of the subject is then estimated from the exercise stage attained and the final pulse count (see Table 3.15). The CHFT is perhaps a little safer than the two preceeding submaximal procedures, because the initial intensity of effort is only 60% of the individual's anticipated aerobic power, and the test is invariably halted at a pulse count corresponding to 70% of maximal oxygen intake, regardless of the subject's age or physical condition.

The CHFT was designed originally to be a simple, self-administered motivational tool (Bailey, Shephard, Mirwald, & McBride, 1974; Bailey, Shephard, & Mirwald, 1976), and it can still be scored in a simple, categoric fashion (see Table 3.16). However, there have been numerous attempts to develop multiple regression equations that would allow prediction of maximal oxygen intake based on the subject's body mass, the peak rate of stepping, the corresponding heart rate, and the subject's age (Shephard, Thomas, et al., 1991). For example, Jetté et al. (1976) proposed the equation

$$\dot{V}_{O_2max} = 42.5 + 16.6(E) - 0.12(M) - 0.12(f_h) - 0.24(A),$$

where E is the oxygen cost of the age- and gender-specific stepping rate in liter/

min, M is the body mass in kilogram, f_h is the final heart rate in beats/min, and A is the age in years. Provided that the heart rate is measured accurately (e.g., by means of an electrocardiogram), the stepping rhythm is accurately maintained, and the subject lifts the body's center of mass the full height of the staircase at each stepping cycle, the CHFT can be interpreted using either the Åstrand prediction formula or a multiple regression of the type described. The error of prediction seems no better and no worse than that of other submaximal procedures for estimating aerobic power (Shephard, Thomas, et al., 1991). Given a typical adult population, the coefficient of correlation between any of the CHFT prediction formulae and the maximal oxygen intake, when measured directly on a treadmill or a step test, ranges from 0.70 to 0.80. Individual CHFT predictions have a coefficient of variation of 10% to 15%, relative to direct measurements. In consequence, little can be said about an individual's personal fitness based on a single, submaximal evaluation. On the other hand, the systematic error relative to direct measurements is fairly small, so that *averaged* data provide a useful measure of the overall level of aerobic fitness in a large population sample.

The main distinction between the CHFT multiple regression equation and the PWC_{170} or the I. Åstrand prediction procedure is that the CHFT regression relies much more on the attained exercise level and much less on the individual's heart rate. Thus, problems of anxiety and habituation are minimized, and if it is necessary to palpate the pulse rate rather than obtain an accurate ECG record, a small counting error has less influence on the subject's calculated aerobic power. Tests using the Jetté formula suggest that the resulting CHFT score is usually capable of detecting a 10% to 20% aerobic training response even in an individual subject, possibly because any errors in a given person's predicted maximal oxygen intake remain relatively constant from test to test (Jetté, Mongeon, & Shephard, 1982).

Those involved in the mass testing of fitness in schoolchildren have commonly used a battery of performance tests, including the times required to run distances of 50 m (an expression of anaerobic power) and 300 to 1,500 m (an expression of aerobic power; Disch, Frankiewicz, & Jackson, 1975; Shephard, 1982b) and such measures of muscle strength, endurance, and coordination as push-ups, pull-ups, sit-ups, a shuttle-run, and a standing broad jump or vertical jump (AAHPERD, 1980; CAHPER, 1980; Reiff, 1980; J.C. Ross, 1989). In the testing of adults, Balke (1954) and Cooper (1968) suggested that aerobic fitness could be assessed according to the distance run during 15 or 12 min, respectively (see Table 3.16). However, the results achieved in performance tests depend heavily on environmental conditions (heat, wind, rain, and hardness of running surface), physical aptitude, recent practice of the required gymnastic skills, motivation, body size, and fatness rather than health-related fitness (G.R. Cumming, 1971, 1978; Drake, Jones, Brown, & Shephard, 1968; Drake et al., 1969; Shephard & Lavallée, 1978). Thus, some authors have distinguished the concept of performance-related fitness (the prime determinant of test-scores in the gymnasium or on the track) from that of health-related fitness (Pate & Shephard, 1989). Motivation to maximal effort is important to both the reliability and the validity

Table 3.15

Interpretation of Canadian Home Fitness Test Scores Based on Attainment of Age-Specific Test Stage and Pulse Count in First 5-15 s of Recovery

Age (yr)	5-15 sec pulse count (original scoring)		
	First stage—undesirable fitness level	Second stage—minimum fitness level	Second stage—recommended fitness level
15-19	>30	>27	<26
20-29	>29	>26	<25
30-39	>28	>25	<24
40-49	>26	>24	<23
50-59	>25	>23	<22
60-69	>24	>23	<22

Norms proposed by Fitness Canada 1986[a]

Age (yr)	15-19		20-29		30-39		40-49		50-59		60-69	
Gender	M	F	M	F	M	F	M	F	M	F	M	F
Excellent	7ᵇ ≤ 25	6 ≤ 28	7 ≤ 26	5 ≤ 25	6 ≤ 24	5 ≤ 26	5 ≤ 21	4 ≤ 23	4 ≤ 20	3 ≤ 22	2 ≤ 16	2 ≤ 19
Above average	7 26-27	6 ≥ 29 5 27	7 27-29	5 26-28	6 25-27	5 27-30	5 22-24	4 24-26	4 21-22	3 23-24	2 17-18	2 20-21
Average	7 28-30	5 28-29	6 26-28	5 29-30 4 26	6 28-29	4 25-27	5 25-26	4 27-28 3 24-25	4 23-24	3 25-26	2 19	2 22-23
Below average	6 26-29	5 30-31	6 29-30	4 27-29	5 25-27	4 28-29	5 27-28 4 24-25	3 26-27	4 25-26 3 23	3 27 2 23-24	2 20	2 24
Poor	6 ≥ 30 5 ≥ 30	5 ≥ 32 4 ≥ 30	6 31-34 5 ≥ 29	4 30-32 3 ≥ 29	5 28-31 4 ≥ 28	4 30-31 3 ≥ 28	4 26-29 3 ≥ 26	3 28-29 2 ≥ 26	3 24-26 2 ≥ 25	2 25-29 1 ≥ 25	2 21-26 1 ≥ 24	2 25-29 1 ≥ 24

Note. Adapted from Fitness Canada (1983) by permission.
[a]Based on Canada Fitness Survey of 1981.
[b]Bold numbers indicate final stepping stage completed.

Table 3.16
Prediction of Maximal Oxygen Intake From Distance Run in 12 min

Distance run (km)	Maximal oxygen intake	
	[μmol/(kg·s)]	[ml/(kg·min)]
<1.6	<21	<28
1.6-2.0	21-25	28-34
2.0-2.4	25-31	34-42
2.4-2.8	31-39	42-52
>2.8	>39	>52

Note. Adapted from Cooper (1968) by permission.

of performance test scores. It is acceptable to demand (if difficult to obtain) maximal effort when testing schoolchildren who are involved in a regular gymnastic program, but it can be hazardous to make similar demands on a sedentary, older population when little is known about preexisting medical conditions. Indeed, there are recorded instances where tests of this type have provoked sudden death in middle-aged adults who attempted to attain specific scores in order to retain their jobs. There have been proposals to assess the aerobic power of senior citizens from observations of habitual walking speed (Bassey, Fentem, MacDonald, & Scriven, 1976; Cunningham, Rechnitzer, & Donner, 1986). This approach avoids the possibility of allegations that the test procedure has provoked a heart attack or a musculoskeletal injury, but unfortunately, there is only a very weak correlation between habitual walking speed and direct measurements of maximal oxygen intake (r = 0.3-0.4).

BODY FATNESS.   Large-scale field assessments of body fatness have commonly relied on measurements of excess mass relative to actuarial standards, or ratios of body mass to standing height such as the body mass index (M/H^2). In a developed society, a subject whose body mass has increased over the adult years and whose current body mass exceeds the actuarial ideal has usually accumulated an excess of body fat. Individuals with a body mass index of more than 25 kg/m^2 also have a statistically increased risk of cardiovascular disease. Thus, the average body mass or the average excess mass of a given population reflects the cardiovascular health of that population.

On the other hand, some subjects have a heavy body mass because of strong bones or well-developed muscles. The use of simple height-weight ratios is particularly risky when comparing populations that differ in socioeconomic status or ethnic background. For example, a 1969-1970 study of the Canadian Inuit demonstrated that this population had a large body mass in proportion to height, but this finding was linked to extremely low skinfold readings (Shephard, 1978). Although the body mass index of the Inuit was high in 1970, this was explained by a short stature and good muscular development, not obesity (Shephard, 1978, 1980). Still, even in this particular community, the interpretation of the body mass index has changed over the past 20 years. The population has become acculturated to the sedentary lifestyle of southern Canada, and many of its members have become relatively fat (Rode & Shephard, 1992; see also Figure 3.2), so much so that they are now at increased risk of cardiovascular disease.

IMPACT OF MEASUREMENT ON FITNESS SCORES.   Data collection can be reactive, influencing the results of fitness tests in several ways. If the test requires subject cooperation, motivation, or motor skills, the processes of learning and habituation may at first improve an individual's test scores (Shephard, 1969). However, if tests are repeated frequently, boredom and loss of interest can lead to a deterioration of peak effort. It is less certain how many sessions are needed for a subject to reach a performance plateau for any given type of fitness test or how rapidly learning and habituation dissipate between test sessions.

Test participation may have at least a limited influence on the subsequent lifestyle of those evaluated (Godin, Cox, & Shephard, 1983; Godin, Desharnais, Jobin, & Cook, 1987). For example, the discovery of an abnormal electrocardiogram may encourage smoking cessation, or the onset of severe dyspnea may encourage adoption of a regular exercise program. Such influences are likely to be stronger among randomly tested subjects than among those who have already committed themselves to an exercise program (Godin et al., 1983).

If a high proportion of a community is evaluated, social norms may also be altered. The construction of a modern, indoor swimming pool at a rural primary school was a somewhat unexpected consequence of a semilongitudinal study of exercise and fitness conducted in the Trois Rivières region (Shephard, 1982a). In small, isolated settlements of indigenous peoples, the arrival of a sizeable team of scientists may also import both new ideas and new diseases.

Intrapopulation Differences in Physical Activity

The proportion of the population who are currently regarded as physically active depends greatly on the criterion that is adopted (Shephard, 1986c). Concepts of an active person vary widely between nutritionists (who think in terms of energy expenditures over a 24-hr day), industrial physiologists (who evaluate levels of performance that can be sustained over 8-hr shifts), and investigators who are studying sport or leisure activity (in which the typical duration of an exercise bout is 30 min or less). Thus a nutritionist would regard miners and forestry workers (14-15 MJ/day) as people engaged in heavy work, although this daily energy expenditure could be accumulated by spending no more than 15 kJ/min over an 8-hr shift. An industrial physiologist would regard a task with a steady energy expenditure of 21 kJ/min (or about 4 METS) as heavy work (J.R. Brown & Crowden, 1963). However, 21 kJ/min is in turn a relatively light intensity of leisure activity, particularly for a young adult; some heavy recreational activities demand 60 to 80 kJ/min (Durnin & Passmore, 1967; see Table 3.10, page 103). There seems little relationship between heavy occupational activity and levels of health-related fitness (Allen, 1966), in part because occupational demands are insufficient to have a training effect, and in part because of the countervailing influence of socioeconomic status on leisure activity patterns.

Estimates of the proportion of the North American population who are active in their leisure hours range from 9% to 78%, depending on the criterion applied (Shephard, 1986c). The proportion of "active" individuals decreases progressively to what intuitively seems the realistic lower end of the range as more rigorous standards of involvement are applied. Data from Australia, Canada, Finland, and the United States (Powell et al., 1991; Shephard, 1988b; Stephens & Caspersen, in press) suggest that few adults meet even the minimum level of participation recommended by the American College of Sports Medicine (1990). Only about 10% report involvement in vigorous activity for at least 20 min three or more times a week, although a further third of the population practices leisure activities either less frequently or less vigorously than the recommended minimum for the maintenance of health.

Influence of Age and Gender

The proportion of subjects who are regularly involved in physically active leisure pursuits diminishes as the age of the sample increases (see Table 3.17). There is also a progressive slowing in the vigor of performance of any self-paced task, which apparently begins quite early during childhood. Klimt (1966) found heart rates of 160 to 180 beats/min during the spontaneous play of preschool children, whereas the children attending school sustained heart rates of 150 to 160 beats/min for longer periods. Seliger, Bartunek, and Trefny (1974) noted higher waking heart rates in 12-year-old boys (~90 beats/min) than in 16-year-olds (~80 beats/min). Durnin and Passmore (1967) found that 9- to 11-year-old boys had an energy expenditure of 12.5 kJ/min while walking; the equivalent rate of energy expenditure in a much heavier adult would require a walking speed of up to 6.4 km/h.

Durnin and Passmore (1967) found that the young Scottish girls of that era were as active as boys. However, their female subjects showed a marked decrease of physical activity coincident with the onset of puberty. By the age of 14 years, the girls that they studied were expending only 2.9 kJ/min at their customary rate of walking, and their total daily energy expenditure, 9.6 MJ, was 2.1 MJ less than that of boys of the same age. In Canada, the adverse trend toward reduction of leisure activity among pubertal girls has apparently diminished over the past decade, with a corresponding increase in their PWC_{170} (R. Gauthier et al., 1983).

Both genders may show a precipitous drop in their habitual physical activity when physical education is no longer a required part of the school program (Ilmarinen & Rutenfranz, 1980). There is generally a continuing decline of active leisure over the span of adult life, although there may be some increase in specific

Table 3.17
Percentage of the Canadian Population With an Energy Expenditure
of More Than 12.6 kJ/kg/day and Allocating More Than 3 hr per Week to Leisure
Activity for 9 or More Months per Year

Age (yr)	Energy expenditure (>12.6 kJ/kg/d)				Time (>3 hr/week for 9-12 month)			
	Men 1981	Men 1988	Women 1981	Women 1988	Men 1981	Men 1988	Women 1981	Women 1988
15-19	42%	69%	41%	39%	70%	92%	71%	85%
20-24	33	47	23	26	63	80	57	80
25-44	27	33	18	20	53	81	55	80
45-64	19	30	13	20	47	77	49	77
65+	27	42	17	23	59	75	54	69

Note. Data from Canada Fitness Survey (1983); Stephens and Craig (1990).

pursuits, such as gentle walking and gardening, among older people (Montoye, 1975). Retirement may temporarily encourage a general increase of active leisure pursuits. The Canada Fitness Surveys of 1981 and 1988 (Canada Fitness Survey, 1988; Stephens & Craig, 1990) noted that relative to immediately succeeding cohorts, there was a small increase in the percentage of people over the age of 65 years with a high level of leisure energy expenditure (and, in the 1981 survey, there was also an increased percentage of such individuals who allocated a substantial amount of time to their leisure activity). Conceivably, this may in part have been a sampling artifact, because a substantial proportion of inactive subjects were excluded from the oldest cohort. However, more detailed longitudinal observations using heart rate recorders have also suggested that some subjects do indeed increase their physical activity at least temporarily with the new found leisure of retirement (Shephard, 1987b). Moreover, a comparison of the data from the 1981 and the 1988 surveys suggests that over the past decade, the proportion of active to inactive individuals has increased much more among the elderly than among younger individuals (Stephens & Caspersen, in press).

Reports of vigorous physical activity are 50% more likely from men than from women (Stephens & Caspersen, in press), but it is less clear whether there is a corresponding gender difference in energy expenditures. Most of the survey instruments that have been used to assess physical activity patterns in large populations were designed to elicit typical male activities, and it may be that the questions asked have neglected the domestic tasks that still fall largely to women in most societies. If the classification of active and inactive individuals is based on the duration of leisure activity, rather than the reported intensity of effort (see Table 3.17), then there seems no great difference in the proportion of active subjects between the two genders. Moreover, the proportion of active individuals appears to have increased more rapidly for women than for men over the past decade (Stephens & Caspersen, in press).

Effects of Socioeconomic Status

Active physical leisure is reported more frequently by people of good education and high socioeconomic status (see Table 3.1, page 84; Canada Fitness Survey, 1983; Shephard, 1986c; Stephens & Caspersen, in press). Indeed, if such statements are representative of participation, then the advantage of education and higher level of employment is enough to cancel out any benefit that the lower social classes might otherwise derive from occupational physical activity or a greater involvement in physically demanding household chores.

Nevertheless, repetition of the Canada Fitness Survey (see Table 3.1) shows that the education gap in reported patterns of active leisure has narrowed in Canada over the past decade (Stephens & Craig, 1990).

Secular Trends

When an epidemic of cardiovascular disease was first deduced from British mortality statistics (J.N. Morris, 1951), the progressive loss of physical activity was suspected to be a major etiological factor. However, during the period of growing mortality (1930-1948), there had been little investment in the automation of British factories, few of the British population owned television sets, and during the war years (1939-1945), even the minority who owned cars were unable to obtain gasoline to drive them. Therefore, the dominant factor must have been some other environmental change, probably the growing consumption of cigarettes.

Nevertheless, by the early 1970s, questionnaire data suggested that much of the population living in the large cities of the developed world had adopted a very sedentary use of free time. Negative factors included a progressive migration of the population from single-family dwellings in small towns to cramped, highrise accommodation in busy urban centers, access to or personal ownership of a car from an early age, and opportunities for both children and adults to watch an ever-growing number of television channels. By the mid 1970s, students in both Canada (Shephard et al., 1975) and the U.S. (Sherif & Rattray, 1976) were spending 20 to 30 hours a week watching television. Plainly, earlier generations of children had passed much of this time in playing physically active games. In the same years (J.N. Morris, Chave, Adam, Sirey, & Epstein, 1973), only 18.5% of a large sample of British executive class civil servants were spending 15 min or more a day in vigorous aerobic exercise (i.e., activities demanding an energy expenditure >31 kJ/min). In Saskatoon, vigorous exercise was defined more modestly as walking 1.6 km or more, jogging, playing tennis or squash, or swimming four or more pool lengths; only 14% of adult men and 9% of adult women reported taking such exercise four or five times a week, although 26% of men and 27% of women were vigorously active two or three times a week.

The U.S. President's Council on Physical Fitness and Sports (1973) found that 45% of a random sample of 3,875 adults were taking no deliberate exercise. Walking and cycling were the most commonly reported pursuits among U.S. citizens who were active, both activities being slightly more prevalent in metropolitan than in nonmetropolitan areas.

Daytime heart rate recordings on smaller samples of the urban population have confirmed the generally low level of habitual physical activity suggested by these self-reports. K.L. Andersen (1967) found daytime average heart rates of 110 beats/min in Norwegian industrial workers and 100 beats/min in office workers. I. Åstrand (1960) observed average heart rates of 108 beats/min in Swedish housewives. In the U.S., Friedman, Rosenman, and Brown (1963) found workers with average heart rates of only 85 to 86 beats/min; Goldsmith and Hale (1971) noted averages of 86 to 94 beats/min for working policemen; and Brunner (1969) reported an average of 95 beats/min for young housewives. In Toronto, the only daytime activities for many individuals of working age were occasional short walks and climbing of a flight of stairs (Shephard, 1967); in 65-year-old subjects, readings averaged 90 beats/min in men and 80 beats/min in women (Sidney & Shephard, 1977b).

During the past two decades, the governments of many developed countries have made vigorous efforts to reverse the trend toward a sedentary lifestyle. Until recently, it has been difficult to determine whether such advocacy has had a positive effect, because succeeding surveys of physical activity have used different methods of assessment. However, this situation is changing. The Canada Fitness Survey used comparable questions in 1981 and 1988 (Canada Fitness Survey, 1983; Stephens & Craig, 1990), and the Ontario government has been using a consistent activity questionnaire (Fitness Ontario, 1983) regularly since November 1978 (although it is arguable that changing social norms may have altered responses to the same measuring instrument). Available data from Canada, Finland, the former German Democratic Republic, and the United States suggest that in recent years there has been a modest overall increase in the proportion of individuals who exercise regularly in their leisure time (see Figure 3.2, page 97), with a subsequent plateauing of interest (Stephens & Caspersen, in press). Finnish data further suggest that in recent years there has been a decrease in the proportion of people walking or cycling to work (Stephens & Caspersen, in press). Likewise, in Ontario the number of adults who reported cycling as a leisure activity during the month of June dropped from 23% in 1979 to 13% in 1983. On the other hand, the construction of urban cycling trails may now be encouraging an opposite trend in some North American cities. Although there are rational explanations of the changes in the activity recommendations and targets that have been adopted recently by governmental health-promotion agencies, skeptics may well draw negative inferences from these downward revisions and the change of emphasis from a more active population to a healthy, overall lifestyle.

During the past two decades, the energy cost of occupational activity has decreased steadily in the developed countries, as the population has moved from blue-collar, heavy industrial work to tertiary-sector office employment. At the same time, the average reduction of family size, replacement rather than repair of worn items, the introduction of labor-saving domestic equipment, and the use of disposable household goods have all contributed to a dramatic reduction in the duration and energy cost of domestic chores.

Indigenous Populations

When the IBP study was first envisaged in the early 1960s, the subsistence activities of some indigenous, agricultural populations required quite high levels of daily energy expenditure (see Tables 3.18 & 3.19). However, even then, the average expenditures were lower than the data suggested, because participation in vigorous hunting activities was only necessary 2 or 3 days a week and not all community members participated. Lammert (1972) recorded the heart rates of Inuit living on the west coast of Greenland. When on board a motorized fishing launch, the subjects' heart rates approximated normal resting levels, but readings of 120 to 140 beats/min were noted when the same men were tracking seals by kayak.

Godin and Shephard (1973a) noted that some Inuit who had chosen to live in a polar settlement still had physically demanding employment. Garbage collection under snowy conditions had an energy cost of 27 to 33 kJ/min, ice delivery demanded 21 to 22 kJ/min, and the manual unloading of supplies from aircraft and ships also demanded 21 kJ/min. Many of the women who were living in the village also faced fairly vigorous tasks, including the cleaning and preparing of skins. Household duties were performed with a minimum of equipment, and there was little furniture. Moreover, most of the younger women carried babies of up to 3 years of age on their backs in the traditional amauti. In contrast, Ekblom and Gjessing (1968) showed low average heart rates among the indigenous population of the lush Easter Islands: 102 and 86 beats/min in two outdoor laborers, 90 beats/min in a fisherman; and 87, 91, and 101 beats/min, respectively, in three housewives.

During the past two decades, the secular trend toward decreased physical activity has been quite marked among those indigenous populations that previously had high daily energy expenditures. For example, among the Inuit of Igloolik (69°40' N), there has been a transition from life in igloos and tents, and hunting by dog-sled, which demanded an average energy expenditure of 15.4 MJ/day in 1970 (see Table 3.19), to watching television and video programs all day in a 3-bedroom house in 1990 (Rode & Shephard, 1992). Even demanding tasks within the village have gradually disappeared, with the introduction of a modern water supply and sewage disposal system, the use of mechanical cargo-handling equipment, and the purchase of domestic equipment and furniture.There has also been a progressive shift from "natural" to store-purchased food. Unfortunately, these changes of lifestyle have been associated with an increase in the prevalence of the chronic diseases of modern civilization, such as diabetes and atherosclerosis (Reichley et al., 1987; Szathmary & Holt, 1983).

Table 3.18
The 24-hr Energy Expenditure of Males in Various
Indigenous and Agricultural Populations

Population	Energy expenditure (MJ/day)
Baganda peasants (Uganda)	8.4
Brazilian villagers	10.5
East Javan villagers	4.2-6.3
Guatemalans	
Agriculturalists	16.2
Horsemen	17.9
Carpenters/masons	14.8
Dairymen/herdsmen	13.2
Foremen	11.6
Ibo, Nigeria	9.8
Inuit hunters, Igloolik	15.4
Settlement workers, Igloolik	14.0
Greenland	13
Indian tribes	7.8-13.0
Israeli Kurds	12.9
Yemenites	12.7
Jamaican farmers	13.6
Kalahari bushmen	8.9
!Kung bushmen	9.0
Maoris (Cook Islands)	7.7-9.2
New Guinea villagers	9.6
Negev Bedouin	5.7-11.1
Phillipine villagers	7.0

Note. Data from Shephard (1978); Andersen et al. (1988).

Physical Activity and Overall Lifestyle

Habitual physical activity shows surprisingly little relationship to other types of
health behavior. One reason is that many large-scale surveys have failed to
distinguish participation in health-related physical activity from the enjoyment
of sports with other appeals such as excitement, competition, or social interaction
(Shephard, 1986c, 1989b). The Canada Fitness Survey (1983) found that among
subjects over the age of 20 years, the percentage of current smokers increased
from 37% in those subjects who were classed as active to 42% in those who
were classed as sedentary. Likewise, the proportion of subjects who slept 7 to
8 hr a night declined from 70% in the active group to 63% in those who were
sedentary, and the proportion who were eating a good breakfast declined from
51% in active to 43% among inactive individuals.

Table 3.19
The 24-hr Energy Expenditure of Traditional Inuit Hunters of Igloolik

Activity	Energy expenditure (MJ/day)
Caribou hunting	
Winter	16.1
Summer	16.3
Fishing	
Ice	16.9
Summer (by kayak)	18.6
Seal hunting	
Boat	14.4
Floe edge	10.6
Ice hole	14.6
Walrus hunting	15.4
Average for 8 types of hunting	15.4

Note. Adapted from Godin and Shephard (1973a) by permission.

Intrapopulation Differences in Health-Related Fitness

The adequacy of current levels of health-related fitness has generally been assessed relative to life expectancy. Arguably, the quality of life is much more important; whereas an increase of physical activity and a resulting increase of aerobic fitness can add perhaps 2 years to the life expectancy of a middle-aged man (Paffenbarger, 1988), it can add much more to the quality-adjusted life expectancy, particularly by helping to sustain independence in the later years of retirement (Shephard & Montelpare, 1988).

Body mass is usually gauged relative to actuarial norms, and in most developed societies a substantial percentage of the population currently exceeds such norms (see Table 3.20). Corresponding standards can be deduced for skinfold readings (see Table 1.2, page 18; Shephard, 1982b) and for measurements or predictions of body fat. There are also published tables of norms for aerobic power, but these reflect mainly the distribution of values as seen in current populations (Bailey et al., 1976). If emphasis is placed on the maintenance of independence in the face of progressive aging, then optimal health-related fitness would maximize the function of the heart, muscle, and major joints to the fullest extent possible without increasing the prevalence of serious musculoskeletal injuries and exercise-induced cardiac emergencies. In most developed societies, optimization would require at least a 20% improvement over current levels of function.

Influence of Age and Gender

Age comparisons of measurements such as maximal oxygen intake are complicated by an increase of stature during childhood and a decrease in both stature

Table 3.20
Percentage of North American Population Exceeding
Desirable Standards of Body Mass and Body Fat by 10% or More

Age (yr)	Canada[a] Men Mass	Canada[a] Men Fat	Canada[a] Women Mass	Canada[a] Women Fat	United States[b] Men (mass) (60/62)	United States[b] Men (mass) (71/74)	United States[b] Women (mass) (60/62)	United States[b] Women (mass) (71/74)
20-29	42%	28%	28%	30%	25.5%	24.4%	21.6%	22.3%
30-39	54	42	45	46	30.3	34.7	34.5	30.9
40-49	63	50	56	56	34.4	37.4	39.0	39.8
50-59	63	47	66	64	36.7	34.8	49.8	46.6
60+	63	50	67	63	35.5	33.3	56.2	49.6

Note. Data from Shephard (1986c); Blair, Kannel, et al. (1989).
[a]Canadian data assessed relative to 1959 standards of Society of Actuaries.
[b]U.S. data assessed relative to values observed in National Health and Examination Survey for men and women aged 20-29 years.

and the proportion of lean mass to total body mass with aging. Unfortunately, there is no standard method of adjusting data for differences of body size (see the appendix). Maximal oxygen intake and muscle strength are closely correlated with body mass and height during the preadolescent years (Shephard et al., 1980). If data are expressed per kilogram of body mass, function declines sharply over the latter part of childhood (Bailey, 1974; Shephard, 1982a). On the other hand, if results are expressed relative to height^2 (an approach that some have argued is dimensionally correct; Von Döbeln, 1966), then there is little change of aerobic power during adolescence.

The effects of senescence—a progressive decrease of stature, a loss of mineral from the bones, and a decrease in the density of lean tissue—all have implications for the determination of optimum body mass. From an actuarial point of view, the optimal body mass increases slightly as a person ages (Andres, 1985). The resting blood pressure also apparently increases with age (see Table 3.21; Whelton, 1985), but it is unclear whether this is a normal response. Certainly, such an increase is not seen among indigenous populations that have a simpler lifestyle (e.g., Solomon Islanders, [Page, Damon, & Moelleriag, 1974] and Navajo Indians [DeStephano, Coulehan, & Kennethewiant, 1979]). This highlights the difficulty in distinguishing normal components of the aging process from incipient pathological changes, such as atherosclerosis and arteriosclerosis.

Most cross-sectional surveys show a progressive loss of aerobic power, muscle strength, and flexibility with aging (Canada Fitness Survey, 1983; Shephard, 1986c). For example, Shephard (1966b) collected his own step-test data for 505 men and 156 women in Toronto and compared them to corrected results from a

Table 3.21
Effect of Age on Systolic and Diastolic Blood Pressure (mm Hg)

Age (yr)	Males		Females	
	CFS	CHS	CFS	CHS
7-9	100/68	95/60	99/66	95/60
10-12	105/70	100/68	103/69	100/67
13-14	110/71	110/68	108/71	111/67
15-19	117/75	118/71	110/72	111/70
20-29	122/78	125/76	110/72	113/71
30-39	121/80	125/78	111/74	114/73
40-49	125/84	125/80	118/77	116/75
50-59	125/83	128/82	123/79	124/78
60+	137/83	138/84	136/82	138/82

Note. Data from Canada Fitness Survey (CFS) (1983); Canada Health Survey (CHS) (1982).

total of 6,633 nonathletic men, 286 Scandinavian women, and 211 U.S. women (see Figure 3.8). Subsequent research, both in Canada (see Table 3.22) and elsewhere, has not substantially changed the average findings. Over ages 25 to 65 years, aerobic power declines from 45-50 ml/(kg·min) to 25-30 ml/(kg·min) in men, and from 35-40 ml/(kg·min) to 25-30 ml/(kg·min) in women. As age increases, a progressive weakening of the quadriceps muscle also widens the gap between cycle ergometer and step-test assessments of maximal oxygen intake (see Table 3.22).

Secular trends and intercohort differences of environment and activity patterns undoubtedly contribute to the age-related changes observed in cross-sectional surveys. It is likely that the oldest cohorts were more active than their successors for much of their lives, thus reducing the apparent impact of aging on scores for the various components of health-related fitness. However, the average 60-year-old is also likely to have a lower level of physical activity than a 20-year-old, so that the apparent changes over the 40-yr interval are a complex interaction of aging and short- and long-term trends in habitual activity. If subjects involved in a longitudinal survey are initially well trained but allow their levels of habitual activity to decline as the study continues, there may appear to be a very steep aging effect on health-related fitness over 10 or 15 years. Indeed, some studies have reported such rapid losses of aerobic power that subjects would have had values of zero before they reached 60 years of age! On the other hand, if a sedentary middle-aged person enrolls in a longitudinal study and is then stimulated to begin vigorous training, there may appear to be no aging response for up to 10 years (Kasch, Wallace, Van Camp, & Verity, 1988). The true effect of aging is most likely to be observed if the training volume remains constant. At least for aerobic power (Shephard, 1988a), the rate of loss of aerobic power of an

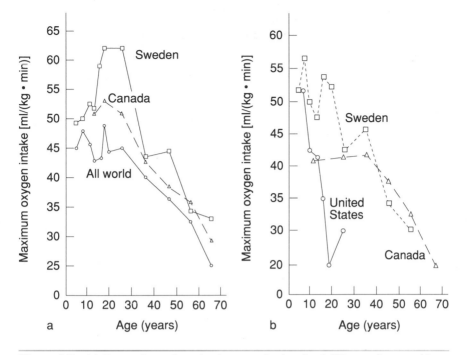

Figure 3.8   (a) Comparison of maximal oxygen intakes for 6,633 men from a wide range of developed countries, 505 Torontonians, and 1332 Scandinavians (mostly from Sweden). (b) Comparison of maximal oxygen intakes for 156 female Torontonians, 286 Scandinavians, and 211 Americans. For sources of data and individual corrections applied, see Shephard (1966b). *Note.* Adapted from Shephard (1977a) by permission.

active person (about 0.29 μmol/[kg·s], or 0.4 ml/[kg·min] each year of adult life) seems to be a little slower than that observed in sedentary individuals (about 0.41 μmol/[kg·s], or 0.55 ml/[kg·min] per year), although it is conceivable that the latter group have exaggerated their inherent rate of aging by becoming more sedentary as they become older.

The method of expressing data is controversial when comparing fitness scores for men and women (Drinkwater, 1984). Men are, on average, 10 cm taller than women, which inevitably gives them an advantage over women on most tests of physical performance. Aerobic power and muscular strength are commonly standardized per unit of body mass, and this is probably a fair basis of assessment when the work to be performed involves displacing the body mass against gravity. However, the composition of the body mass that is used to "normalize" the data differs between the two sexes; breast tissue increases the proportion of body fat and a lighter bone structure means a lower density of lean tissue in the female. Use of a height standard overcomes some of these difficulties, but as in younger age groups, it is unclear whether maximal oxygen intake should be standardized in terms of height^2 or height^3 (see the appendix). Men have 10% to 20% higher

Table 3.22
**Data on Aerobic Power of Canadian Subjects As Predicted
From Nomogram of I. Åstrand (1960)**

Age (yr)	Toronto, step test		Saskatoon, step test		Saskatoon, cycle[a]	
	Male	Female	Male	Female	Male	Female
10-12[b]	46.9 ± 6.0 (n = 30)	37.3 ± 4.0 (n = 33)	–	–	–	–
15-19	48.8 ± 7.9 (n = 61)	–	47.2 (n = 102)	39.2 (n = 144)	42.5	33.7
20-29	47.0 ± 7.6 (n = 129)	38.2 ± 3.9 (n = 34)	40.1 (n = 104)	37.3 (n = 138)	36.3	30.6
30-39	39.5 ± 6.9 (n = 106)	38.6 ± 4.7 (n = 16)	37.1 (n = 163)	34.6 (n = 152)	32.4	28.1
40-49	34.7 ± 8.2 (n = 98)	35.1 ± 10.5 (n = 38)	33.8 (n = 84)	31.8 (n = 93)	27.0	24.4
50-59	33.0 ± 6.4 (n = 71)	31.6 ± 8.8 (n = 22)	32.3 (n = 68)	31.2 (n = 88)	25.7	21.9
60-69	26.8 ± 2.8 (n = 10)	24.1 ± 5.5 (n = 13)	30.7 (n = 33)	30.2 (n = 56)	22.5	18.9

Note. All values expressed in ml/(kg·min) STPD.
[a]*n* as for step test in Saskatoon.
[b]Submaximal treadmill test.
Reprinted from Shephard (1977a) by permission.

standardized scores for most health-related fitness measurements (Drinkwater, 1984), except the sit-and-reach test of flexibility (where women have a substantial advantage, in part because of more flexible joints and shorter legs).

Some of the female deficiency of aerobic power is plainly due to a lower blood hemoglobin level (an average of 2.16 mmol/L, or 138 g/L, compared to an average of 2.44 mmol/L, or 156 g/L in well-nourished males). It remains unclear how much of the gender difference in aerobic power and muscle strength is caused by differences in hormonal secretions and muscle fiber dimensions. The female disadvantage may reflect little more than the different social roles of men and women and their unequal opportunities to develop health-related fitness.

Geographic Factors

Thirty years ago, W.H.M. Morris (1967) organized an epidemiological study of the prevalence of ischemic heart disease based on the assumption that farmers had a higher level of habitual energy expenditure than their city-dwelling peers. Durnin and Passmore (1967) likewise cited the example of a Swiss mountain goatherd who had a daily energy expenditure of 21 MJ. However, more recent studies have shown that levels of health-related fitness are uniformly higher in urban than in rural areas (McPherson & Curtis, 1986; Seliger, 1970; Shephard, 1982b, 1986c; Shephard et al., 1974; Steplock, Veicsteinas, & Mariani, 1971; see Table 3.23). In the case of rural children, the primary explanation of their current poor physical condition is probably that much of their leisure time is now spent in school buses, being driven to and from consolidated schools. Other factors affecting both children and adults from rural areas include the mechanization of modern farm work, the low socioeconomic status of most rural communities in North America, and limited facilities for sport and recreation in rural areas.

Reported levels of physical activity increase on moving from east to west across Canada (McPherson & Curtis, 1986) because of climatic factors and associated gradients of socioeconomic status. Canada's Health Promotion Survey (1988) found that 32.5% of the Québec population over the age of 15 years were

Table 3.23

Comparison of Body Fat (Skinfold Thickness in mm *or* % Body Fat) and Aerobic Power [in mmol/s and L/min *or* μmol/(kg·s) and ml/(kg·min)]

Population	Skinfold/ body fat		Aerobic power			
	Urban	Rural	Urban	Rural	Urban	Rural
Alberta			(mmol/s)	(mmol/s)	(L/min)	(L/min)
Boys			2.38	2.16	3.20	2.90
Girls			1.61	1.51	2.16	2.03
Czechoslovakia	(%)	(%)	(μmol/[kg·s])	(μmol/[kg·s])	(ml[kg·min])	(ml[kg·min])
Boys 12 yr	19.8	16.7	35.0	32.0	47.0	43.0
15 yr	13.7	13.8	34.1	33.0	45.8	44.4
Girls 12 yr	22.9	20.9	28.5	27.3	38.3	36.7
15 yr	19.4	19.5	26.6	26.0	35.8	34.9
Quebec	(mm)	(mm)	(μmol/[kg·s])	(μmol/[kg·s])	(ml[kg·min])	(ml[kg·min])
Boys	5.6	6.1	45.1	40.8	60.6	54.9
Girls	8.4	7.6	36.8	31.5	49.4	42.4
Italians	(%)	(%)	(μmol/[kg·s])	(μmol/[kg·s])	(ml[kg·min])	(ml[kg·min])
Men 20 yr	20.0	14.0	37.9	30.5	51	41
50 yr	24.0	18.2	27.5	26.0	37	35
Women 20 yr	26.0	26.5	30.5	25.3	41	34
50 yr	28.0	31.3	21.6	23.1	29	31
South African Bantu			(μmol/[kg·s])	(μmol/[kg·s])	(ml[kg·min])	(ml[kg·min])
Venda			30.1	29.7	40.5	39.9
Pedi			31.2	28.0	41.9	37.6

Note. Data from Shephard (1978).

never or seldom active, but in British Columbia only 19.8% of subjects gave this response. In contrast, the percentages of those reporting physical activity three or more times a week were 45.9% and 60.6% for the two provinces, respectively.

Effects of Socioeconomic Status

Although the reported participation in formal programs of active leisure shows a substantial correlation to socioeconomic status (Canada Fitness Survey, 1983; Stephens & Craig, 1990; see Table 3.1, page 84), perhaps because of the compensating physical demands of manual occupations, the correlation of health-related fitness to social class is less clearly established.

Secular Trends

Secular trends in health-related fitness are difficult to assess because of differences in both sampling and measurement techniques from year to year. Canadian men have apparently shown little change of relative body mass over the past 4 decades (Canada Fitness Survey, 1983; Pett & Ogilvie, 1956), but older women were substantially heavier in 1956 than they were during the Canada Fitness Survey of 1981, reflecting the current female tendency to thinness. It is unclear whether women have lost body fat or lean tissue mass over this period. Between 1966 and 1981, older Canadian girls showed a substantial gain in physical working capacity and thus in predicted maximal oxygen intake (see Table 3.24; also R. Gauthier et al., 1983; Howell & MacNab, 1968). Scores for performance-related fitness also improved over the same period, both in Canada and the United States (AAHPERD, 1980; CAHPER, 1980), although some of these gains may have occurred because the students gained experience at the required test procedures year by year.

Among indigenous populations, levels of fitness have been decreasing, although there have been relatively few attempts to document such a trend. A mixed longitudinal–cross-sectional survey of the population of Igloolik demonstrated a progressive deterioration in most measures of health-related fitness over the past two decades (Rode & Shephard, 1992; Shephard & Rode, 1985; also see Figure 3.3, page 99); this trend is apparently an expression of acculturation to the adverse, sedentary lifestyle of southern Canada.

Fitness and Activity Patterns

From our underlying model (see Figure 1.1), we might anticipate a correlation between health-related fitness and habitual activity patterns. But in urban samples, the relationship is sometimes relatively weak (Godin & Shephard, 1985). This may reflect the difficulty of measuring physical activity patterns accurately, or it may indicate that few people in developed societies are very active (Montoye, 1975; Shephard, 1986c), rather than proving a lack of impact of physical activity on health-related fitness. Generally, those who used complicated questionnaires to assess physical activity have seen only a limited relationship. Thus, Montoye

Table 3.24
Trends in Health-Related Fitness Among the General Populace of Canada

Age (yr)	Body mass index (kg/m²)				Age (yr)	Predicted aerobic power [ml/(kg·min)]*			
	Men		Women			Boys		Girls	
	1954	1981	1954	1981		1966	1981	1966	1981
20-29	23.8	24.0	22.3	21.9	7-9	38.4	41.3	33.8	36.8
30-39	25.5	25.1	23.6	23.5	10-12	40.2	41.8	33.4	37.5
40-49	25.8	26.0	25.5	24.5	13-14	42.3	43.3	30.0	35.9
50-59	25.9	26.0	26.9	25.7	15-19	40.9	43.7	29.0	36.8
60+	25.7	26.5	27.0	25.8					

Note. Data from Pett and Ogilvie (1956); Canada Fitness Survey (1983); Howell and MacNab (1968); Gauthier et al. (1983).
*Estimated from PWC_{170}.

(1975) found quite small differences in blood pressure (137/78 vs. 140/81 mm Hg) and average skinfold thickness (20.9 vs. 23.1 mm) between the most active and the least active people living in Tecumseh, Michigan. Similarly, the Canada Fitness Survey (1983) showed only marginal, activity-related variations in most indices of health-related fitness (Shephard, 1986c; see Tables 3.12 & 3.13). On the other hand, substantial differences in maximal oxygen intake were seen when the activity of populations was categorized using simple questionnaires (Bailey, Shephard, et al., 1974; Bailey et al., 1976; Shephard & McClure, 1965).

Few surveys of indigenous populations have been large enough to permit classification of individuals by activity patterns. However, a substantial difference in aerobic power and a smaller difference in skinfold readings were seen between Inuit who engaged regularly in hunting and sedentary members of the same community (see Table 3.25; Shephard, 1980).

Interpopulation Differences in Physical Activity and Health-Related Fitness in Adults

Interpopulation comparisons of physical activity and health-related fitness are still severely hampered by a lack of representative samples. Even when surveys have been coordinated by a single observer (e.g., the Seven Countries Study; Keys, 1980), intersample differences have apparently arisen as much from interlaboratory differences in methodology as from differences in phenotype.

Table 3.25
Comparison of Skinfold Thicknesses and Aerobic Power
Between Inuit of Igloolik With Differing Patterns of
Acculturation and Habitual Physical Activity

| | Skinfold (mm) | | Aerobic power | | | |
| | | | (μmol/[kg·s]) | | (ml/[kg·min]) | |
Population	Summer	Winter	Summer	Winter	Summer	Winter
Hunters	5.0	6.4	45.8	45.5	61.5	61.1
Transitional	6.1	6.7	44.4	44.4	59.7	59.7
Settled	6.6	7.7	41.4	40.6	55.6	54.5

Note. Reprinted from Rode and Shephard (1973) by permission.

Physical Activity Patterns

In developed societies, daily energy expenditures have traditionally ranged from a little over 6 MJ a day for senior citizens living an almost totally sedentary life in a residential care institution through 10 to 11 kJ a day in office workers to around 15 kJ a day in farmers, coal miners, and forestry workers (Durnin & Passmore, 1967). However, automation has greatly reduced the energy demands of the last three occupations.

Some authors have suggested that traditional indigenous populations need a high level of physical activity for their survival in a hostile environment. However, much depends on the nature of the terrain (e.g., flat or hilly), the richness of the local fauna and flora, the need to transport small children and domestic equipment from one campsite to another, and the degree of exposure to advanced technology (see Table 3.26). For example, the highland Lufa have a much greater aerobic power than the lowland Kauls in New Guinea, and Canadian Inuit who follow the traditional, migratory lifestyle have far-above-average levels of aerobic fitness. The observer must sometimes rise early to avoid making erroneous judgments about daily energy expenditures, because many tropical populations complete their daily chores before the day becomes hot, taking a long siesta just at the time the observer is searching for evidence of their physical activity. In some instances, the introduction of intermediate technology, such as power saws and rotary cultivators, has increased the speed of work without reducing the hourly energy expenditure (Edholm, 1970). But in general, the introduction of modern power equipment has reduced the need for high rates of physical activity (Rode & Shephard, 1992).

In the pleasant climate of Easter Island, 24-hr heart rate recordings suggested that many of the indigenous population did little vigorous physical activity, in keeping with their low levels of aerobic fitness; indeed, the estimated 24-hr

Table 3.26
Health-Related Fitness of Young Adult Males From Selected
Populations in Countries Less Developed Than Industrialized North America

Population	Excess mass* (kg)	Skinfold (mm)	Body fat (%)	Aerobic power (μmol/[kg·s])	Aerobic power (ml/[kg·min])
Arabs (Chaamba)		6.2			
Australian aborigines		6.6			
Canadian Inuit		5.6		42.0	56.4
Chilean Indians				36.5	49.1
East African Dorobo				34.2	46.0
Easter Islanders	0.0			31.3	42.0
Ethiopians	-10.7			28.1	37.7
	-13.0	6.0		29.7	39.9
Israeli Kurds	-0.4			36.0	48.4
Yemenites	+2.5			39.0	52.4
Jamaicans	-5.3			35.0	47.0
Malayan Temiars				39.6	53.2
Mexican Tarahumara					
runners			11.1	46.9	63.0
nonrunners			17.9	28.9	38.9
New Guinea Kauls				39.6	53.2
Highland Lufas				49.9	67.0
Tukisenta-Lagaip		5.0		33.6	45.1
Nigerian Yoruba					
active	-3.7			41.3	55.5
inactive	-4.0			34.2	45.9
Peruvian Quechua		6.3		36.7	49.3
Russian Kirghiz				25.2	33.9
South African					
Bantu	-4.7	5.6		35.6	47.9
Kalahari		4.6		35.0	47.1
Tanzanians					
active	-1.2			42.6	57.2
inactive	-4.1			35.1	47.2
Trinidadian Negroes	-1.3	7.9		28.5	38.3
East Indians	-3.4	10.6		29.3	39.4
American Navaho Indians				32.7	44.0
Venezuelan Warao		5.9		38.1	51.2
Zairian Hoto	-6.7			31.8	42.7
Twa	-7.7			35.3	47.5

Note. Data from Shephard (1978).
*Relative to actuarial norms.

energy expenditures for this population were lower than those for urban office workers (Ekblom & Gjessing, 1968). Likewise, the physical activity of East African nomads was rated as only moderate (Shaper, 1970). Boshoff (1965) suggested that Ugandan farmers worked only 3.5 hr a day. In more recent years, many of the men from the rural communities of central Africa have migrated to large urban centers or to the gold and diamond mines of South Africa, augmenting the traditional responsibilities of the women villagers in caring for children and tending an agricultural small-holding. Groups such as New Guinea highlanders, Tarahumara Indian runners, and Inuit hunters traditionally have had very high daily energy expenditures, matching or exceeding those of the heaviest industrial work (see Table 3.18, page 135). But even when a particular habitat demands a high daily energy expenditure, this often takes the form of sustained bouts of moderate intensity activity, so that a large increase of aerobic fitness does not necessarily result. For example, in the early 1970s, it was common for Inuit hunters to continue a chase for several days with little interruption if the hunting conditions were particularly favorable (Shephard, 1978, 1980). The total energy expenditure amounted to the very high figure of 15 to 16 MJ/day, but averaged only 10 to 11 kJ/min.

Body Composition

Representative data for Canada and the United States, together with the results of large surveys in other leading industrial nations (Shephard, 1986c), show that a substantial portion of the world's population currently has a body mass index, an average skinfold thickness, and a waist-hip skinfold ratio that exceed the limits recommended for cardiovascular health (see Tables 3.24 & 3.27). For instance, Renold (1981) found that in the U.S., 31% of young men, 23% of young women, 57% of old men, and 68% of old women applying for life insurance had a body mass that was at least 10% above the actuarial ideal value. Bray (1979) noted that 14% of American men and 24% of American women exceeded the actuarial standard by the clinically important margin of 20%.

In the U.K., the proportion of people who exceed the 20% ceiling seems to be somewhat lower than in North America (respective values for men and women being 6% and 8% in the age range 15-29 years, 18% and 17% at 30-49 years, and 18% and 32% at 50-65 years; James, 1976). The Seven Countries Study (Keys, 1980) provides other comparative data for men living in developed countries of varying wealth. The percentages of men having a body mass 10% above the actuarial ideal were 2% in Japan, 11% in Greece, 13% in the Netherlands, 15% in Finland, 19% in Yugoslavia, 32% in the U.S., and 33% in Italy. A slightly different ranking was observed in terms of the percentage of the population having excessive skinfold measurements: 2% in Japan, 11% in Greece, 14% in Finland, 28% in Italy, 29% in Yuogoslavia, 32% in the Netherlands, and 63% in the U.S.

In contrast, available data for the average body mass of populations living in the less industrialized countries have shown, until recently, a substantial deficit

Table 3.27
Average Skinfold Thicknesses for Male Subjects Aged 40-45 Years
in Arbitrary Samples From Selected Developed Countries

Country	Skinfold thickness (mm)
Finland	
East	13
West	16
Greece	
Corfu	16
Crete	14
Italy	
Crevalcore	23
Montegiorgino	15
Roma	26
Japan	15
Netherlands	24
U.S. (railworkers)	33
Yugoslavia	
Dalmatia	15
Slavonia	15
Velikakrsna	13
Zrenjanin	23

Note. Data from Keys (1980).

relative to North American actuarial norms (see Table 3.26). Skinfold readings have also been much lower than those in developed societies (Shephard, 1978), with a correspondingly low prevalence of cardiovascular disease (Sarvotham & Berry, 1968). The educated elite for many years have provided an exception to this generalization in countries such as India (Shah, Shah, & Panse, 1968). Now, with the loss of their traditional patterns of subsistence and a rapid acculturation to a sedentary (and often an urban) lifestyle, many indigenous populations are becoming grossly obese (Greksa & Baker, 1982; Rode & Shephard, 1992).

Aerobic Power

The majority of population data on aerobic power has been for small, nonrepresentative samples, such as volunteers for fitness tests or those entering exercise programs. Shephard (1966b) reviewed the world literature and assembled data on 6,633 men who were regarded as nonathletic. Other large samples have been accumulated by Hollmann and Hettinger (1976), Seliger (1970), and Shvartz and Reibold (1990).

Bailey, Shephard, Mirwald, & McBride (1974), Montoye (1975), and the Canada Fitness Survey (1983) all attempted to test representative samples of

North American men and women, but the generality of their conclusions was limited by low response rates. The aerobic power of participants in all of these studies was lower than in the widely quoted but selected series reported by P.O. Åstrand (1952) and I. Åstrand (1960). It is possible that Swedes are somewhat more active and thus fitter than North Americans, but it is worth comment that the scores seen in the Canada Fitness Survey were higher than those of an unselected population of Swedish military recruits (Jonsson & Berggren, 1979). The Canada Fitness Survey scores were also somewhat higher than those obtained in Czechoslovakia (Seliger, 1970) and West Germany (Hollmann & Hettinger, 1976).

The aerobic power of populations in some less developed societies is apparently quite low (see Table 3.26), which may be a reflection of a low level of habitual activity (see Table 3.18). However, other potential contributing factors include difficulties in obtaining a maximal performance from members of noncompetitive societies (particularly when the investigator does not speak the local language), questionable methods of allowing for interpopulation differences of body size, malnutrition (a deficient intake of protein or energy from an early age), and the adverse consequences of diseases such as malaria (which may result in extremely low blood hemoglobin levels). Despite these potential handicaps, a number of indigenous groups, including the Canadian Inuit, Chilean Indians, Israeli Yemenites, Tarahumara runners, New Guinea Kauls, active Nigerian Yoruba, active Tanzanians, and Venezuelan Warao, show higher average figures than would be expected in young North American adults (see Table 3.26). Their data reflect a more active lifestyle, a much lower burden of body fat, and in some groups, the necessity of traversing rough or mountainous terrain in the course of daily living.

Lean Tissue Mass and Strength

Skinfold estimates of lean tissue mass based on the Canada Fitness Survey data (Shephard, 1986c) are lower than the lean mass of middle-class British subjects calculated from the hydrostatic weighing data of Womersley and Durnin (1977). However, in view of differences in both subject selection and methodology, it is not clear whether there is a real difference in average lean body mass between Canada and Europe (Shephard, 1986c).

Interpopulation comparisons of handgrip strength are hampered because of differences in measuring instruments, and there have been few representative surveys of adults. Particularly in women, the Canada Fitness Survey (1983) recorded somewhat higher grip strengths than those reported by Montoye (1975) in his study of Tecumseh. The number of sit-ups and push-ups performed in 1 min by young men in the Canada Fitness Survey (1983) was similar to that reported in an earlier generation of U.S. army recruits (Banks, 1943). Comparisons of sit-ups and push-ups between American (AAHPERD, 1980) and Canadian children (CAHPER, 1980) are largely invalidated by differences in details of technique (Shephard, 1986c; Shephard & Lavallée, 1978). Earlier comparisons between the U.S. and Europe suggested that European children had better scores on all tests except the softball throw, where U.S. students had much greater experience (Campbell & Pohndorf, 1961).

Blood Pressure and Serum Cholesterol

A substantial amount of data on blood pressure and serum cholesterol levels is now available, in part as a result of the Seven Countries Study (see Table 3.28). Blood pressure readings from the Canada Fitness Survey (1983) were lower than those in most of the cities participating in the Seven Countries survey. The Canadian values also fell below average figures in the U.S. National Health Examination Study (Stamler, 1973) and the Danish Supermarket Survey (Schnor & Hansen, 1976). This discrepancy is not due to a selective exclusion of hypertensives from the Canadian study. It probably arose because the Canada Fitness Survey made measurements in the relaxed setting of the subjects' homes (M.A. Young et al., 1983), whereas most of the other data was obtained in a medical setting. Comstock (1957) also found low average blood pressure readings when he conducted a representative household survey in the southern U.S.

Blood pressure and serum cholesterol seem generally related in middle-aged adults. The highest values for both variables are found in regions such as eastern Finland (Keys, 1980), which traditionally has consumed a high-fat diet, and low values occur in regions where the consumption of fat is restricted by tradition or poverty (e.g., Japan and parts of the former Yugoslavia).

The majority of population data refers to young adults, although there have been some comparisons of growth and aging between developed and less industrialized countries (Shephard, 1978; Shephard & Pařízková, 1991).

Interpopulation Differences in Physical Activity and Health-Related Fitness in Children

The large amount of time that young children spend in watching television now seems general among the populations of developed societies (Alderson & Crutchley, 1990; Shephard et al., 1975; Sherif & Rattray, 1976). Though two decades ago, the children of some indigenous groups, such as the Canadian Inuit, had very high levels of aerobic fitness and little body fat, this advantage diminished as their families moved to urban settlements and gained access to video programs and satellite television (Rode & Shephard, 1992).

Body Composition

Differences in stature are sometimes seen even between apparently well-nourished populations. In Canada, children of francophone origin have been typically smaller than those from English-speaking provinces (Demirjian, Jenîcek, & Dubuc, 1972; Shephard et al., 1975), but this discrepancy seems to have had a socioeconomic rather than a phenotypic basis; it has gradually disappeared with improved economic conditions and a reduction of average family size among

Table 3.28
Blood Pressure and Serum Cholesterol Levels in Subjects Aged 40-45 Years
(Males, Unless Otherwise Specified)

Country	Blood pressure (mm Hg)	Serum cholesterol (mmol/L)	Author
Canada (M/F)		5.48/5.50	Hewitt et al., 1977
Finland			
East	141/87	6.87	Keys, 1980
West	133/80	6.43	Keys, 1980
Finns (M/F)		7.21/7.00	Aromaa et al., 1975
Lapps (M/F)		7.29/6.95	Aromaa et al., 1975
Greece			
Corfu	130/81	5.00	Keys, 1980
Crete	131/80	5.13	Keys, 1980
Israel			
Civil servants		5.30	Goldbourt et al., 1985
Europeans (M/F)		5.43/5.15	Kark et al., 1985
Asiatics (M/F)		5.27/5.30	Kark et al., 1985
N. Africans (M/F)		5.09/4.95	Kark et al., 1985
Italy			
Crevalcore	136/84	5.03	Keys, 1980
Montegiorgino	128/78	4.98	Keys, 1980
Roma	135/86	5.37	Keys, 1980
Japan			
Tanushinaru	120/68	4.33	Keys, 1980
Ushibuka	126/75	4.20	Keys, 1980
Netherlands	140/90	6.04	Keys, 1980
South Seas			
Palau (M/F)	113/70 113/75		Lovell, 1967
Saipan (M/F)	126/78 125/78		Lovell, 1967
United Kingdom			
M	132/84	6.00	Mann et al., 1988
F	130/81	5.60	Mann et al., 1988
London (M/F)	130/83	6.03/5.89	Slack et al., 1977
United States			
Railroad		6.07	Keys, 1980
Lipid Clinics (M/F)		5.31/5.31	Lip. Res. Clin., 1984
Yugoslavia			
Dalmatia	136/85	4.72	Keys, 1980
Slavonia	130/79	5.08	Keys, 1980
Velikakrsna	124/78	3.99	Keys, 1980
Zrenjanin	126/80	4.40	Keys, 1980

Note. See Keys, 1980, for details of references. Data taken in part from Keys (1980).

the Québeçois (Landry et al., 1980; Shephard, 1986c). Similarly, the Japanese were once considered a small race, but this characteristic has changed rapidly as the wealth of most Japanese families has grown to match and even to exceed that of their North American counterparts (Asahina, 1975).

Poor nutrition among the children of developing countries generally leads to a stunting of growth, but with extreme malnutrition, the size of the child may also be small in relation to height (Waterlow, 1986; see Figure 3.9). As in developed societies, interpopulation differences of body build seem to be determined more by socioeconomic factors than by ethnic group (Pařízková, Merhautova, & Prokopec, 1972; Shephard & Pařízková, 1991). Interpopulation comparisons of adolescents are further complicated by the later maturation of those from less well-nourished communities (Shephard, 1982a).

Until recently, the children of indigenous populations and developing societies have been much smaller than those living in developed nations, but recently there

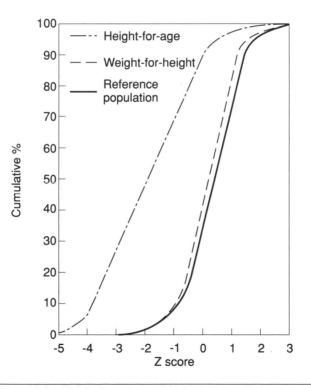

Figure 3.9   Cumulative distribution of Z scores in an undernourished population, which includes stunted individuals but is free of wasting malnutrition, and in a well-nourished reference population. Note that the weight-for-height curve of the malnourished sample conforms to the line for a well-nourished sample, but that the height-for-age distribution is displaced to the left. *Note.* Based on Waterlow (1986); reprinted from Shephard (1991b) by permission.

has been a strong secular trend to a reduction of this differential (Skrobac-Kaczynski & Lewin, 1976).

Aerobic Power

An early review found that the children of developed societies had remarkably uniform aerobic power readings, 35 to 37 μmol/(kg·s), or 48 to 50 ml/(kg·min), in boys and around 30 μmol/(kg·s), or 40 ml/(kg·min), in girls (Shephard, 1971b; Shephard, Allen, Bar-Or, et al., 1968). Recent studies from China (Chen, 1991), Colombia (Spurr, Barrac-Nieto, & Reina, 1991), and Cuba (Arbesu, 1991) all reported maximal oxygen intakes in these ranges. In contrast, and perhaps because of an insufficient intake of protein, values were substantially lower for Algeria (Dekkar, 1991) and Argentina (Narvaez-Pérez, D'Angelo, & Zabala, 1991).

Over the past two decades, there has been some improvement of scores in both the U.S. and in Canada (Shephard, 1986c), apparently a result of governmental encouragement of physical activity and the improvement of physical education programming in schools.

In the 1970s, levels of aerobic fitness were particularly high among Canadian Inuit children, but these values have regressed toward those of children in developed societies as the level of habitual activity has diminished in the circumpolar regions (Rode & Shephard, 1992).

Other Measures of Health-Related Fitness

The percent body fat found in the children participating in the Canada Fitness Survey (1983) was a little lower than in some U.S. surveys, but substantially greater than in the representative sample of Czechoslovakian students studied by Seliger (1970). The Czechoslovakian students also had a somewhat greater lean mass per centimeter of height than the Canadians (Shephard, 1986c), with a matching advantage in handgrip force (Seliger, 1970).

Perhaps because the North American students were more familiar with the test procedures, the number of speed sit-ups they performed was appreciably larger than that of German and Israeli students studied by Ruskin (1978) and the Scottish students examined by Watkins, Farrally, and Powley (1983).

In terms of flexibility, Canadian students were marginally inferior to the Dutch students examined by Kemper and Verschuur (1982), although the performance of the latter group may have been influenced favorably by their involvement in a longitudinal study of fitness.

Interpopulation Differences in Physical Activity and Health-Related Fitness in the Elderly

Although there have been almost no interpopulation comparisons of physical activity and aging, it seems logical that differences in activity patterns will appear, dependent on the attitude of specific societies toward their elders, the nature of the habitat, and the need for individuals to continue agriculture or hunting activities in order to assure their survival.

The 1970 survey of the Igloolik Inuit suggested that the age-related deterioration of aerobic power had a more convex form than would be anticipated in a developed society (Shephard, 1978, 1980). This reflected a persistence of vigorous activity through later middle age, but a steep decline of activity when the younger generation assumed their parents' hunting responsibilities. This hypothesis found some support in the change toward patterns of aging commonly seen in developed societies as physical activity declined among the younger members of the community (Shephard & Rode, 1985; see Figure 3.3, page 99).

Body Composition

Perhaps because they have a greater desire to retain a youthful appearance, the age-related increase of body fat is lower among Canadian and American adults than among Europeans (Shephard, 1986c).

Some indigenous populations see obesity as a status symbol, and in such groups wealthy people show a large increase of body fat with age. But the average person in such communities has a somewhat marginal nutrition, very low skinfold readings, and a body mass far below the actuarial ideal. This situation has changed with acculturation, but because the young are usually the most acculturated, and acculturation is a recent phenomenon, the young are often now more obese than their elders.

Aerobic Fitness

The limited data do not suggest any substantial differences in the rate of aging of aerobic fitness between developed populations (Shephard, 1966b; Shvartz & Reibold, 1990). Given that a part of the age-related loss is attributable to a decrease of habitual physical activity, differences may emerge if some societies are more successful than others in promoting physical activity among their senior citizens. The atypical pattern of aging seen in the traditional Inuit (Shephard & Rode, 1985) has been discussed previously.

Other Measures of Health-Related Fitness

There are some difficulties in comparing the effects of aging on blood pressures because of differences in measuring techniques, but it is generally agreed that blood pressures rise less with age in southern Europe and Japan than in North America and northern Europe. Blood pressure measurements, echocardiograms, and postmortem studies all show a low incidence of hypertension and atherosclerosis in developing and indigenous societies (Alekseev, 1991; Astakhova et al., 1991; Hart-Hansen, Hancke, & Moller-Petersen, 1991; Naimark et al., 1991).

Population data also suggest no great differences in the aging of grip strength between Czechoslovakia and North America (Seliger, 1970; Shephard, 1986c). There are no useful data on flexibility or other aspects of health-related fitness for elderly populations outside of North America.

Priorities for Future Comparative Research

Gaps in current knowledge make our attempts at intra- and interpopulation comparisons of physical activity patterns and health-related fitness somewhat frustrating. However, before embarking on any massive international comparisons, it is necessary to decide whether the observers should focus on physical activity patterns, health-related fitness, or both. Issues of sampling and the standardization of methodology also require more attention. Furthermore, it is important that the size of intra- and interpopulation differences in activity patterns and fitness needed to realize the various health benefits discussed in chapter 5 be determined.

Issues of Sampling

Much of the available information on health-related fitness has been gathered on small samples of healthy, relatively active young men. Before strong generalizable conclusions can be drawn about relationships between physical activity, health-related fitness, and overall community health, repeated tests on large, representative samples of national populations must be made. Those who are assessed must include women and men, covering the full spectrum of ages and drawn from regions that represent a variety of physical and sociocultural environments.

Incomplete sampling, particularly of older subjects, is inevitable, and it is necessary to develop better methods of adjusting population data to allow for the bias introduced by the selective omission of the diseased, those in lower socioeconomic groups, and those with adverse lifestyles.

Standardization of Methodology

There remains an urgent need to standardize the methodology that is used to assess both physical activity and health-related fitness. Too many of the apparent interpopulation differences are attributable to small differences in the methods of measurement. Before interpopulation comparisons can be made with confidence, investigators must agree on procedures. It must also be demonstrated that different observers can reach the same results when testing a common pool of subjects.

Uniform procedures are needed for skinfold measurements. Preferably, data should be reported in skinfold units, because interpopulation differences in the density of lean tissue preclude the development of a sole equation for the prediction of body fat from either skinfold data or hydrostatic weighing (Shephard, 1990c).

Twenty-five years after the International Biological Programme Working Party (Shephard, 1978; Shephard et al., 1968a, 1968b), there is still a need for a common protocol to determine aerobic power. Agreement is required on such fundamental issues as the choice of apparatus (treadmill, cycle ergometer, or step test), the duration of warm-up, the number and duration of test stages, and criteria for defining maximal effort.

The measurement of muscle strength and endurance also requires agreement on both apparatus and technique. Flexibility is thought to be an important component of health-related fitness in older individuals, but there is no consensus on which movements are critical to continued health, on the correlation of sit-and-reach test scores and the extent of flexibility at other joints (Shephard et al., 1990), or on the appropriate warm-up period prior to assessment of flexibility.

Surveys of resting blood pressures still lack a common protocol for such key items as the posture of the subject, the length of the preliminary rest period, the site and dimensions of the measuring cuff, the rate of cuff deflation, the indicator of the diastolic reading (i.e., a muffling of the Korotkov sounds, Phase 4, or their disappearance, Phase 5), and the familiarity of the subject with the observer and the measurement situation (Shephard, Cox, et al., 1981; M.A. Young et al., 1983). Equally, techniques for determining blood glucose and lipid profiles must be carefully standardized from laboratory to laboratory (Hewitt et al., 1977).

Performance-type tests may seem simple to carry out, but even if such measurements are useful in the context of population health, there is a pressing need for surveys to adopt absolutely identical techniques under closely matched environmental conditions (Shephard, 1978, 1986c; Shephard & Lavallée, 1978). Finally, there must be a standardization of techniques for measuring the effects of covariates, such as smoking habits and exposure to air pollutants.

Clinical Significance of Differences

It is agreed that an increase of body fat, a reduction of maximal oxygen intake, an increase of systemic blood pressure, the development of an abnormal electrocardiogram during vigorous exercise, a poor glucose tolerance curve, a high total-serum-cholesterol concentration, and a low ratio of HDL-cholesterol to total cholesterol are all adverse changes in health-related fitness. In a few people, gross abnormalities in these variables clearly indicate a poor prognosis. But in most members of a sedentary population, functional deterioration is small, and the associated small increase of risk is statistical rather than predictive of the health outcome of the individual. The combination of a number of adverse findings generally has a worse prognostic significance than does a single adverse measurement, but there is no agreement on how data should be combined to yield a single prognostic index. Furthermore, the various adverse characteristics that could be corrected by an increase of physical activity interact (perhaps additively) on the individual's prognosis along with inheritance, age, and negative lifestyle habits such as cigarette smoking.

There is a need to establish clearer dose-response relationships between changes in individual and combined fitness variables and resulting levels of community health. Should estimates of community health be based on mean values for leisure activity or on the various determinants of health-related fitness, treating both types of data as continuous variables? Alternatively, should we also examine those members of various populations that fail to meet certain arbitrary threshold criteria? Making decisions on such questions is an important prelude to proposing future demographic comparisons, whether in terms of sample size or methods of data collection and analysis.

4
Chapter

Aerobic Fitness: Nature or Nurture?

A fundamental belief of those promoting health-related fitness has been that personal scores for the various indices of aerobic power could be augmented by regular participation in an appropriate aerobic training program. On the other hand, those who select and prepare endurance athletes have commonly argued that top competitors inherit from their parents specific characteristics that give them a substantial advantage in distance competition.

The Genetic Component of Aerobic Fitness

A clearer understanding of the magnitude of genetic effects is important for both the sport scientist and for the person interested in health promotion. Depending on the duration of an event, the success of endurance athletes depends on their aerobic power (absolute, in weight-supported sports, but relative, if body mass must be displaced against gravity), their ability to exercise for long periods at close to maximal oxygen intake, their reserves of fuel, and their efficiency in translating energy consumption into physical work. Most information on the inheritance of traits that favor endurance performance relates to relative aerobic power, a value that is also of interest in the context of cardiovascular health.

Evidence of Genetic Effects From Population Statistics

Shephard (1978) suggested that a rough estimate of the contributions of athletic selection and rigorous training to the development of a high level of relative aerobic power could be derived from the mean and standard deviation of the data observed in the general population. A value of perhaps 48 ± 8 ml/(kg·min), or 36 ± 6 μmol/(kg·s), is typical for healthy young men in industrialized nations

(Shephard, 1978). How readily could an international-class distance competitor be discovered simply by an exhaustive search of such a population? The aerobic power of an outstanding cross-country skier can be as high as 70 μmol/(kg·s), or 94 ml/(kg·min) (P.O. Åstrand & Rodahl, 1986), at least 5.5 standard deviations (SD) above the population mean. Rigorous selection might bring to light a person with an aerobic power 4 SD above the population mean; assuming that the extreme upper limit of the distribution conformed closely to a normal curve, a value of 60 μmol/(kg·s), or 80 ml/(kg·min) might be discovered. But the remaining advantage of the cross-country skier (a further 10 μmol/[kg·s], or 30% of the total difference from an average person) must be attributed to rigorous training.

Unfortunately, this simple calculation is less definitive than it might at first appear. Even if the assumption about the normality of the distribution curve is warranted when seeking individuals who are 4 SD above the population mean, both the mean and the SD of the base data are inevitably biased, because they are derived from a volunteer sample. Moreover, much of the observed variance of aerobic power in the base population is environmental rather than genetic in origin. Thus, in the study conducted by Shephard and Callaway (1966), 36% of the interindividual variation in a simple measure of aerobic fitness could be explained in terms of subjects' responses to a single question on personal patterns of habitual activity (see chapter 3). At best, population data suggest that healthy adults have a capacity to respond to aerobic training beyond any advantage of constitution that they may have inherited, but the extent of this potential response is unclear.

Twin Studies

Many authors have adopted the classical twin methodologies of quantitative genetics in an attempt to pursue the issue of nature versus nurture (Bouchard & Malina, 1983; Klissouras, 1971) in the inheritance of aerobic power. In some reports, the distinction between identical and nonidentical twins has been weakened by accepting inspection of physical characteristics rather than making a rigid genetic scrutiny.

Assumptions inherent to such analyses (Bouchard & Malina, 1983) were (1) that the mean aerobic power was similar for the two types of twin (Christian, 1979), (2) that the shared environment of pregnancy was unimportant in reducing later inter-twin differences in aerobic performance, and (3) that other sources of variance, whether attributable to environment, including diet and habitual physical activity (Engström & Fischbein, 1977; Bouchard et al., 1986), or to methodological factors, were similar for identical twins, nonidentical twins, and the general population. The majority of such studies made no allowance for possible interactions between environment and inheritance. Except in the rare instances where the twins had been separated by adoption immediately after birth, calculations were thus largely invalidated by problems arising from a commonality of family environment.

Because of the many limitations inherent in twin methodology and the very small sample sizes, estimates of the percentage of aerobic power that can be attributed to inheritance have been highly unstable, ranging from 0% to near 100% (see Table 4.1). Some twin studies have estimated the heritability of individual components in the oxygen transport chain, but the data have again shown considerable instability. For instance, T.D. Adams et al. (1985) and Fagard, Van den Broeke, Bielen, and Amery (1987) concluded that after allowing for the effects of body size, genetic factors had little influence on cardiac volumes, whereas Bouchard et al. (1986) concluded that after adjustment for relevant factors, about 50% of the variation in oxygen pulse (the oxygen transported per heartbeat) was due to inheritance.

Studies of Entire Families

Some more recent studies have been based on path analyses of entire families, taking into account the closeness of kinship between individual family members (Lesage, Simoneau, Jobin, LeBlanc, & Bouchard, 1985; Pérusse, C. LeBlanc, & Bouchard, 1988; Pérusse et al., 1987). This approach has facilitated the use of much larger subject groups, spanning a wide range of environmental conditions. It has also been possible to compare the respective maternal and paternal contributions to aerobic power and to investigate the placental transmission of relevant personal characteristics.

On the other hand, it has been necessary to impose a hierarchical cause-and-effect structure on the available data (Schull, 1990). Moreover, the methodological component of the overall variance has tended to be larger and less consistent in community surveys than in the smaller-scale twin studies. Furthermore, adoption of a familial approach does not eliminate the danger that environmental differences may be inversely related to the closeness of kinship.

In general, familial studies have indicated a lesser heritability of fitness than did the earlier investigations that examined monozygous and dizygous twins. In terms of the familial resemblance in aerobic power per kilogram of body mass, the ratio of variance between nuclear families to within nuclear families (including any adopted children) is about 1.3, whereas the ratio between to within siblings is about 1.5. Likewise, in terms of PWC per kilogram of body mass, the variance ratio is 1.4 for adoptive siblings and about 1.8 for biological siblings. The importance of the family environment or positive assortative mating, as opposed to a true genetic influence, is shown by a substantial correlation of aerobic power and physical working capacity between marriage partners.

Genetic-Environmental Interactions

The initial endurance fitness of a subject reflects the combined influence of genetic endowment, habitual patterns of physical activity, and the influence of inheritance on the response to such physical activity.

Bouchard and his associates suggested that although inheritance makes only a small contribution to the initial fitness status of the individual, genetic factors

Table 4.1

Estimates of the Proportion of Variability in Aerobic Power Attributable to Inheritance

Test	Author	Proportion	Type of study
Aerobic power (μmol/[kg·s], ml/[kg·min])			
	Klissouras, 1971	94%	Monozygous, dizygous twins
	Howald, 1976	0	Monozygous, dizygous twins
	Weber et al., 1976	51	Monozygous, dizygous twins (7% due to environment-gene interaction)
	Komi & Karlsson, 1979	0	Monozygous, dizygous twins
	Lesage et al., 1985	10-20	Family studies (maternal effect 20%, paternal 0%)
	Bouchard et al., 1986	40	Siblings—twins and brothers (estimated 25% after corrected for common environment)
Physical working capacity, PWC$_{150}$			
	Bouchard et al., 1984	0	Family studies
	Pérusse et al., 1987		(20% transmissibility, no maternal effect)
Canadian Home Fitness Test			
	Pérusse et al., 1988	0	Family studies (28% transmissibility, no maternal effects)
90-min aerobic capacity			
	Bouchard et al., 1986	60	Siblings—twins and brothers

are major determinants in the magnitude of the response elicited in deliberate training studies (Bouchard, 1990, 1992). Thus, Lortie et al. (1984) found that when a group of subjects participated in a common aerobic training program, the observed gains of maximal oxygen intake ranged very widely from 7% to 87%. Surprisingly, and contradictory to much other research, gains were said to be independent of the subject's initial training status. The evidence of Lortie et al. (1984) is theoretically strengthened by their use of an experimental rather than a cross-sectional design, but the fact that some people responded more to training than others could still reflect unrecognized or unmeasured differences in initial patterns of physical activity, initial levels of aerobic fitness, or subsequent program compliance rather than a major genetic-environmental interaction.

A second study from the same laboratory (Prud'homme, Bouchard, LeBlanc, Landry, & Fontaine, 1984) examined 10 pairs of monozygotic twins. Endurance training induced gains of aerobic power ranging from 0% to 41%, and 77% of the variation in response was found to be common to the twin pairs (Bouchard, 1990). Therefore, this data was interpreted as strong evidence that genetic factors influence the training response, although again the confounding influence of household similarities in habitual physical activity, diet, and other aspects of initial status may not have been fully excluded.

Other Potential Mediators of Genetic Effects

There are many other potential mediators of genetic influence. Inheritance might determine the basic motor skills that allow a person to train effectively; it might influence the patterns of habitual physical activity that a subject chooses to adopt voluntarily; and it might alter the impact of physical activity or aerobic fitness on health status.

Pérusse, Tremblay, LeBlanc, and Bouchard (1989) estimated that some 20% of the variance in population levels of habitual activity was genetically determined and a further 6% was culturally transmitted, but that—surprisingly—inheritance had no influence on the likelihood of participation in competitive sports.

More than half of the variance in HDL-cholesterol is thought to be genetically determined, in this case with clear pointers to a specific controlling genome (Pérusse, Després, et al., 1989). Changes in the lipid profile during participation in an apparently common training program have shown a strong resemblance between pairs of monozygous twins (Després et al., 1988), although once more, the confounding influences of a common home environment have yet to be ruled out.

Specific Markers of Genotype

Attempts to link aerobic fitness to specific markers of genotype, such as blood groupings, leucocyte antigens, and enzyme polymorphisms, have generally proven negative (Chagnon, Allard, & Bouchard, 1984; Couture, Chagnon, Allard, & Bouchard, 1986; Shephard, 1978), as have studies looking for associations between aerobic fitness and variations in DNA sequencing.

Further investigation is still hampered, because as yet only 1% to 2% of the human genome can be identified with certainty (Schull, 1990). One recent report found that the seven genotypes of phosphoglucomutase-1 could account for 6% of the variance in response to aerobic training (Bouchard, 1992). Given the number of physiological and biochemical variables that could exert an influence on physical condition, there is a correspondingly high potential of a complex polygenic inheritance, and negative findings are, perhaps, not surprising.

Any response-determining combination of genetic factors probably interacts in a complex fashion with the influences of environment and personal lifestyle. Nevertheless, the nature and extent of genetic influences on aerobic fitness will ultimately be elucidated through the demonstration of an association between certain structures in the gene exons or introns and a high base level of aerobic power or a large increase of maximal oxygen intake with training.

Characteristics of Endurance Athletes

Given that inheritance makes a relatively small contribution to aerobic power and other physiological characteristics of the endurance athlete, the observed differences between the superb competitor and the average person must reflect largely the outcome of rigorous training. Thus, a review of the standards achieved by national and international competitors in different athletic disciplines (Shephard, 1978) may be useful in indicating both the type of training most likely to maximize aerobic fitness in those individuals who are currently sedentary, and the potential magnitude of response. However, the analysis must not be pursued too rigorously, because most athletes train at a level that is far beyond the tolerance of the sedentary person from either a physical or a psychological standpoint.

Successful competitors in most endurance sports have shown a trend toward an increase of maximal oxygen intake and other measures of aerobic fitness over the present century, although the physiological gains have been smaller than the performance gains seen on the track or in the pool. Thus, when comparing data for the various athletic disciplines, it is preferable to look at results that are homogenous with respect to both level of competition and the year of evaluation (see Table 4.2). Now that sports have been ranked in terms of their apparent aerobic demand, it is possible to analyze how the physiological characteristics of competitors in the aerobic disciplines have changed in recent years.

Sports With a High Aerobic Demand

There is consensus that the highest values of relative aerobic power are observed in male, international-class, cross-country skiers. One reason is that competitions are of longer duration than those for many other types of sport. In swimming, for example, even the 1,500-m event is completed within 15 min (Gullstrand, 1992). Likewise, most rowers compete for only 7 to 8 min. A second factor augmenting aerobic demand in cross-country skiers is that the task is widely distributed over the muscles of the legs, arms, and back.

Table 4.2
Maximal Oxygen Intake of Top National Competitors in Selected Sports at the Time of the International Biological Programme Survey

Sport	Men µmol kg·s	Men ml kg·min	Women µmol kg·s	Women ml kg·min	Female disadvantage
Alpine skiing	51	68	39	52	24%
American football	45	60			
Archery	44	59*	30	40	32
Badminton	41	55			
Baseball	39	52			
Basketball	44	59	33	44	25
Biathlon	58	78			
Boxing	41	55			
Canoeing	52	70			
whitewater	45	60	36	49	18
Cross-country skiing	66	82	47	63	23
Cycling (1,000 m)	49	66			
(4,000 m)	57	76			
(30-50 km)	58	78	47	63	19
Decathlon	43	58			
Fencing	44	59	32	43	27
Field hockey	47	63			
Figure skating	44	59	36	49	17
Golf	40	54			
Gymnastics	45	60	32	43	28
Handball	46	62			
High-jumping	44	59			
Ice hockey	43	58			
Judo	36	49			
Miscellaneous throwing events	41	55	28	38	31
Netball			34	45*	
Orienteering	57	77	45	60	22
Pentathlon	55	74	37	50	32
Rowing	55	74			
Rugby football	37	50			
Running (400 m)	50	67	42	56	16
(800-1,500 m)	59	79			
(3 km-10 km)	61	82	46	62	24
(42 km)	57	76			
Sailing	37	50			
Ski jumping	46	62*			
Soccer	49	66			

(continued)

Table 4.2 (*continued*)

Sport	Men (µmol kg·s)	Men (ml kg·min)	Women (µmol kg·s)	Women (ml kg·min)	Female disadvantage
Softball			33	45*	
Speed-skating	59	79	39	53	33
Swimming	52	70	43	58	17
Table tennis	45	61*	32	43*	30
Volleyball	42	56	38	51	10
Weight-lifting	42	56			
Wrestling	42	56			

Note. Data from Shephard (1978); other values from Butts (1985) and Reilly and Secher (1990) marked with asterisk.

Selecting those athletic disciplines in which male international competitors have peak aerobic powers of over 52 µmol/(kg·s), or 70 ml/(kg·min), we may infer that other classes of competition with a high aerobic demand include biathlon, canoeing, cycling, orienteering, pentathlon, rowing, running distances of 800 m to 42 km, speed-skating, and distance swimming (see Table 4.2).

At the time of the IBP survey, the aerobic power of female competitors was 16% to 33% less than that of male competitors (Shephard, 1978). This difference probably reflects not only inherent physiological differences between the two sexes (Drinkwater, 1984), but also a number of sociocultural influences that had to this time discouraged women from participation in many types of aerobic training, with a resultant decrease in the pool of female athletes available for selection. Two observations support the important influence of cultural factors: (1) In the 1970s and early 1980s, the gender-related difference in aerobic power was least in swimming and volleyball, sports which were then particularly popular with women, and (2) over the past 2 decades the gender difference in aerobic power has narrowed progressively with changes in socially accepted gender roles.

Some investigators have speculated that within 1 to 2 decades, women may outperform men in certain types of aerobic event. However, the rapid gains in female records during the past few years had their counterpart among an earlier generation of male competitors, and it is likely that the future gains of female athletes will be smaller as they also approach their potential ceiling of performance.

Cross-Country Skiers

Typical cross-country ski competitions are 15- or 50-km events for men and 10-km events for women. The course is covered at an average speed of about 5 m/s, so that a 15-km event is completed in about 50 min. Many competitors tolerate exercising at or near their maximal oxygen intake during the ascent of hills, with recovery periods of somewhat less intense activity during the subsequent descents (Eisenman, Johnson, Bainbridge, & Zupan, 1988). Top-level competitors currently spend about 700 hr/year in preparing for cross-country ski competitions (Bergh & Forsberg, 1992), training on skis during the winter and on roller skis and skiing treadmills in the summer.

P.O. Åstrand & Rodahl (1986) cited one male competitor in a 15-km cross-country skiing event who had demonstrated an aerobic power of 70 μmol/(kg·s), or 94 ml/(kg·min). Bergh and Forsberg (1992) noted that there were substantial interindividual differences of body mass between successful competitors. They argued that the variation of aerobic power among cross-country skiers was minimized if results were expressed per $kg^{2/3}$ of body mass. Uphill treadmill-running values in the more commonly adopted per kilogram units averaged 61 μmol/ (kg·s), or 82.0 ml/(kg·min) for world-class male competitors in the 1960s and 63.2 μmol/(kg·s), or 84.9 ml/(kg·min) in the 1970s. Using an uphill skiing test, which probably increased results by about 3% relative to treadmill running, the average figure for the 1980s (64.9 μmol/[kg·s], or 87.2 ml/[kg·min]) was not greatly improved relative to the 2 previous decades.

The corresponding values for female world-class Nordic skiers, who compete over 10-km distances, currently approach 56 μmol/(kg·s), or 75 ml/(kg·min), (P.O. Åstrand & Rodahl, 1986; Bergh & Forsberg, 1992). The gender-related discrepancy in the aerobic power of top cross-country competitors has thus dropped from 23% to 11%-12% over the past 2 decades.

Important determinants of cross-country skiing performance other than aerobic power include two measures of the efficiency of energy usage: the fraction of the maximal oxygen intake used at a given skiing speed and the years of racing experience (Bergh & Forsberg, 1992; Niinimaa et al., 1979).

Runners

Runners are traditionally classified into sprinters, middle-distance competitors (800-1,500 m), and long-distance runners (5,000 m and more). In terms of relative aerobic power, runners who compete over distances of 3 to 10 km are those who achieve the next highest values to cross-country skiers (Boileau, Mayhew, Riner, & Lussier, 1982; Svedenhag & Sjödin, 1984). The duration of their events ranges from 7 min for a 3-km race to 27 min for a 10-km run.

DiPrampero (1992) suggested that the world-record times for distances in this range were slightly faster than would be predicted based on the biomechanics of running, assuming a full exploitation of the anaerobic capacity and use of 100% of aerobic power throughout the race. However, diPrampero based his calculations on a peak aerobic power of only 55 μmol/(kg·s), or 74 ml/(kg·min), which is about 10% too low for the current generation of male distance runners. Given the more reasonable current value of 61 to 62 μmol/(kg·s), or 82 to 83 ml/(kg·min) for an international winner (Péronnet & Thibault, 1989; Snell, 1990), the work performed by the runner implies usage of 90% to 92% of maximal oxygen intake during the race. It is accepted that distance runners of both sexes can use a large fraction of their aerobic power (Wells, Hecht, & Krahlenbuhl, 1981), but this estimate still seems a little high for a prolonged bout of exercise. It may be that the oxygen cost of running is reduced relative to the assumed theoretical value by such factors as the grouping of runners (Kyle, 1979; Yamaji & Shephard, 1987) and an increase in the mechanical efficiency of running relative to that of laboratory subjects (Conley & Krahlenbuhl, 1980).

Making measurements over the range 80 to 240 min, diPrampero (1992) estimated that the usable percentage of aerobic power equaled $90.5 - .091t$, where t was the duration of the run. Extrapolation of this formula to shorter events implies that a runner is able to use 88% of aerobic power for a 27-min race. Péronnet and Thibeault (1989) proposed the alternative formulae of $100 - 5 \ln(.14t)$ for women and $100 - 5.6 \ln(.14t)$ for men. Their equations predict usage of 93.4% and 92.6% of peak aerobic power in women and men, respectively, throughout a 27-min race.

The usable percentage of aerobic power shows increasing interindividual differences as the running distance is extended. diPrampero (1992) commented that if the duration of activity was increased to 100 min, the usable fraction of peak aerobic power ranged from 72% to 88% in different individuals. He predicted that this would result in a 30-min interindividual variation in marathon running times.

Plainly, if a race continues for half an hour or longer, the aerobic capacity, or the ability to continue operating at close to maximal aerobic power, is crucial to success. Snell and Mitchell (1984) suggest that a well-developed capillary network and an increase of local metabolic potential are important determinants of aerobic capacity. To this list, the present author would add the development of sufficient strength in the active muscles to minimize external compression of the local blood supply. Strength training becomes increasingly important as the race distance is shortened.

The preferred pattern of training varies with the competitive distance. Interval training allows event-specific training over short distances, but for the longer events, continuous training allows a greater total volume of training to be undertaken before the onset of fatigue or overtraining (Snell, 1990).

Speed Skaters

There is relatively little available information concerning the physiology of the speed skater (Geijsel, 1980; Geijsel, Bomhoff, van Vezen, de Groot, & van Ingen Schenau, 1984). Typical durations of competition range from 2 min 25 s for a 1,500-m race to 13 min 48 s for 10-km events. The participant's preparation is complicated, because many athletes compete in both short and long distances. The highest reported aerobic power, 59 μmol/(kg·s), or 79 ml/(kg·min), was observed when a male 10-km competitor was running uphill on a treadmill. Even international competitors are able to attain only 90% to 95% of their treadmill maxima while skating (Ekblom, Hermansen, & Saltin, 1967).

Under firm ice conditions, a large fraction of the total energy usage is expended in overcoming air resistance. For instance, when skating at a speed of 10 m/s, 47% of the energy expenditure is due to air resistance and the remaining 53% to gravitational and inertial factors. Friction at the skate blades is only a minor concern (diPrampero, Cortilo, Mognoni, & Saibene, 1976). Thus, if the competitor is able to skate in a crouched position (adopting a trunk angle of 20°-30°), it is advantageous to have not only a large relative aerobic power, but also large absolute values (e.g., 3.7 mmol/s, or 5.5 L/min, in the most successful member of the group studied by Ekblom et al., 1967). However, if the ice becomes soft, a heavy person is then at a significant disadvantage, which discourages the participation of massive individuals in speed-skating competitions. Typical weights range from 67 to 77 kg for men and from 60 to 61 kg for women (Quinney, 1990).

On-ice training is frequently limited by difficulty in obtaining the use of a skating rink. Thus, a typical regimen combines sport-specific training with running, cycling, and roller skating (Bedingfield & Wronko, 1981). Strength training is also important, particularly for the person who competes over various distances.

Orienteering Competitors

Orienteering is another sport that is associated with a high relative aerobic power. The average build of the successful competitor is similar to that of a distance runner (72 kg for men and 58 kg for women; Reilly & Secher, 1990).

The typical orienteering course covers rough wooded and hilly terrain. Completion of a competition demands about 1.5 hr of running for men and 1 hr for women. As with cross-country skiing and cross-country running, one may presume that energy usage approaches 100% of aerobic power when hills are climbed, with some metabolism of accumulated lactate when descending slopes (Staab, Agnew, & Sicionolfi, 1992). Training follows the principles associated with distance running.

Rowers

The absolute maximal oxygen intake of a male competitor may be as high as 4.5 to 4.7 mmol/s, or 6.1 to 6.3 L/min (Hagerman, 1984; Secher, 1990, 1992). The weight of the rower and boat is supported by buoyancy, and part of the drag is attributable to the mass of the boat (e.g., a minimum weight of 14 kg for a double-scull single-rower craft) rather than that of the rower. There are now lightweight categories of rowing competition (with respective maximal body masses of 72.5 kg for men and 59 kg for women). But in open categories where there is no restriction on the body mass of the rower, the sport attracts mainly heavy, powerful individuals. The weights of the leading competitors currently average 94 kg for men and 79 kg for women. The aerobic power per unit of body mass [48 to 52 μmol/(kg·s), or 65 to 70 ml/(kg·min) in men and around 45 μmol/(kg·s), or 60 ml/(kg·min) in women] is thus less impressive than the absolute maximal oxygen intake, and the individual's rowing performance is better related to absolute than to relative aerobic power. Interestingly, the variance of aerobic power among rowers is minimized if data are expressed in ml/min per $kg^{2/3}$ of body mass.

Measurements of aerobic power that are made on the water, or when operating a well-designed rowing ergometer, do not differ substantially from those recorded during uphill treadmill running. However, compared to most sedentary subjects, rowers are able to develop a large fraction of their treadmill aerobic power while operating an arm ergometer. This raises the question, why does the combination of arm and leg exercise demanded by rowing not increase maximal oxygen intake substantially above the values observed on the treadmill? The most likely explanation is that the centrally limited pumping ability of the heart has already been realized during treadmill exercise. However, there have also been suggestions that maximal rhythmic exercise of the arm muscles induces a general vasoconstriction, thus limiting maximal perfusion of the leg muscles (Klausen, Secher, Clausen, Hartling, & Trap-Jensen, 1982).

The force resisting motion of the craft is approximated by $kV^{1.95} M^{0.56}$, where V is the average forward velocity and M is the mass of the boat-plus-rower (Secher & Vaage, 1983). It might be anticipated that the energy cost of propulsion would be proportional to the third power of speed, but in practice the cost rises to $V^{2.4}$, because part of the energy expenditure at any given speed is attributable to the cost of operating the sliding seat mechanism and the resultant reaction on the motion of the boat (Secher, 1990).

A summer regimen of continual aerobic training yields better competitive results than a program in which bouts of anaerobic training are introduced in the weeks immediately preceding a major rowing competition (Secher, 1990). In some countries, such as Canada, it is difficult to maintain training on the water throughout the year, but the aerobic power of the rower can be well maintained over the winter season if an appropriate dry-land training program is developed (Wright, Bomba, & Shephard, 1976).

Canoeists and Kayakers

The canoeist faces some of the mechanical constraints experienced by the rower, although the lack of a sliding seat precludes any major use of the leg muscles in propulsion. The craft is usually lighter than a rowing skiff, and this factor reduces the optimal body mass. The typical top male competitor has a weight of around 80 kg (Reilly & Secher, 1990).

Classic races cover distances of 500 m to 10,000 m. Times for the 10,000-m event are clearly in the aerobic range (about 45 min). Top-level canoeists have quite large absolute values of aerobic power—3.9 to 4.2 mmol/s, or 5.3 to 5.6 L/min (Shephard, 1987c; Tesch, 1983). Given a body mass of 80 kg, this equates to a relative maximal oxygen intake of 52 μmol/(kg·s), or 70 ml/(kg·min). One male canoeist is reported to have attained a relative value of 63 μmol/(kg·s), or 85 ml/(kg·min), while he was exercising on the treadmill (Dransart, as cited in

Shephard, 1987c), but unfortunately he was able to realize only 77% of this total when using an arm ergometer. Whitewater contests (Fry & Morton, 1991; Shephard, 1987c; Sidney & Shephard, 1973; Vaccaro et al., 1984) involve a much larger component of anaerobic activity than normal canoeing, and the aerobic power of the contestants is correspondingly lower.

Typically, the well-trained kayaker can develop almost 90% of the treadmill oxygen intake when operating an arm ergometer or kayak simulator. This is in marked contrast to the 70% of maximum that can be realized by an inexperienced, sedentary subject.

Cyclists

Compared to sedentary individuals, top-level cyclists can attain higher peak oxygen intakes when operating a cycle ergometer or when cycling on a treadmill than during uphill treadmill running (Burke, Faria, & White, 1990; Faria, 1984; White, Quinn, Al-Dawabi, & Mulhall, 1982). Track races in cycling are quite brief (1-5 min), and thus the aerobic power of 1,000-m and 4,000-m competitors is a little lower than that of athletes who are involved in some of the longer contests. One sample of male East German, national-class, 4,000-m competitors had an average aerobic power of 56.5 $\mu mol/(kg \cdot s)$, or 76 ml/(kg·min) (Neumann, 1992).

Road events typically last for 2 to 4 hr, although some contests are much longer (e.g., the Tour de France covers 5,000 km and lasts for 23 days). Competitors in the 2- to 4-hr road events have a slightly higher average aerobic power (58 $\mu mol/$ [kg·s], or 78 ml/[kg·min]) than the 4,000-m racers. However, in part because the effort of cycling is sustained mainly by a relatively small group of muscles (i.e., the quadriceps), it is difficult to develop more than 70% of aerobic power over an extended race. Perhaps for this reason, Krebs, Zinkgraf, and Virgilio (1983) found that relative aerobic power made no contribution to the prediction of 40-km cycling times after due allowance had been made for years of cycling experience. As in other protracted sports, the ability of the long-distance cyclist to match aerobic capacity closely to aerobic power is likely an important ingredient in competitive success (I.E. Faria, Faria, Roberts, & Yoshimura, 1989). Despite the assumption of constancy of mechanical efficiency in cycling, in practice, the mechanical efficiency also varies widely from 19.6% to 28.8%. The main reason for the high efficiency of peak performers is that with experience, cyclists are able to develop high pedal speeds without engaging in extraneous, inefficient body movements (Ryschon & Stray-Gunderson, 1991).

Regardless of the distance that is covered, the effort of the racing cyclist is expended mainly against air resistance. For example, if a 50-km course is completed over 62 min, air resistance accounts for 82% and rolling resistance for only 7% of the total energy expended. Drafting, cycling behind another cyclist, can reduce the energy cost by 27% at a speed of 40 km/hr (McCole, Claney, Conte, Anderson, & Hagberg, 1990).

Large cyclists have a lower ratio of frontal area to body mass (Swain, Coast, Clifford, Milliken, & Stray-Gunderson, 1987), particularly if the bulk is concentrated in the lower half of the trunk (Miller & Manfredi, 1981). In theory, the competitive cyclist would gain some advantage from a large body size and a high absolute aerobic power. But in practice, the body mass is unremarkable, and average values decrease from 76 kg in 1,000-m competitors to 72 kg in road competitors (Neumann, 1992).

The training plan of the cyclist may include distance work, race pace, and sprinting segments. The exact combination depends on the particular event. Conconi, Borsetto, Casoni, and Farrari (1984) emphasized anaerobic threshold training (70%-80% of maximal oxygen intake) in their preparation of a 1-hr-world-record holder. But if the training places an excessive emphasis on anaerobic preparation, the aerobic power may diminish (Neumann, 1992). The total volume of distance training undertaken can amount to as much as 35,000 km/year (about 700 hr/year). Depending on details of the training plan (Neumann, 1992), aerobic power can vary by as much as 9 $\mu mol/(kg \cdot s)$, or 12 $ml/(kg \cdot min)$ over any given competitor's year (i.e., an 18% training effect). Given also that an international-class cyclist is unlikely to become totally sedentary at any point in the year, this observation reinforces the view that a substantial part of the endurance athlete's performance capability is acquired rather than inherited.

Triathlon Competitors

Participants in triathlon events (Daniels, 1992) must undertake a combination of 3.8 km of swimming, 180 km of cycling, and a marathon run. They have maximal oxygen intake values rather similar to those reported for long-distance swimmers, cyclists, and runners (Holly, Baranard, Rosenthal, Applegate, & Pritikin, 1986).

Types of Aerobic Training

There is considerable specificity in the response to aerobic training. The optimum tactic for endurance athletes is thus repeated practice of the disciplines in which they intend to compete. This leads not only to a specific development of aerobic power, but also to enhancement of the mechanical efficiency and psychomotor performance of the required skills. The primary drawbacks of this advice are the potentials for boredom and overtraining injury.

Athletes with the largest relative maximal oxygen intakes typically compete over periods of 15 to 60 min, and the majority prepare themselves for such events by concentrating their training at or near the anaerobic threshold (70% to 80% of maximal oxygen intake) for at least 2 hr a day. The size of fluctuations in aerobic power over the course of the year support the view that much of the high levels of attainment seen in the endurance competitor is a result of training rather than the selection of those who are particularly well endowed.

If an athlete is preparing to compete in events of less than 10- to 15-min duration, then there is a greater need for sprint training and increased muscle mass, whereas if the intent is to compete in events demanding more than 1 hr of exercise, the ability to sustain the aerobic capacity at close to maximal aerobic power becomes a major determinant of success. Peripheral training is important to aerobic capacity, but it is unclear whether this reflects predominantly a development of muscle capillaries, muscle enzyme systems, or muscle strength.

Sport Training and the Average Person

It is quite possible for the average person to develop aerobic fitness by means of the individual and team sports already discussed. Participation in many common team sports, such as soccer (Berg, LaVoie, & Latin, 1985) and ice hockey (Daub et al., 1983), has only a minimal impact on the player's maximal oxygen intake. Nevertheless, such activities sometimes reduce the heart rate during submaximal exercise (Daub et al., 1983). The health significance of intensity-specific changes of performance has yet to be clarified.

Features of sport that have a positive impact on the motivation of some people include the challenge of preparation for and participation in competition (Kenyon, 1968), peer praise, and the companionship of the team or competitive environment, the last being a well-recognized feature even of Masters' competitions for older adults (Kavanagh, Lindley, Shephard, & Campbell, 1988). Data presented by Paffenbarger (1988) suggest that for any given total weekly energy expenditure, the health benefit of sport participation is somewhat greater than that of less vigorous forms of aerobic activity (see Figure 4.1).

However, there are significant practical barriers to regular participation in most types of sport. Costly facilities and equipment are needed, events often take place

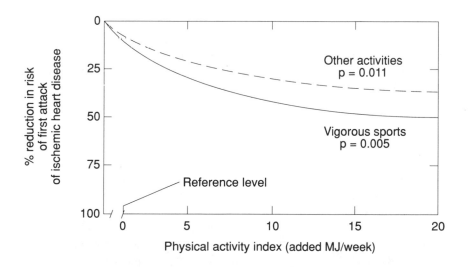

Figure 4.1   A comparison between the health benefit of regular participation in sports and other forms of aerobic activity. Data for Harvard alumni, followed longitudinally for 16 years. *Note*. Adapted from Paffenbarger (1988) by permission.

at a distant site (which increases the participant's opportunity cost for a given dose of exercise; Shephard, 1989a), and an amateur team may not gather on a very regular basis for either play or practice. Team sports are particularly expensive in terms of land use, and the demand for playing space would be prohibitive if everyone wanted to participate on a regular basis (Shephard, 1986a). Many sports carry a much higher musculoskeletal injury rate than simple aerobic activities such as rapid walking (MacIntosh, Skrien, & Shephard, 1972). It is also very difficult to regulate the intensity of physical activity during play. Energy expenditures vary with the personality of the participant and the skill of team members or opponents. For some subjects, the physical demands of participation and the associated emotional excitement may present a risk of heart attack (Blimkie et al., 1977), whereas in others, the small dose of training that is obtained may be inadequate for any health benefit. Depending on the sport chosen, there also may be rather specific training of one body region, sometimes at the expense of loss of condition in other parts of the body. Finally, children are frequently selected out because of disadvantageous body build (Shephard, Lavallée, et al., 1978), older participants become discouraged by deteriorating performance, and many of the sports that are practiced at school or university have a rather limited carry-over value into adult and family life (Ilmarinen & Rutenfranz, 1980; Telama, 1978, 1991).

Some indication of the relative aerobic training values of different types of sport can be obtained from tables of energy cost (e.g., Durnin & Passmore, 1967), although much depends on the vigor with which a given activity is pursued. The aerobic points system (Cooper, 1968) was one attempt to make simplified information on energy costs accessible to the general public, though critical review suggested there were a number of limitations. Specifically, there were some important discrepancies between the points awarded by the system and the energy usage found in most tables of energy costs, and there were uncertainties regarding the relative point values appropriate to short but intense activity and prolonged but more moderate bouts of exercise (Massie, Rode, Skrien, & Shephard, 1970).

Continuous Aerobic Activity

Continuous aerobic activity is the most commonly adopted choice of middle-aged adults who wish to improve their physical condition. The exercise may be derived from fast walking, slow or moderate jogging, cycling, swimming, cross-country skiing, skating, canoeing, rowing, or other enjoyable activities that use a relatively large muscle mass. Many of the proposed activities can be pursued by the family, which appeals more to the introverted individual than to the extrovert (Massie & Shephard, 1971). The ideal program has minimal needs of costly facilities and equipment. Some activities such as walking, canoeing, and skiing can be combined with other pursuits and interests that enhance the participant's motivation (e.g., the study of urban architecture, a review of the local fauna and flora, or an appreciation of the beauty of the wilderness; Laakso & Telama, 1979; Telama, 1991).

In a country with a continental climate, one disadvantage of outdoor pursuits is the constraint imposed by sharp seasonal changes of environmental temperature. Permanent facilities, such as outdoor swimming pools, may be used for only a few weeks each year, minimizing their cost-effectiveness (Shephard, 1986a). The participant who wishes to sustain a year-round program must have an alternative training plan for extremes of temperature; for example, the principal aerobic activity may change from jogging to swimming during very hot periods of the summer, or to rope-skipping in the basement during the coldest weeks of the winter. If there is a radical change in the pattern of exercising, it is important to recommence the program at less than the previous intensity of training in order to avoid musculoskeletal problems.

Because individual activities usually have no immediate class leader, it is important that a person choosing this approach either has strong, personal motivation (the internal locus of control noted by Rotter, 1975) or reports regularly to an exercise specialist (e.g., by the completion of activity diary sheets or use of a computerized activity record). The usual recommendation is that subjects exercise just below the lactate threshold, at 60% to 70% of their maximal oxygen intake. This intensity of effort will be perceived as "somewhat hard" (i.e., a rating of 13 units on the original scale of Borg, 1971). It will induce moderate sweating and a little breathlessness (although the person should still be able to talk). The overall exercise session should leave a participant no more than pleasantly tired on the following day. If aerobic power has been determined in the laboratory, the aerobic component of the exercise prescription can also be translated into a set walking pace (e.g., the subject should cover 1.6 km in 15 min; Kavanagh, 1992). On mastering the skill of carotid pulse counting, the subject can adjust the intensity of activity to keep such values at 60% to 70% of their heart rate reserve.

From the viewpoint of overall health, the main disadvantage of a continuous training regimen is that the participants often neglect to strengthen their muscles and to increase the flexibility of their joints. Ideally, the exercise session should begin with some gentle stretching exercises and be supplemented by muscle-strengthening activities. One possibility is to carry and swing some weights when walking (Graves, Pollock, Montain, Jackson, & O'Keefe, 1987; Owens, al-Ahmed, & Moffat, 1989). The subject may purchase a pair of hand-held weights, but the impact of such a tactic upon oxygen consumption or muscle strength is small. It is equally possible to strengthen the arms and shoulders by swinging a well-loaded brief-case on the walk to and from work or by carrying the groceries home from a neighborhood store, although ideally an approximately equal load should be carried by each arm.

Interval Training

Interval training was popularized by the German cardiologist H. Reindell before World War II. When preparing young endurance athletes, he advocated that 30-

to 70-s periods of activity at heart rates of about 180 beats/min should be followed by recumbent recovery periods that were long enough to allow the competitor's heart rate to drop to 120 beats/min. He postulated that during the recovery phase, the heart rate decreased faster than the cardiac output (Reindell, Roskamm, & Gerschler, 1962), so that the subject's myocardial function was stimulated by a transient increase of stroke volume. Many subsequent studies of interval training have been complicated by use of the supine position to facilitate measurements of cardiac output, and some authors (e.g., P.O. Åstrand & Rodahl, 1986) have denied that the stroke volume rises immediately following exercise. However, D.I. Goldberg and Shephard (1980) were able to obtain data during and immediately following seated cycle ergometry. They noted that if exercise was followed by a period of loadless pedalling (in order to sustain venous return), there was a 29% increase of stroke volume in the first 30 s after exercise, and the stroke volume was greater than during exercise even 216 s after the activity had ceased. Given that the force of quadriceps contraction impedes local muscle blood flow to a much greater extent during cycle ergometry than during running, this does not necessarily prove that the stroke volume would increase immediately following a short bout of jogging. Possibly, the 29% increase in stroke volume generated when using the cycle ergometer does no more than compensate for the restriction of quadriceps flow during the active phase of the experiment. In support of this view, D.I. Goldberg and Shephard (1980) noted that the increase of stroke volume following exercise was greatest in those having the lowest levels of fitness and thus, by inference, the greatest likelihood of perfusion limitation due to local muscular weakness.

Other investigators have used various lengths of exercise bout and recovery interval (Shephard, 1982b; Wilt, 1968). Recumbent recovery has also been replaced by slow walking, on the basis that mild exercise speeds the clearance of lactate from the active muscles (Hermansen & Stensvold, 1972). The physiological stress imposed by a modern interval training regimen depends largely on the exercise-recovery sequence that is adopted. If the active intervals are very short (5-10 s), then the energy needs during the active phase are satisfied from anaerobic reserves (i.e., phosphagen and the oxygen content of the myoglobin and tissue fluids). Such a regimen seems likely to develop the subject's anaerobic power rather than his or her aerobic condition. If very intensive 30- to 60-s bouts of exercise or longer periods (2-3 min) of near-maximal activity are employed, then there is a large accumulation of lactate (I. Åstrand et al., 1960). Such a regimen can give a competitive middle-distance athlete experience exercising at racing pace, although the main stimulus is then to the development anaerobic capacity rather than aerobic mechanisms. Indeed, there have been suggestions (Snell, 1990) that the adoption of such a regimen may impair the subject's aerobic power and/or capacity.

Regardless of the theoretical influences of interval work on stroke volume, most data show a similar development of aerobic power in response to either continuous training or moderate-length, moderate-intensity interval training, provided that an equivalent amount of work is performed in each type of program

(Eddy, Sparks, & Adelizi, 1977; Poole & Gasser, 1985; Pyke, Ewing, & A.D. Roberts, 1978). The main disadvantage of interval training is that it takes longer to complete, an adverse feature for many time-conscious exercisers. On the other hand, an interval training regimen with an extended recovery period may be helpful in allowing patients with effort-induced angina pectoris to reach a useful intensity of training without developing debilitating chest pain (Kavanagh & Shephard, 1975).

DeBusk, Stenestrand, Sheehan, and Haskell (1990) recently explored another variant of conditioning exercise, comparing three 10-min a sessions a day to one daily session of 30 min. They argued that busy people might find repeated short bouts of activity more practicable than a single extended session. Such a regimen could also be useful to those with very low levels of aerobic fitness who could not tolerate 30-min, undivided sessions. DeBusk et al. (1990) found that the 10-min sessions yielded heart rates above the usually accepted training zone for an average of 1.9 min and within the training zone for 7.7 min, compared to periods of 10.4 min above and 16.3 min within the training zone during the longer sessions. Sweating was noted by only 65% as opposed to 84% of subjects, so adoption of the divided regimen might save the participant time spent in showering. The rating of perceived exertion for the 10-min session averaged 11.2 units on the Borg (1971) scale, as opposed to 12.2 units for the 30-min session. Over 8 weeks of observation, the increase in maximal oxygen intake under the modified program (1.8 μmol/[kg·s], or 2.4 ml/[kg·min]) was about half of that realized in the usual 30-min exercise sessions (3.3 μmol/[kg·s], or 4.4 ml/[kg·min]).

Circuit Training

Circuit training (Gettman & Pollock, 1981; R.E. Morgan & Adamson, 1965) is normally undertaken to develop muscular strength. Although the heart rate may be quite high, this reflects the influence of resistance exercise rather than a high overall energy expenditure (Hempel & Wells, 1985). A series of 8 to 12 exercise stations are established, each requiring use of a particular muscle group to complete an assigned task. At each station, the exerciser executes the required movement 8 to 10 times (repetitions, or reps) at a substantial fraction (50%-60%) of the maximal force that can be developed with one repetition of the particular task. If a high level of strength is desired, the subject completes several circuits of the stations at each training session.

Resistance exercises are a useful adjunct to aerobic training. The latter often does little more than sustain function in the most active muscle groups and may be associated with a loss of lean tissue from other parts of the body. However, the subject must observe the precautions appropriate to muscle training.

There is no fundamental reason why aerobic exercises cannot be incorporated into a training circuit—for example, the participant could undertake 10-min periods of activity on a cycle ergometer, a stair-climbing device, and a rowing ergometer between the stations that are designed to increase muscle strength.

However, unless the stations have a heavy aerobic emphasis, the gains of maximal oxygen intake under a circuit training program are likely to be smaller than those for continuous or interval training (MacDonald, 1983; Roskamm, 1967).

Calisthenics

Traditional forms of gymnastics had a very low level of energy expenditure. Indeed, Weiss and Karpovich (1947) found that the most vigorous of 40 such exercises demanded an oxygen consumption of no more than 0.6 mmol/s, or 0.8 L/min. Such activities may nevertheless serve as a useful warm-up before a session of vigorous aerobic exercise. They can also contribute to arousal and an increased awareness of the need for physical activity, if they are introduced as short fitness breaks at the worksite (LaPorte, 1966; Shephard, 1986b).

The extent of any aerobic conditioning achieved by calisthenics alone depends mainly on the cadence that is set by the instructor. With a sufficiently forceful pattern of movement, it is possible to induce some gains in cardiorespiratory performance as well as increases in strength and flexibility (Andrew, Brooker, & Brawley, 1974; Cox, Shephard, & Corey, 1981). The typical class time, nevertheless, is relatively short for aerobic benefit. Adults spend at most 13 to 17 of a nominal 30 to 40 min in activities that are intense enough to have a cardiovascular training effect, and gains in health-related fitness are often disappointing (Bassey, Patrick, Irving, Blecher, & Fentem, 1983; Cox et al., 1981; Shephard et al., 1979). If a major impact on either aerobic power or body composition is desired, participants must supplement class sessions by exercising at home.

Calisthenics classes for children may induce an even smaller amount of training-related physical activity. Peak heart rates of about 160 beats/min are common, but these may not be sustained long enough to have any training effect (Verabioff, 1981). Some studies have shown that almost all of the nominal class hour is occupied in changing, receiving instructions, and awaiting an opportunity to use specific items of apparatus (Goode et al., 1976; Marshall, Conjer, & Quinney, 1983; Verabioff, 1981). Moreover, the long-term influence on attitudes can be quite negative, and a high proportion of students stop exercising in the first year after leaving required school programs of physical education (Ilmarinen & Rutenfranz, 1980).

Aerobics classes for adults commonly use vigorous, stimulating, and rather loud music, the tempo of the exercises being set by the beat of the music. Such activities appeal most to the extrovert who has a boring job and is looking for an external source of arousal; they are less appreciated by the introvert holding a stressful job (Massie & Shephard, 1971). The need to attend group sessions at fixed times and places puts a significant constraint on both recruitment and program compliance, to the extent that very few Canadians report participating in such activities (Canada Fitness Survey, 1983; Stephens & Craig, 1990). If they are offered a worksite program, employees may be reluctant to remain after work because of car-pool arrangements or family responsibilities. If a community program is developed, most participants will face a substantial opportunity cost in travelling to and from the gymnasium (Shephard, 1992h).

The Canadian 5BX and 10BX plans are personal programs of progressive exercise that combine 5 min of daily calisthenics with 6 min of stationary running or a longer period of outdoor aerobic activity, such as running or walking (Orban, 1962). The energy cost of the program, averaged over the normal 11-min session, is progressively increased from 33 to about 70 kJ/min as the condition of the participant improves (Brown, 1965). Thus, the intensity of the prescribed activity is sufficient to provide an effective cardiovascular stimulus (Kappagoda, Linden, & Newell, 1977), although by modern standards, the session duration is rather short. In contrast to most aerobic programs, 5BX and 10BX programs also encourage some development of muscular strength (Malhotra, Sen Gupta, & Joseph, 1973).

Aerobic Dance

Aerobic dance classes are, in essence, a variant of aerobic calisthenics. Gains in aerobic power can be as large as those for a comparable intensity, frequency, and duration of jogging (Milburn & Butts, 1983; Vaccaro & Clinton, 1981; Williford, Blessing, Scharff, Keith, & Barksdale, 1990). Some authors have suggested that aerobic dance induces an excessive number of injuries to the lower limbs, but an epidemiological study (Garrick, Gillian, & Whiteside, 1986) found that such fears were exaggerated. The risk of injury is lower in low-impact programs, but unfortunately the training response is also reduced (McCord, Nichols, & Patterson, 1989).

It is possible to get considerable aerobic stimulation from vigorous participation in traditional types of activity, such as square and country dancing, and even disco dancing (Léger, 1982). Again, the format of the activity provides opportunities for body movement and social contact, a combination that is valued more by the extrovert than the introvert.

Other Options

The typical energy expenditure when using a minitrampoline is in the range 10 to 13 μmol/(kg·s), or 14 to 17 ml/(kg·min) (J.F. Smith & Bishop, 1988). Several authors have suggested that use of this type of equipment can improve cardiorespiratory condition in older adults (Gerberich, Leon, McNally, Serfass, & Edin, 1990; Hartung & Kirby, 1980; J.R. White, 1980), although one study found no such benefit (Edin et al., 1990).

Rope-skipping is another simple indoor option. The energy cost does not vary greatly with the speed of skipping and can be as high as 28 to 37 μmol/(kg·s), or 38 to 50 ml/(kg·min) (Quirk & Sinning, 1982). However, if there is a sudden change from outdoor exercise to skipping on a hard, basement floor, there is a substantial injury rate (Buyze et al., 1986).

Aquabics, or aerobic exercises performed in a swimming pool (Kirby, Sacamano, Balch, & Kriellaars, 1983; Lawrence, 1981; Sheldahl, 1986; Shephard,

1985c), is particularly useful as a means of offering aerobic exercise to the obese and those with joint problems. The energy expenditure can be varied as required by changing the depth of the water, the speed of movement, and the size of any movement-resisting paddles that are carried. Running through water can offer a good aerobic stimulus, depending on the skill of the runner (J.H. Green, Cable, & Elms, 1990; Yamaji, Greenly, Northey, & Hughson, 1990). Because of the subject's lower core temperature and the facilitation of venous return, gains in aerobic power can be similar to those made on dry land, despite the typically lower heart rate when exercising in the water (Avellini, Shapiro, & Pandolf, 1983).

Normal wheelchair ambulation usually does not offer a sufficient aerobic training stimulus to maintain the physical condition of those who have spinal cord injuries (Shephard, 1990c). Appropriate options for individuals in this category include arm ergometry and wheelchair ergometry. Both means of training yield rather similar gains in physical conditioning (Boldin & Lundegren, 1985), and gains made on the arm ergometer are transferable to wheelchair ambulation (Sedlock, Knowlton, & Fitzgerald, 1988).

Physiological and Biochemical Effects of Aerobic Training

Aerobic training induces changes that within a few hours affect acute responses to a single bout of vigorous exercise (Blomqvist & Saltin, 1983). Distinction may be drawn between these early "regulatory" changes, which are mediated by neural and hormonal mechanisms, and later "structural" adaptations (Holmgren, 1967a), although both contribute to a progressive increase in maximal oxygen intake.

Magnitude of Overall Response

Typically, the final gain in aerobic power is between 5% and 30%. However, the magnitude of response varies with the initial aerobic fitness of the subject, the pattern of training that is adopted (Pollock, 1973; Shephard, 1965, 1968b, 1975), the proportion of slow-twitch muscle fibers (Rusko & Rahkila, 1983), and the subject's persistence with the training program. When subjects have been initially deconditioned by bed rest or some medical condition and their dose of exercise has been increased progressively over years rather than weeks, gains in maximal oxygen intake have sometimes been as large as 100% (Saltin et al., 1968; Shephard, 1981; see Figure 4.2).

Particularly after high-intensity interval training, there is also an increased tolerance for anaerobic effort. This reflects alterations of tissue-buffering capacity and increases of muscle enzyme activity (Gollnick & Hermansen, 1973), a greater tolerance for muscle pain and dyspnea, and the physical consequences of an increased lean-tissue mass. Thus trained subjects are able to undertake prolonged bouts of exercise at levels much closer to their maximal oxygen intake than those who are untrained, and they show a corresponding increase of aerobic capacity.

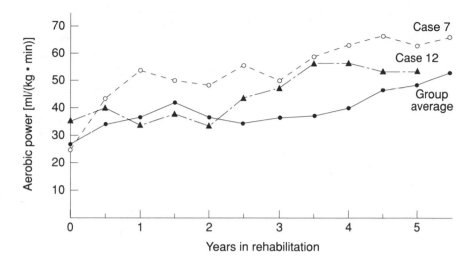

Figure 4.2 Increase in maximal oxygen intake during progressive endurance training. Average curve for 14 postcoronary patients who trained for a marathon race; individual lines are for 2 subjects who showed an exceptionally large response. *Note.* Adapted from Shephard (1981) by permission.

Training may also increase the mechanical efficiency of exercise, particularly in older subjects, so that more work can be accomplished for a given oxygen delivery (Mertens et al., 1978). In addition to choosing more economical movement patterns and developing specific skills, the subject may show a better coordination of overall muscular contraction, a more effective relaxation of antagonists, a better control of body sway, and sometimes a reduction of respiratory work rate, the last being associated with a more efficient pattern of breathing.

Cardiac Performance

A variety of regulatory and structural responses can augment cardiac performance as training proceeds; changes include a slowing of resting heart rate and thus an increase of heart rate reserve, an increase of stroke volume both at rest and during exercise, and an increase in the physical dimensions of the heart.

HEART RATE. Perhaps the most obvious and earliest of the training-induced changes is a decrease of heart rate (Scheuer & Tipton, 1977), both at rest and at a fixed intensity of submaximal exercise. Khosla and Campbell (1982) classified marathon runners into three groups, depending on their race times, and found resting heart rates of 51, 63, and 68 beats/min for the best, average, and poorest performers, respectively. Schoenfield, Keren, Birnfield, and Sohar (1981) and Laird and Campbell (1988) also reported substantial inverse correlations between resting heart rates and aerobic fitness. Pollock (1973) noted that the conclusion drawn from 19 reports was that aerobic training decreased the heart rate by 6.6 beats/min under resting conditions and by 3.9 beats/min during maximal exercise.

The main reason for the development of a resting bradycardia seems to be increased parasympathetic nerve activity (Raab & Krzywanek, 1966; M.J. Smith, Hudson, Gratitzer, & Raven, 1989), possibly reflecting a change in the bradycardic activity of the arterial baroreceptors (Gwirtz, Brandt, Mass, & Jones, 1990). The acetylcholine content of the atria also increases, and excised atrial muscle from aerobically trained animals has a low intrinsic rate of contraction (Nylander, Sigvardsson, & Kilbom, 1982; M.J. Smith et al., 1989). During exercise, these changes may be further modulated by a reduced drive from the peripheral metaboreceptors of strengthened muscles (Mitchell & Schmidt, 1983) and alterations in the numbers or the sensitivity of the cardiac beta-adrenergic receptors, particularly as the heart hypertrophies (Brundin & Cernigliaro, 1975; H.K. Hammond, White, Brunton, & Longhurst, 1987; Jost, Weiss, & Weicker, 1989).

Bradycardia decreases the cardiac work rate and also facilitates perfusion of the myocardium (Scott, 1967), both changes improving the relative oxygen supply to the heart muscle.

STROKE VOLUME.   The stroke volume, both at rest and at all levels of physical activity, is increased by aerobic training (H.J. Green, Jones, & Painter, 1990; Wolfe & Cunningham, 1978). The improved ventricular performance reflects, in part, an increase of ventricular preloading; this is secondary to an increase of peripheral venous tone, an increase in plasma volume of up to 10% (Convertino, 1991; Holmgren, 1967a), and a faster peak lengthening rate of the left ventricle during diastole (Fagard et al., 1989; Matsuda et al., 1983). There is also an increase of myocardial contractility (Krzeminski, Niewiadomski, & Nazar, 1989; G.S. Morris, Baldwin, Lash, Hamlin, & Sherman, 1990), with an increase of cardiac ejection fraction for any given conditions of pre- and afterloading of the ventricles (Molé, 1978). Finally, there is usually some reduction of blood pressure, and thus of afterloading (Tipton, 1984, 1991).

Aerobic training per se does not have a great influence on the dimensions of the skeletal muscles (Saltin, Henriksson, Nygaard, & Andersen, 1977), but if resisted exercises are included in the conditioning program, then a progressive hypertrophy of the skeletal muscles occurs. As the skeletal muscles become stronger and contract at a smaller fraction of their maximal voluntary force, there is a lesser, exercise-induced rise of blood pressure (Lind & McNicol, 1967). This reduces both afterloading and the cardiac work rate at any given intensity of exercise, so that it becomes easier to sustain stroke volume at high external work rates (Bunc, Heller, Moravec, & Sprynarova, 1989; Niinimaa & Shephard, 1978).

CARDIAC OUTPUT.   Given that aerobic training induces a substantial increase of stroke volume, and at most a minor decrease of maximal heart rate, the overall cardiovascular response to an endurance conditioning program is an increase of maximal cardiac output. Given also that cardiac output is the primary determinant of oxygen transport, it is not surprising that the gains in maximal cardiac output and maximal oxygen intake are closely correlated (Rowell, 1974).

During submaximal exercise, a combination of some increase in muscle capillarity, less compression of the muscle blood vessels during the active phase of muscle contraction, and an increase of sarcoplasmic enzyme activity may allow the aerobically trained subject to sustain a given oxygen consumption with a smaller increase of cardiac output (Clausen, Klausen, Rasmussen, & Trap-Jensen, 1973).

CARDIAC VOLUME. The large hearts of international-class endurance athletes are well documented (George, Wolfe, & Burggaf, 1991; Marganroth & Maron, 1977; Rost & Hollmann, 1983, 1992; Shapiro, 1987), as is the cardiac hypertrophy that occurs with valvular stenosis. It is less clear how far similar adaptations of ventricular dimensions occur in response to the more modest aerobic training efforts of the average adult (Snoeckx et al., 1983).

Endurance training seems to favor an increase of left ventricular diastolic dimensions rather than an increase of wall thickness (Cohen & Segal, 1985), and indeed Mickelson, Byrd, Bouchard, Botvinik, and Schiller (1986) found no relationship between heart size and 10-km or marathon-running performance. Hagan, Laird, and Gettman (1985) pointed out that, whereas marathon runners appeared to have large hearts when volumes were expressed per kilogram of body mass, much of this advantage reflected no more than a low level of body fat. When the data were expressed per unit of lean tissue, only the interseptal thickness was increased.

Depending on the intensity of aerobic training, and possibly the genetic characteristics of the individual participant (Landry, Bouchard, & Dumesnil, 1985; Lortie et al., 1984), some myocardial hypertrophy may occur nevertheless (Blomqvist & Saltin, 1983; Hickson, Kanakis, J.R. Davis, Moore, & Rich, 1982; Shapiro, 1987), particularly in the posterior ventricular wall and septum (Cox, Bennett, & Dudley, 1986; Northcote, McKillop, Todd, & Canning, 1990; Snoeckx et al., 1982; Tharp, Thorland, Johnson, & Peter, 1986; Wolfe, Cunningham, & Boughner, 1986). Such changes facilitate the development of a large stroke volume in the well-trained person.

Changes in Blood and Arteriovenous Oxygen Difference

In the early stages of aerobic training, expansion of the plasma volume may cause a relative anemia, that is, a decreased blood hemoglobin concentration despite a normal total hemoglobin (H.J. Green et al., 1984; H.J. Green et al., 1987; J.H. Ross & Attwood, 1984). This limits the trainee's maximal arteriovenous oxygen difference.

As endurance training continues, there is a gradual increase of erythropoiesis (Schmidt, Maasen, Trost, & Böning, 1988; Szygula, 1990), but red cell formation may still be hampered by low iron stores in bone marrow and a low serum ferritin (Clement & Amundson, 1982; Fredrickson et al., 1980; Weight & Noakes, in press). Other factors exacerbating the tendency to anemia include visceral hemorrhage (Eichner, 1989; J.G. Stewart et al., 1984), a more ready deformation of red cells (Lorlin, Beck, & Kinnear, 1979), an increase of red cell fragility (Puhl et al., 1981), and (in runners) an increase of hemolysis as red cells pass through the blood vessels of the feet (Newhouse & Clement, 1988; O'Toole, Hiller, Roalstad, & Douglas, 1988) with a resultant decrease of serum haptoglobins (Spitler, Alexander, Hoffler, Doerr, & Buchanan, 1984). Because the average age of the red cells decreases during endurance training (Brodthagen et al., 1985), the 2,3-diphosphoglycerate level rises (Smalley, Runyan, & Puhl, 1981; Veicsteinas et al., 1984), the oxygen affinity of the hemoglobin decreases (Mairbäurl, Humpeler, Schwaberger, & Pessenhofer, 1983), and individual cells also may have a below-normal hemoglobin content.

The maximal arteriovenous oxygen difference is generally widened a little by aerobic training (Roskamm, 1973; Simmons & Shephard, 1971a). Given that the maximal oxygen extraction of the working muscles is fairly complete even in an untrained subject, any increase of arteriovenous difference should not be attributed to an enhanced activity of aerobic enzymes in the skeletal musculature. Rather, it reflects a change in the distribution of peripheral blood flow during maximal effort (Simmons & Shephard, 1971a). In particular, blood is redirected from the skin and viscera, where little oxygen would be extracted, to the working muscles, where oxygen extraction is almost complete.

Any acute, exercise-induced increase of fibrinolytic activity lasts for only a few minutes, and this response is not consistently enhanced by aerobic training (Bourey & Santorio, 1988). However, there have been suggestions that the platelets are less active and thus clump less readily after a subject has participated in an aerobic conditioning program (R.B. Davis, Boyd, McKinney, & Jones, 1990; Rauramaa & Salonen, in press; Sinzinger & Virgolini, 1988).

Blood Pressure

As discussed further in chapter 5, training tends to reduce the resting blood pressure by 0.7 to 1.3 kPa, or 5 to 10 mm Hg (Tipton, 1984, 1991). In conjunction with the slower heart rate, this change decreases the double-product (systolic pressure × heart rate, an approximate measure of the work of the heart). The afterloading is also reduced, which allows a larger stroke volume for a given ventricular effort.

Because of training-induced improvements of myocardial contractility or an increased coronary blood flow, the aerobically trained subject may be able to develop a higher, peak systolic blood pressure during exercise. This type of response is particularly likely if myocardial function was initially limited by ischemia (Kavanagh, Shephard, Chisholm, Qureshi, & Kennedy, 1979). The increased peak stroke volume usually leads to some increase in the peak pulse pressure.

Microcirculation and Coronary Perfusion

Debate continues on the ability of aerobic training to augment the perfusion of either cardiac or skeletal muscle (Kavanagh, 1989; Laughlin, McAllister, & Delp, in press). Among postulated responses are regulatory and structural changes that would increase the cross-sectional diameter of large or small arteries and veins and increase the number of capillaries per gram of muscle.

Animal-training experiments have demonstrated a number of responses likely to improve oxygen delivery to the heart muscle, including increased dimensions of the coronary arterial tree (Haslam & Cobb, 1982; Ho, Roy, Taylor, Heusner, & Van Huss, 1983; Stevenson, 1967; D.P. Thomas, 1985), capillary proliferation (Mattfeldt, Krämer, Zeitz, & Mall, 1986), an increase of total capillary length (Rakusan, Wicker, Abdul-Samad, Healy, & Turcz, 1987), greater capillary density (Tamaki, 1987), and an enhanced collateral blood flow (demonstrated by Eckstein, 1957, but not by Schaper, 1982). In general, such gains are uniform throughout the myocardium, although one study of endurance-trained rats reported a response localized to the right ventricular wall.

Most observations on human subjects have failed to demonstrate any significant changes in the coronary vasculature during aerobic training (Pearl, 1987). Nevertheless, the slower heart rate of the well-trained person allows a relative extension of the diastolic phase of the cardiac cycle, when most of the left ventricular perfusion occurs (Scott, 1967). Thus, even if a moderate dose of aerobic training has no direct influence on coronary vascular dimensions, the combination of a prolonged diastolic phase and a reduction of cardiac work rate may substantially improve the ratio of coronary blood flow to myocardial oxygen demand.

Other factors that may further improve myocardial perfusion in the aerobically trained individual include an altered coronary vascular response to vasoactive substances, changes in endothelium-mediated vasoregulation, and alterations in the mechanisms governing the concentration of intracellular free-calcium ions in endothelial and vascular smooth muscle cells (Laughlin et al., in press). Endurance training blunts endothelium-mediated vasodilatation in the large coronary arteries and has little effect on the response of small arteries, but it enhances the vasodilator response in the critical region of the resistance-sized coronary arterioles.

There is generally some increase in the capillarity of skeletal muscle in response to aerobic training. Gains are largest around the muscle fibers that are most involved in the training program (Shephard & Plyley, 1992).

Respiratory Performance

The effects of aerobic training on the respiratory system must generally be inferred from rather unsatisfying cross-sectional data. Comparisons of well-trained athletes with sedentary individuals show only minor differences in static lung volumes, respiratory muscle strength, mechanical characteristics of the lungs and airways, and pulmonary diffusing capacity (Shephard, 1987b).

A large vital capacity has been described among participants in sports that develop the shoulder muscles (e.g., rowing) and in swimming, where a large lung volume confers the advantage of buoyancy. Endurance training does not enhance vital capacity unless specific resistance exercises are introduced to strengthen the respiratory muscles (Leith & Bradley, 1976); but it may increase the endurance of the chest muscles and thus minimize the loss of respiratory performance that would otherwise follow a prolonged bout of exercise (Coast, Clifford, Henrich, Stray-Gunderson, & Johnson, 1990).

Aerobic training also seems to reduce the time required to reach a steady level of ventilation at the onset of exercise, the ventilatory on-transient (Beaver & Wasserman, 1970; Bunc, Heller, & Lesso, 1988), and it lowers the steady-state ventilation rate at any given level of oxygen consumption. The ventilatory demands of effort are decreased in a well-conditioned person because of (1) an overall increase of muscular efficiency, (2) a centrally mediated decrease in ventilatory drive (Miyamura & Ishida, 1990), (3) a possible reduction in the sensitivity of the carotid chemoreceptors or their central connections (Byrne-Quinn, Weil, Sodal, Filley, & Grover, 1971; B.J. Martin, Sparks, Zwillich, & Weil, 1979), and (4) a lesser production of lactate in severe effort, due to a faster on-transient, the ability to undertake a given task at a smaller fraction of maximal oxygen intake, and an improved perfusion of the working muscles.

The increase in peak respiratory minute volume roughly parallels the training-induced gain in aerobic power. Pollock (1973) noted an average 9.8% increase of peak ventilation in 18 aerobic-training studies. Robinson and Kjellgaard (1982) found that after 20 weeks of aerobic training, there was a strengthening of the expiratory muscles, reflected in a 14% increase in maximal expiratory pressures. Top endurance athletes can develop respiratory minute volumes as large as 160 L/min. Such a level of ventilation would be uneconomic for an untrained individual, because respiratory efforts would have surpassed the cross-over point (Shephard, 1966a), where the cost of any additional ventilation exceeds the resulting increase in oxygen delivery (see Chapter 3).

The cross-over point is displaced to a progressively higher respiratory minute volume during aerobic training, because of the increase of peak pulmonary blood flow and an associated augmentation of peak pulmonary diffusing capacity (Anderson & Shephard, 1968b). Nevertheless, well-trained individuals are driven closer to the functional limits of the system with respect to (1) the capacity to generate inspiratory pressures, (2) inspiratory muscle fatigue during prolonged effort, (3) expiratory collapse of the airways, and (4) incomplete alveolar-arterial equilibration in pulmonary capillaries with a rapid transit time (Dempsey & Babcock, in press).

Body Fat

The percent body fat is potentially reduced by an aerobic training regimen, provided that the exerciser does not counter the added energy expenditure with an increased intake of food. Pollock (1973) noted that in 18 adult studies of such training, body fat decreased by an average of 0% to 3.8%; in general, losses were greater after long periods of walking than after shorter periods of jogging (Pollock, Dimmick, Miller, Kendrick, & Linnerud, 1975). Sidney, Shephard, and Harrison (1977) found that 3 months of aerobic training reduced the estimated percent body fat of 65-year-old subjects by an average of 2.7%, without any need for deliberate dietary restriction. In these experiments, the average skinfold thickness decreased by 3.3 mm, corresponding to some 75% of the increment of subcutaneous fat that had occurred over the adult life of these subjects (see Table 4.3).

A substantially increased energy expenditure is needed to induce such responses, and a minimal aerobic exercise prescription with no control of diet may have little effect on a person with established obesity. Any exercise-induced changes of body composition reflect not only the energy cost of the activity that is undertaken, but also possible small, upward adjustments of postexercise metabolism (Gore & Withers, 1990; J.O. Hill, in press), postprandial metabolism, and basal metabolic rate (Butterfield & Tremblay, in press; J.O. Hill, in press) relative to dieting without exercise. Fat loss seems to occur more readily in men than in women (Murray, Shephard, Greaves, Allen, & Radomski, 1986; Després, in press), perhaps because of gender differences in fat metabolism, and is facilitated if the subjects are exposed to a cold environment during the exercise sessions (O'Hara, Allen, Shephard, & Allen, 1979). In men, the fat loss occurs selectively from the trunk, particularly the abdomen (Després, Bouchard, Tremblay, Savard, & Marcotte, 1985; Schwartz et al., 1991), whereas in women, the larger portion of any fat loss is from the hips and thighs.

Fat loss may result in a decrease of body mass, and if so, the training-induced increase of relative oxygen intake, Δ μmol/(kg·s), will be larger than the absolute gain, Δ mmol/min. More commonly, an exercise-centered program leads to the preservation, or even a gain, of lean tissue, so that the total body mass is unchanged. Unfortunately, this point is rarely understood by clinicians, many of whom still watch for a weight loss as evidence of a favorable response from the patient enrolled in an exercise program (Sidney et al., 1977). It is unclear how much influence the increase of lean mass has on the increase in resting metabolic rate as participation in the exercise regimen continues.

Table 4.3
Decrease of Skinfold Thickness and Estimated Loss of Percent Body Fat With Participation of 65-yr-old Subjects In Self-Selected 14-Week Training Program

Variable	Self-selected regimen			
	HF,HI[a]	LF,HI[a]	HF,LI[a]	LF,LI[a]
Skinfold[b] (mm)	3.1	1.9	2.9	1.4
Percent body fat	2.7	2.4	2.0	1.9

Note. Reprinted from Sidney et al. (1977) by permission.
[a]HF, high-frequency; LF, low-frequency; HI, high-intensity; LI, low-intensity; [b]Average of 8 skinfolds.

Both the size and the triglyceride content of individual fat cells are reduced by aerobic training (A.W. Taylor, 1979), although the total number of fat cells remains unchanged (Salans, Horton, & Sims, 1971; Tremblay, in press). Sedentary individuals already mobilize large amounts of fat during exercise, so aerobic training may induce only slightly increased lipolysis of body fat deposits (Stefanik & Wood, in press). The sensitivity of the beta-adrenergic receptors increases, particularly in lean subjects, so that more free fatty acids are liberated in response to a given secretion of catecholamines (Gollnick, 1971; Tremblay, in press), but this change is offset by a reduced secretion of catecholamine. The activity of the adipose tissue lipoprotein lipase is also increased, as is insulin-stimulated glucose transport. These responses facilitate the clearing of triglycerides from the bloodstream after eating and speed the replenishment of body fat stores, thus reducing the risks of diabetes and atherosclerosis (Vranic & Wasserman, 1990).

Muscle

Aerobic training causes only limited gains in skeletal muscle size even in the active muscles (Jansson & Kaijser, 1977; Nygaard et al., 1977; Saltin et al., 1977; Sidney et al., 1977). Gains in muscle force are also limited, and muscles not involved in the training program may even lose strength (Harmon, Maughan, & Nimmo, 1987). But at the cellular level, skeletal and cardiac muscle show changes in a variety of proteins, including contractile, regulatory, structural, and metabolic proteins (Faulkner, Green, & White, in press).

Individual skeletal muscle fibers show some hypertrophy through an increase in the number of myofibrils, but there is no significant increase in the total number of muscle fibers. The link between regular physical activity and the hypertrophy of skeletal muscle seems to be related to the development of tension, although details of the mechanism are far from clear. The increase in fiber cross-sectional area apparently arises from a decrease of catabolism rather than an enhancement of protein synthesis (Watt, Kelly, Goldspink, & Goldspink, 1982). Typically, the individual who has completed a program of aerobic training shows an increase in the relative number and size of Type I (slow-twitch) fibers and an abundance of sarcolemmal mitochondria close to the capillaries (Crenshaw, Friden, Thornell, & Hargens, 1991; Howald, 1982). A purely aerobic training program may cause a decrease in Type II (fast-twitch) fiber area (Harmon et al., 1987).

Vigorous aerobic training also leads to a proliferation of capillaries between muscle fibers, in regions where a sharing of vascular supply can occur. Several months of moderate aerobic training increase muscle capillarity by at least 20% to 30% (Ingjer, 1979; Klausen, Andersen, & Pelle, 1981; Sexton, Korthuis, & Laughlin, 1988; Shephard & Plyley, 1992), and gains of 40% to 50% are possible with more rigorous conditioning (Ingjer, 1979). There is disagreement as to whether aerobic training increases muscle myoglobin content; Nemeth, Chi, Hintz, and Lowry (1982) saw such an effect, but Jansson, Sylvén, and Sjödin (1982) did not.

An increase in the activity of aerobic enzymes slows muscle glycogen utilization and lactate accumulation. Over 2 to 4 months of progressive aerobic exercise, the activity of aerobic enzymes in the muscle fibers increases by 20% to 40% (Gollnick & Hermansen, 1973; Henriksson & Reitman, 1977; Howald, 1975, 1982). It is unlikely that enzyme changes contribute greatly to endurance performance when the subject is undertaking a large-muscle task; such activities are limited primarily by the pumping ability of the heart (see chapter 2). However, the enzymatic changes redirect metabolism from carbohydrates to fats, thus conserving intramuscular glycogen stores. This process is enhanced by the increased capillary-fiber ratio. Repeated bouts of aerobic exercise also increase muscle lipoprotein lipase activity and thus the ability of the skeletal muscle fibers to transport fatty acids into the cells. This further conserves local reserves of carbohydrates and delays the onset of metabolic acidosis during aerobic exercise (Stefanik & Wood, in press).

Skeletal System

The biomechanical forces imposed by repeated bouts of aerobic exercise alter the metabolism and the structure of the various types of connective tissue in the skeletal system (A.C. Vailas & J.C. Vailas, in press). Given the difficulties in measuring the forces imposed on the system, inferences regarding the effects of such exercise have been drawn from the resultant structural changes. The amount of connective tissue is commonly proportional to the applied force, and its architecture is determined by the axis along which the force is applied.

However, the response of connective tissue to a training regimen is also modified by biological factors:

1. Age—The deterioration of bone structure in a woman occurs most readily if she is inactive during the perimenopausal years, and in both sexes, aging increases the risk of osteoporosis
2. Diet—The synthesis of hydroxyproline requires an adequate intake of vitamin C, and body reserves of calcium and vitamin D are also important to bone formation
3. Endocrine status—Aerobic training that is pushed to the point of hypogonadism has a negative effect on the bone health of young women (Drinkwater et al., 1984; Drinkwater et al., 1986), and hormone replacement therapy is an important adjuvant for those who are suffering from postmenopausal osteoporosis
4. Environment—For example, exposure to sunshine facilitates the synthesis of vitamin D

Regular physical activity enhances not only anabolic but also catabolic activity, so that there is a faster turnover of connective tissue. Thus, participation in a marathon race may lead to increases in plasma levels of amino acids such as hydroxyproline. It is thought that physical activity accelerates the resorption of mature collagen, but the formation of younger protein proceeds more rapidly

(Karpakka, Väänänen, Orava, & Takala, 1990; Suominen & Heikkinen, 1975), thus decreasing the cross-linkages between the collagen fibrils that would otherwise impair elasticity (A.C. Vailas & J.C. Vailas, in press; Viidik, 1973). At the same time, the strength of the tendons increases (Kiiskinen & Heikkinen, 1975), and they become more firmly attached to bone (Tipton, Matthes, & A.C. Vailas, 1977). Animal experiments suggest that these changes occur more readily in males than in females (A. Adams, 1966).

The joint capsule becomes more flexible (Chapman, DeVries, & Sweezey, 1972) and articular cartilages become thicker and more resilient to compression as a result of regular aerobic training (Holmdahl & Ingelmark, 1948). There is no evidence that reasonable use of a joint predisposes it to osteoarthritis, even over many years (Lane et al., 1986; Panush & D.G. Brown, 1987). Indeed, the flexibility that is important to continued independence seems better conserved in old people who continue to follow a program of regular exercise (Bassey, Morgan, Dalloso, & Ebrahim, 1989).

Bones are also strengthened by moderate aerobic training (E.L. Smith, Smith, & Gilligan, 1990), due to stimulation of local osteogenesis, increased mineral and hydroxyproline content (Kiiskinen & Heikkinen, 1975), increased density (D.W. King & Pengelly, 1973; Zylstra, Hopkins, Erk, Hreshchyshyn, and Anbar, 1989), and enhancement of their architecture through the development of new trabeculae (Ross, 1950). However, responses are less than anticipated in those who follow a weight-lifting regimen (Heinrich et al., 1990), particularly if the amount of aerobic training is excessive (Bilanin, Blanchard, & Russek-Cohen, 1989; Michel, Block, & Fries, 1989).

The stimulus for these changes comes in part from the force of muscle contraction, but for maximal benefit, body mass or some external load must be displaced against gravitational forces.

Central Nervous System

Some types of motor activity correlate positively to the academic performance of young children, although it is difficult to be certain of the direction of the relationship; higher levels of cognition may facilitate performance of the required training program, rather than the converse (J.R. Thomas, Salazar, & Landers, in press). Volle, Shephard, et al. (1982) and Volle, Tisal, et al. (1982) demonstrated that higher academic marks were achieved by primary-school children who were given additional physical education classes, relative to their peers who were not. They noted an apparent link between academic achievement and gains in psychomotor processing. Even if further research eliminates the suggestion of a causal relationship between regular aerobic exercise and enhanced mental performance, these observations remain an important argument to counter those who claim that a school curriculum is too crowded to allow the investment of additional time in physically active pursuits.

Available information suggests that movement speeds are faster in fit than in sedentary individuals, particularly in old age. Active individuals have faster scores on a variety of psychomotor and cognitive tests (Hollmann, in press). Such apparent benefits of regular endurance exercise perhaps could be explained by the mutual association of factors that optimize sensory-motor function, such as socioeconomic status, intelligence, motivation, and pattern of reactions (a focus upon the signal rather than the response). Nevertheless, there is some longitudinal data suggesting that training can induce this type of response (Spirduso, 1980; Tomporowski & Ellis, 1986).

Metabolic and Hormonal Responses

Aerobic training induces important changes both in the resting levels and in the response of many hormonal systems, including changes in the secretion, binding, metabolism, and excretion of potent compounds. We shall here concentrate on changes in catecholamines and metabolic, fluid-regulating, and reproductive hormones; a full discussion is offered in Shephard, 1983a.

CATECHOLAMINES.   Resting concentrations of noradrenaline and adrenaline are generally unchanged by aerobic training (Richter & Sutton, in press). During exercise, there is usually a reduced secretion of catecholamines (Hartley, 1975), in part because the individual has become habituated to the sensations of exercise. Because of an increase in peak power output, the aerobically trained person can also undertake a given task at a lower relative intensity of stress; however, if reactions are tested at a fixed percentage of maximal aerobic power, the catecholamine response is little affected. There are important alterations in the number and sensitivity of receptors in many parts of the body. For instance, aerobic training substantially increases the sensitivity of adipocytes to catecholamines (Richter & Sutton, in press).

METABOLIC REGULATION.   Glucose tolerance is substantially improved with aerobic training. A large part of the observed change reflects an upward shift in the sensitivity or density of the tissue-insulin receptors (Vranic & Wasserman, 1990). Aerobic training increases the binding of insulin in formerly sedentary subjects (Shephard, 1983a), thus decreasing fasting concentrations of insulin (Richter & Sutton, in press). However, binding is decreased during exercise, and the output of catecholamines at a given power output is also reduced (Shephard, 1983a), so that blood insulin levels are usually higher after aerobic training at a fixed work rate (Bloom, Johnson, Park, Rennie, & Sulaiman, 1976; Hartley et al., 1972). In contrast, there is less increase of the opposing glucagon level in trained than in untrained subjects.

Prolonged, vigorous exercise causes a substantial secretion of growth hormone in primarily sedentary subjects, increasing blood levels of fatty acids as intramuscular glycogen stores become depleted (Shephard & Sidney, 1975). But aerobic training usually lessens the output of growth hormone at a given intensity of effort, possibly because alternative pathways for the mobilization of fatty acids are exploited after such conditioning.

Cortisol also contributes to the mobilization of fat and protein, stimulating hepatic gluconeogenesis and conserving muscle glycogen. The response to aerobic training depends on the intensity of the program; moderate training increases plasma cortisol levels, but overtraining leads to exhaustion and depletion of glucocorticoids (Shephard & Sidney, 1975).

The thyroid hormone can also play a role in the mobilization of fatty acids during prolonged exercise, probably by enhancing the normal lipolytic response to noradrenaline. Thyroxine turnover may be increased after a program of aerobic training (Terjung & Winder, 1975), and free thyroxine levels also are also usually increased, although apparently without an increase in resting metabolic rate. But in females who exercise to the point of amenorrhea, the level of T3 may be reduced.

FLUID-REGULATING HORMONES.   Changes in the plasma concentrations of fluid-regulating hormones contribute to the rapid expansion of plasma volume that accompanies aerobic training (H.J. Green et al., 1990). During vigorous aerobic exercise, a fall of venous pressure reduces renal flow, liberating renin, increasing the output of angiotensin and stimulating secretion of aldosterone by the adrenal cortex (Shephard, 1983a). This hormone stimulates the retention of sodium and potassium ions, which encourages an expansion of plasma volume. Aerobic training also speeds the hepatic clearance of aldosterone from the bloodstream (Frenkl, Györe, Meszaros, & Szeberenyi, 1980).

Reproductive Hormones

In men, a decrease in resting levels of plasma testosterone and in women, the appearance of hypothalamic hypogonadism (Prior, 1990) in part reflect an alteration in the body's balance of anabolism and catabolism. With very heavy endurance training, there is a reduction in plasma testosterone levels in men, and possibly a temporary decrease in sperm count and fertility (Prior, 1990). In women, the disturbance of reproductive hormone secretion may lead to amenorrhea, or an abbreviated luteal phase of the menstrual cycle, with abnormally low serum-progesterone levels.

These hormonal changes apparently represent the body's attempt to avoid conception and pregnancy when protein and energy intake do not meet the demands imposed by physical activity. The responses are influenced by the intensity of effort, any associated stress (e.g., thermal or emotional), and the total increase of energy expenditure relative to the available food supply. An adverse combination of these various stimuli leads, in both sexes, to a suppression of the gonadotropin-releasing-hormone pulse generator in the hypothalamus (Loucks, in press; Warren, in press). Clinical consequences include temporary infertility, a loss of bone mineral, which may have more long-lasting consequences for bone health, and (in women) a loss of the beneficial influence of estrogens on lipoproteins, which leaves the affected individuals more vulnerable to ischemic heart disease.

Immune Responses

A moderate dose of aerobic training can reduce any adverse response of the immune system to a given bout of exercise (Shephard, Verde, et al., 1991). On the other hand, a period of high-intensity training, pushed to the point of over-training, can have a number of negative consequences for the immune system (Mackinnon, 1992). It reduces the ratio of CD-4 (helper) to CD-8 (suppressor) T cells, decreases the response of T cells to mitogen stimulation in vitro, decreases the bactericidal activity of monocytes, reduces the levels of complements C-3 and C-4, decreases the synthesis of antibodies, and lowers antiglobulin levels in saliva and blood (Newsholme, in press; Shephard, Verde, et al., 1991). In consequence, the affected individual becomes more vulnerable to bacterial and viral infections (Niemann et al., 1990), and the healing of any injuries is slowed.

A depression of immune responses is most likely to occur if very intensive, prolonged aerobic training is combined with some other emotional or environmental stress (e.g., preparing for a major athletic competition). Another important contributing factor is an inadequate diet, particularly one deficient in glutamine. A high rate of glutamine utilization is essential to a rapid response of lymphocytes when the immune system is challenged (Newsholme, in press). The release of glutamine from muscle is facilitated by increases in blood levels of thyroxine, growth hormone, and endotoxin, but is inhibited by high catecholamine levels. (The influence of aerobic training on blood levels of these hormones has been discussed previously.)

Nature of Training Stimulus

If a training response is observed, it is probably a reaction to functional overload (Pelosi & Agliati, 1968). The immediate response to a single bout of vigorous exercise is a slowing of protein synthesis (Swartman, Cook, & P.B. Taylor, 1978) and an increase of protein catabolism (Bozner & Meessen, 1969; Hatt, Ledoux, Bonvalet, & Guillemat, 1965), the latter being shown by an increase in plasma urea concentration (Kavanagh & Shephard, 1975), an increased excretion of nitrogen in sweat and urine, and the production of carbon dioxide from amino acids—as indicated by the metabolism of labelled leucine and glycine (Rennie, Bowtell, & Millward, in press). Particularly when an exercise bout is sufficiently prolonged to deplete glycogen stores, there is a rapid efflux of alanine and glutamine from muscle, and the loss of the latter appears to limit protein synthesis, both in muscle cells and in the immune system. However, supranormal rates of protein synthesis are observed within 24 hr of a bout of strenuous aerobic exercise (Sobel & Kaufman, 1970). The immediate stimulus to enhanced protein synthesis may be an increased concentration of amino acids in the cytoplasm. Stretching of the cell membrane during overload could also facilitate entry of amino acids into the active fibers (Poortmans, 1978). Catecholamines may activate a protein kinase, removing inhibition of RNA polymerase and allowing the aggregation of ribosomes into polyribosomes, which results in increased protein synthesis (Poortmans, 1978).

Increases in the blood levels of pituitary growth hormone, testosterone, thyroid hormone, and insulin are not essential to hypertrophy, but these hormones may serve as linear amplifiers of the overload-induced changes (Gollnick, 1971). It is probable that the daily nitrogen intake must exceed commonly accepted dietary norms, if anabolic activity is to be maximized.

Variations in the Pattern of Training

The pattern of training to be recommended depends on the individual's objectives. The competitive athlete is usually anxious to maximize performance on the specific day when a major competition is to be held, though both immediate psychosocial health and long-term medical and surgical prospects may be sacrificed in meeting this goal. In contrast, the average, middle-aged person wishes to know the minimum exercise prescription that will assure a reasonable level of health in later years. For older people, there may be a quite narrow margin between a regimen that will satisfy health objectives, yet not exceed a safe ceiling of intensity or duration, and one that could prove dangerous.

The recommendation of an appropriate pattern of training for the average person presupposes a detailed knowledge of dose-response relationships and of the interactions of initial fitness with the intensity, frequency, and duration of the prescribed conditioning activity (see Figure 4.3). Unfortunately, there is little information about patterns of training that will maximize health benefits. Moreover, given the large number of variables involved (Pollock, 1973; Shephard, 1975), it is unlikely that a clear verdict will be forthcoming for many years. Nevertheless, the American College of Sports Medicine (1978, 1990, 1991) and the American Heart Association (1981) each have advanced tentative proposals regarding the optimum intensity, frequency, and duration of exercise training sessions. The recommendations of the American College of Sports Medicine changed substantially from 1978 to 1990, reflecting a clearer distinction between physical performance and health-related aspects of fitness.

Intensity

Many of the current suggestions regarding the optimal intensity of an aerobic training prescription can be traced to the work of Karvonen, Klemola, Virkajarvi, and Kekkonen (1957). These Finnish investigators exercised young, male university students for 30 min a session, 4 to 5 days a week, and found an improvement of oxygen transport when the training heart rate averaged 150 beats/min but not when it was only 135 beats/min. These observations were first interpreted as a need to exercise at 60% of the heart rate reserve (i.e., the difference between resting and maximal heart rate), or 60% of maximal oxygen intake (Hollmann & Venrath, 1963). Erroneously, others spoke of training at 60% of maximal heart rate. Subsequent observations showed that the lactate threshold of the average sedentary subject was reached at 60% to 70% of maximal oxygen intake (McLellan, 1987; Shephard, 1992c). Thus, alternative recommendations for an effective

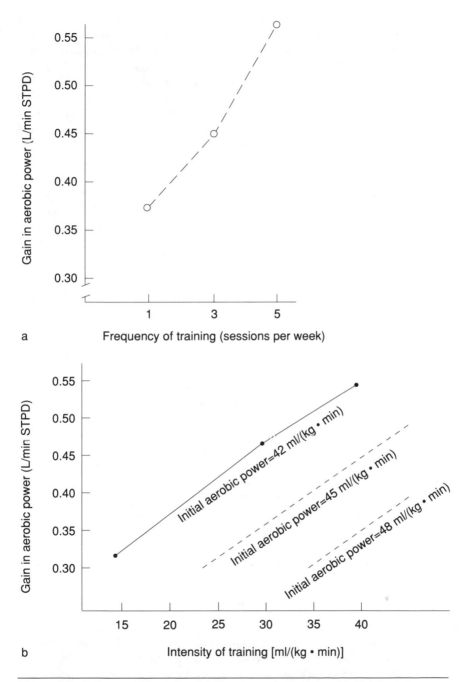

Figure 4.3 Influence of intensity and frequency of exercise and initial fitness on response to training. (a) Effect of frequency if intensity and initial fitness held constant; (b) effect of intensity and initial fitness if frequency held constant. *Note.* Adapted from Shephard (1977a) by permission.

aerobic training stimulus were based on the perceptions of breathlessness (Bakers & Tenney, 1970) and perceived exertion (Purvis & Cureton, 1981) at an intensity of exercise that was just below the lactate threshold, that is, at a level of effort that produced some sweating and some dyspnea but still allowed the subject to converse normally. A third approach, based on the relatively linear relationship of heart rate to the overall perception of exertion on the Borg (1971) scale, sought an intensity of effort that was rated as somewhat hard (13 units).

Shephard (1968b) pointed out that whereas the intensity of training was the most important variable in terms of maximizing the increment of oxygen transport, the response of the cardiorespiratory system to any given intensity of effort was also strongly influenced by the initial aerobic fitness of the individual. This observation has been confirmed repeatedly (American College of Sports Medicine, 1990). Although an intensity just below the lactate threshold might be considered appropriate for the aerobic training of relatively sedentary university students, the response of fit, young athletes is best enhanced by training at 90% to 100% of maximal oxygen intake (Wenger & Bell, 1986). In contrast, quite low intensities of aerobic activity can augment oxygen transport in older, very sedentary subjects. For instance, Oja (1983) and Porcari et al. (1987) both found that fast walking was as effective a method of training as jogging for such persons. Likewise, Sidney and Shephard (1978) observed a slow increment of maximal oxygen intake in 65-year-old subjects who exercised 3 to 4 times a week for 14 weeks at heart rates of no more than 120 beats/min (see the HFLI group in Figure 4.4). Immediately following myocardial infarction, the maximal oxygen intake commonly drops to about 70% of the age-related normal value, and in such individuals even heart rates of 110 beats/min can induce some aerobic training (Kavanagh, 1992).

The immediate circumstances of a given bout of physical activity are important when setting a safe ceiling of exercise intensity. The output of catecholamines and the associated heart rate response to a given intensity of aerobic effort are greatly exacerbated by the excitement of competition (Blimkie et al., 1977; also see Figure 4.5) and other strong emotional stimuli (Shephard, 1981). Both the heart rate response to exercise and the associated perception of effort are further increased by either a high or a low environmental temperature, an awkward working posture, exercise of a small-muscle group, or use of the arms above heart level (e.g., when hammering nails into a ceiling; I. Åstrand, 1971).

Duration

The extent of the training response at any given intensity of exercise is affected by the duration of the bout of activity; in other words, the body tends to respond to the amount of added energy expenditure (American College of Sports Medicine, 1990; Shephard, 1968b; Wenger & Bell, 1986). Prolonged training sessions are necessary to induce left ventricular hypertrophy (Douglas, Hiller, & O'Toole, 1987; Elias, Berg, Latin, Mellion, & Hofschire, 1991; Northcote et al., 1990; Ricci et al., 1982). Marathon preparation is also associated with a decrease of

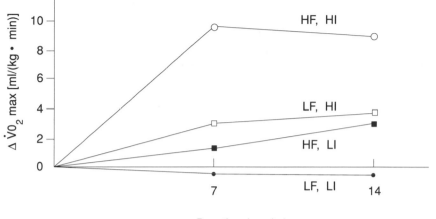

Figure 4.4 Response of 65-year-olds to self-selected, 14-week training regimen. *Note.* Adapted from Sidney and Shephard (1978) by permission. HF, HI = high frequency, high intensity; LF, HI = low frequency, high intensity; HF, LI = high frequency, low intensity; LF, LI = low frequency, low intensity.

both serum cholesterol and systemic blood pressure (Findlay et al., 1987). The lipid profile is favorably influenced by the energy equivalent of jogging 18 to 20 km/week (see Figure 5.1; also Haskell, 1984; Kavanagh, Shephard, Lindley, & Pieper, 1983; P.T. Williams, Wood, Haskell, & Vranizan, 1982).

Although there have been occasional reports of gains in maximal oxygen intake with exercise bouts as short as 5 min a session (Bouchard, Hollmann, Venrath, Herkenrath, & Schlüssel, 1966), most early recommendations specified a minimum duration of 30 min of aerobic activity. Now that the interaction between intensity and duration has been recognized, the recommended duration of aerobic training has shifted to a more flexible 20 to 60 min a session, depending on the intensity of activity (Wenger & Bell, 1986). Gains can be detected with an added energy expenditure of 2 MJ/week, but for maximal cardiovascular benefit, the product of intensity × duration × frequency should be sufficient to assure an added energy expenditure of 8MJ/week (Paffenbarger, 1988). Recent clinical epidemiological studies have emphasized that prolonged sessions of moderate intensity aerobic exercise can make an important contribution to the health of an average adult. Indeed, the largest reductions of morbidity and all-cause mortality have been associated with progression from the lowest levels of aerobic fitness to the next lowest categories of physical condition (S.N. Blair et al., 1989; Leon, Connett, Jacobs, & Rauramaa, 1987).

Frequency

The multiple regression analysis of Shephard (1968b) suggested that increments of aerobic power for any given intensity and duration of effort became progressively

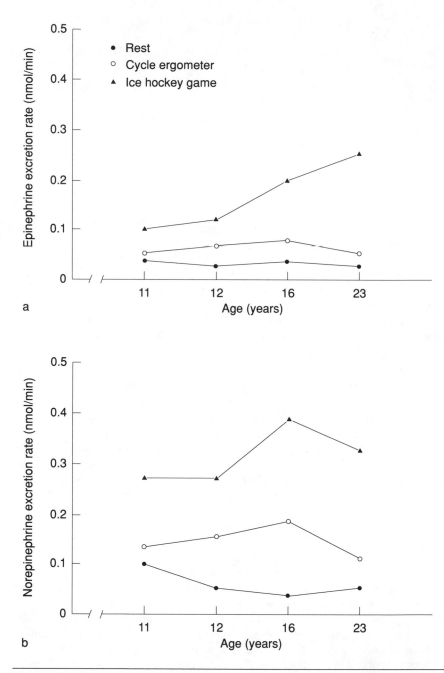

Figure 4.5   Comparison of catecholamine excretion (a. Epinephrine; b. Norepineph-
rine) in response to cycle ergometer exercise and ice hockey game. Comparisons are
for ages 11, 12, 16 and 23 years, with the ice-hockey game becoming progressively
more competitive in the older age categories. Intensity of exercise on cycle ergometer
approximately equivalent to that of hockey game. *Note.* Adapted from Blimkie et al.
(1977).

larger as the exercise prescription was boosted from one through three to five sessions a week. It is generally agreed that gains in aerobic power are small if the subject trains fewer than 2 days/week (Wenger & Bell, 1986), but there may be a plateauing of benefit if subjects train more than 3 sessions a week (Gettman et al., 1976; Pollock, 1973). The thrice-weekly optimum seems logical from the commonly observed biochemical response to a bout of vigorous exercise, that is, a brief initial phase of enhanced protein catabolism, followed by up to 48 hr of enhanced protein synthesis (Booth & Watson, 1985).

Mode

Provided that the intensity, duration, and frequency of exercise sessions are comparable and that the proposed regimen involves sustained vigorous activity by a large-muscle mass (e.g., swimming, jogging, or cross-country skiing), the mode of exercise seems to have little influence on the gains in physical condition that develop during aerobic training (D.C. Lieber, Lieber, & Adams, 1989; Pollock et al., 1975). However, with some patterns of exercise (e.g., arm ergometer training), gains in physical conditioning may have little effect on the performance of work in which other parts of the body are used (Clausen, 1977).

The choice of exercise mode should be based on personal preferences, available equipment and facilities, and (particularly in older subjects) the relative risks of causing new or recurrent musculoskeletal injuries (Kavanagh & Shephard, 1977a; Kavanagh, Lindley et al., 1988). For example, Pollock et al. (1977) found that beginning joggers experienced a substantial increase in the incidence of foot, leg, and knee injuries if they trained for more than 30 min three times a week. Walking is the preferred recommendation for sedentary older adults who wish to augment their daily physical activity. Walking exposes the knees and spine to only about one sixth of the impact stress encountered during jogging (Pascale & Grana, 1989), yet if it is pursued vigorously, walking can induce an equal gain of physical condition. In very old people, the choice of activity must also be tempered by other hazards, including hypotensive attacks and loss of consciousness in water sports, the danger of falls in pursuits demanding rapid reactions and a good sense of balance, and the risk of collisions with opponents or static obstacles during many types of games (Shephard, 1990b).

Time Course

Hickson and Rosenkoetter (1981) suggested that the half-time of the adaptive response in aerobic power to a given intensive aerobic training program (in their experiments, 40 min/session, 6 day/week) was 10 to 11 days. The discrepancy between the speed of this process and the time required for the development of tissue enzymes is a strong argument for a central limitation of aerobic power (see chapter 2). The training process can, of course, continue for much longer than a few weeks, if the intensity of the conditioning stimulus is increased progressively.

Specificity of Aerobic Training

Argument continues concerning the specificity of aerobic training. Any observed response may be specific to the type and intensity of activity, to the postural attitude adopted during exercise, and to the velocity of limb movement.

Type of Activity

There is some transfer of the aerobic training response from a jogging or cycling program to the subject's subsequent performance on a treadmill or cycle ergometer (Wilmore et al., 1980). But much of any increment in aerobic power or improvement in submaximal performance is apparently specific to the type of exercise undertaken during training (C. LeBlanc, Bouchard, Godbout, & Mondor, 1981).

Perhaps because cycling involves a smaller volume of muscle than running does, cycle ergometer training seems more mode specific than a corresponding dose of treadmill training (Fernhall & Kohrt, 1990; Pechar et al., 1974). In contrast to the general population, trained cyclists can sometimes develop a larger peak oxygen intake on the cycle ergometer than on the treadmill (Withers, Sherman, Miller, & Costill, 1981). About 50% of the gains made while training on a cycle ergometer can be transferred to the performance of arm work (Clausen, 1977; Bhambani et al., 1991; Rösler et al., 1985; Silber, McLaughlin, & Sinoway, 1991). The transfer of aerobic training from one leg to the other is even more limited (C.T.M. Davies & Sargeant, 1975; Saltin et al., 1976), and there is almost no transfer of the local gains from arm exercise (whether on an ergometer or against pulleys) to the performance of work by the legs (Grogan & Kelly, 1985; Loftin, Boileau, Massey, & Lohman, 1988; Magel et al., 1975).

Freund, D. Allen, and Wilmore (1986) even found some specificity in the response to treadmill conditioning, commenting that if training had been performed on an incline, then increases in oxygen transport were larger when running uphill than when running on the level. Nevertheless, specificity is not absolute for most large-muscle tasks, and if a minor injury temporarily restricts one type of activity, it is possible to maintain physical condition for several weeks by substituting another form of aerobic exercise (e.g., replacing jogging with an equivalent cycle ergometer program; Moroz & Houston, 1987).

Specificity of Intensity, Posture, and Velocity

There is some evidence that the individual's aerobic training response may be specific to the intensity at which the training has been conducted. Thus, with the usual aerobic type of prescription (i.e., exercise at 60%-70% of maximal oxygen intake), gains are seen more readily in submaximal than in maximal tests (Rogers et al., 1988; Roskamm, 1967).

Adaptation may also be specific to the posture that has been used during training (e.g., supine vs. sitting ergometry; Ray, Cureton, & Ouzts, 1990). Moreover, at least with isokinetic exercise, gains are specific to the angular velocity that has been adopted in training sessions (Kanehisa & Miyashita, 1983; Rösler, Conley, Howald, Gerber, & Hoppeler, 1986).

REASONS FOR SPECIFICITY.   The various manifestations of specificity are most readily understood in terms of the factors limiting aerobic performance. When the large muscles of the legs are active, the main determinant of peak power output is the maximal cardiac output (Shephard et al., 1988a). The training gains observed with repetition of this type of exercise thus reflect a combination of increased preloading of the heart (an increase of blood volume or an increase of peripheral venous tone), enhanced myocardial contractility, reduced afterloading of the heart (through a strengthening of the active muscles and a reduction of systemic blood pressure), an increase of total hemoglobin, and direction of a larger fraction of peak cardiac output to the working limbs.

At first inspection, most of these changes, except the decrease of afterloading associated with stronger muscles, might seem transferable benefits. However, in reality the situation is quite complex. For example, if the exercise tachycardia reflects a stimulation of local metaboreceptors (Mitchell & Schmidt, 1983), then the reduction of heart rate induced by aerobic training could be specific not only to a given limb (Saltin, 1977) but even to certain muscles within that limb. Thus, the consequences of the slower heart rate for peak cardiac work rate, diastolic filling, coronary perfusion, and ultimately myocardial contractility could, in their turn, show limb and muscle specificity.

The performance of arm work is limited in large part by the subject's ability to perfuse the vigorously contracting muscles of the upper limbs (Shephard et al., 1988a; Shephard & Plyley, 1992). Aerobic arm training strengthens the local musculature, facilitating muscle perfusion, and making such exercise more dependent on central cardiac performance (Loftin et al., 1988). However, the stimulus to the heart is quite limited during arm exercise, and the local strengthening of the arm muscles does nothing to facilitate the local perfusion of the legs. Thus, an arm training prescription normally does little to improve the performance of leg work.

Health Benefits

Whereas following a high-intensity aerobic regimen seems the most effective way to achieve a rapid increase of maximal oxygen intake (Sidney & Shephard, 1978), changes in overall body mass, the relative proportions of fat and lean tissue, and other health-related metabolic gains are more closely linked to the total energy expenditure than to the intensity of individual exercise sessions.

Indeed, if the primary goal of the exercise prescription is to control obesity, then a low-intensity aerobic regimen may be the optimal recommendation, because the proportion of fat that is metabolized decreases at exercise intensities greater than 50% of maximal oxygen intake (Christensen & Hansen, 1939). Moreover, a person who is somewhat obese is more likely to persist with moderate than with intense aerobic activity, allowing a greater total increase of energy expenditure during each training session. There may thus be a specificity of programs with respect to their effects on the various aspects of health.

Body Composition and Muscle Strength

The influence of any type of training program on body composition is heavily influenced by the overall daily energy balance. Often, those who begin a conditioning program have some concerns about becoming obese, and they restrict their intake of food energy during the weeks when they are exercising. Certainly, there is little evidence that food intake is increased to counter the increased energy expenditure (Staten, 1991).

Negative Energy Balance

Any tendency toward a negative energy balance is enhanced by exercise, because it reverses the depression of metabolism that is normally seen when food intake is reduced (Molé, Stern, Schultz, Bernauer, & Holcomb, 1989; Wadden, Foster, Letizia, & Mullen, 1990); it may even induce a small but sustained elevation of energy expenditure (Bagley, Berg, Latin, & LaVoie, 1991; Bahr & Sejersted, 1991; Gore & Withers, 1990) for a period after exercise.

If an obese subject induces a negative energy balance while following an exercise program, there will be a progressive loss of both fat and lean tissue (Hill, Sparling, Shields, & Heller, 1987; Zuti & Golding, 1976), although the loss of lean tissue will be less than in those who attempt to correct obesity by dieting only. If energy balance is maintained, an exercise-centered regimen generally induces a small increase in lean mass, despite a 1 to 2 kg decrease in total body mass and a 2% to 3% decrease in body fat (Wilmore, 1983). Even so, the apparent constancy of total lean mass may hide a small increase of mass in the more active muscles and a larger loss of protein from some of the smaller, less involved muscles.

Muscle Strength

At one time, those interested in aerobic training were inclined to avoid exercises intended to develop muscular strength. It was reasoned that muscle-building exercises had so low an oxygen cost that they had no direct influence on the aerobic conditioning process (Josenhans, 1967; Hempel & Wells, 1985). It even was suggested that such exercises might interfere with responses to aerobic training (Dudley & Fleck, 1987; Hortobagyi, Katch, & LaChance, 1991; McCoy, Wiley, Clayton, & Dunn, 1991), either through the resultant metabolic changes or simply by diverting the subject's attention away from the need for cardiac conditioning. It was further argued that resisted exercise could impose a dangerous acute loading on the heart of an older individual, because of an associated rise in systemic blood pressure (Bezucha et al., 1982). Finally, it was argued that by increasing total body mass, muscle building would increase the load to be supported and displaced each day, without offering any matching increment of cardiovascular condition.

More recently, these criticisms have been vigorously challenged (Franklin, Bonzheim, Gordon, & Timmis, 1991). MacDougall, Tuxen, Sale, Moroz, and Sutton (1985) showed that with a suitable limitation of the resisting force, and avoidance of the Valsalva maneuver during contractions, the rise in systemic blood pressure during a formal muscle-building program was no greater than what would be incurred during submaximal cycle ergometry. A simple alternative to formal resistance exercise is to carry small weights in each hand when walking or jogging. This tactic stimulates the development of muscle, tendon, and bone in the arms, but it increases the blood pressure by an average of only 9 mm Hg (Graves et al., 1987) and it leads to only a very small increase in the total energy expenditure—1.8 ml/(kg·min) for 0.9-kg weights, and 2.7 ml/(kg·min) for 1.8-kg weights (Francis & Hoobler, 1986; Owens et al., 1989).

Many of the increases in blood pressure that occur during normal daily life reflect attempts to perfuse muscles that are contracting at an excessive fraction of their maximal voluntary force (Kay & Shephard, 1969). A strengthening of the major muscles thus has the beneficial effect of reducing the severity of such hypertensive episodes. Furthermore, the average person shows an accelerating loss of lean tissue throughout the latter half of adult life (Shephard, 1987a), and unless specific precautions are taken, participants in an aerobic training program seem particularly vulnerable to such losses. Pollock, Foster, Knapp, Rod, and Schmidt (1987) noted a 2-kg loss of lean tissue in a 10-year follow-up of Masters' athletes. Leg circumferences remained unchanged, but arm circumferences diminished significantly. It is important to design an aerobic exercise program so that such losses are checked, if not reversed, because of the implications of muscle weakening for systemic blood pressure, the associated risks of musculoskeletal injury, and the danger that increasing weakness will ultimately preclude undertaking the activities of daily living (Shephard, 1991c).

There have been reports that leg presses can augment the performance of aerobic exercise on a cycle ergometer or a treadmill (Pels, Pollock, Dohmeier, Lemberger, & Oehrlein, 1987). If there has been extensive muscle wasting (e.g., in patients with chronic, obstructive pulmonary disease), then muscle strengthening can certainly contribute to a training-induced increase in maximal oxygen intake (Mertens et al., 1978; Schols, Mostert, Soeters, & Wouters, 1991). However, the usual objective of an aerobic fitness program is an enhancement of overall health and quality of life, rather than simple maximization of aerobic power, so that the other health benefits that have been cited offer stronger grounds for encouraging the maintenance, and even the strengthening, of the major muscles of the body.

Similarly to cardiorespiratory training, muscle strengthening follows the overload principle (Hettinger, 1961). Gains are due more to improved neural coordination than to local hypertrophy (Narici, Roi, Lanoni, Minetti, & Cerretelli, 1989). Perhaps for this reason, the increments of strength are highly specific, not only to a given muscle but also to the joint angle at which contractions have occurred (Hettinger, 1961). It is thus advisable that a muscle training program include resistance exercises throughout the full range of motion at each of the major joints in the body (Graves, Pollock, Jones, Colvin, & Leggett, 1989; Knapik, Maudsley, & Rammos, 1983). The intensity of the training stimulus can be manipulated by varying the magnitude of the opposing resistance, the number of repetitions performed each set, the interval between individual contractions, and the number of sets performed in a session (Fleck & Kraemer, 1987). To avoid adverse circulatory effects (MacDougall et al., 1985), contractions should be held to a moderate intensity (<40% of maximal voluntary force) and carried out at a moderate to slow speed, without impeding normal breathing.

The American College of Sports Medicine (1990, 1991) now recommends that exercise prescriptions for the general public include a circuit of 8 to 10 muscle-strengthening exercises. These should be performed twice a week, completing one set of 8 to 12 repetitions to near-fatigue at each station. Such a regimen is likely to increase the strength of an average fitness-class member by 20% to 25%. Neither a larger number of repetitions each session nor a higher weekly frequency of muscle training is helpful. Neither approach augments strength significantly relative to the standard regimen (Braith et al., 1989), but both options increase a trainee's likelihood of suffering musculoskeletal injuries or dropping out of the program.

The intensity of muscle-strengthening exercise is most easily controlled through the use of sophisticated resistance-training equipment, but if this is not readily available, quite simple forms of resisted activity (for example, calisthenics that require displacement of the body mass against gravity) can provide an effective alternative.

Factors Modifying the Aerobic Training Response

The subject's response to a given combination of intensity, frequency, and duration of aerobic training can potentially be modified by genetic factors, associated muscle strengthening exercises, an adverse environment, psychological influences, pregnancy, young or old age, various clinical disorders, and the administration of certain drugs.

Genetic Factors

The possible influence of genetic factors upon the ability of the individual to respond to a given regimen of aerobic training (Landry et al., 1985; Lortie et al., 1984) has been discussed previously.

Strength Training

Once, it was feared that engaging in resisted exercise would reduce the response to aerobic training (Dudley & Fleck, 1987; Hortobagyi et al., 1991; McCoy et al., 1991). However, in practice, it is possible to combine aerobic conditioning with regular muscle-strengthening exercises, so that the subject's strength is not only maintained but enhanced.

Environment

A cold environment may discourage physical activity, so that populations exposed to a continental climate may show some deterioration of physical condition during the winter months (Rode & Shephard, 1973). Cold weather apparently has little direct influence on the response to aerobic training (Harri, Donnenberg, Oksanen-Rossi, & Hohtola, 1984), except that it encourages the metabolism of fat during the training sessions (Doubt & Shieh, 1991; O'Hara et al., 1979; Shephard, in press-c; Timmons, Araujo, & T.R. Thomas, 1985). If body fat is reduced, there may be a resultant increase in the individual's relative aerobic power.

Warm weather encourages outdoor activity, but if it becomes too hot, physical activity may be inhibited. There are many parallels between heat acclimation and aerobic training, including an increase of venous tone (Tripathi, Mack, & Nadel, 1990), expansion of plasma volume (M.H. Harrison, 1986), earlier sweating for a given increase of body temperature (Buono & Sjoholm, 1988), and a lower increase in core temperature after adaptation (Shephard, 1982b). Thus, it is not surprising that the two stimuli, aerobic exercise and heat, combine to speed and to augment the ultimate physiological adjustments (L.E. Armstrong & Maresh, 1991; Gisolfi, 1973; Inbar et al., 1978). If a subject is required to undertake physical activity in a hot climate, the optimal method of preparation is to carry out a program of aerobic training in natural or artificial heat (Wyndham, Strydom, Benade, & Van Rensberg, 1973).

High-altitude training was much in vogue at the time of the Olympic Games in Mexico City. In retrospect (Saltin, 1992; Shephard, 1974a), little added benefit was gained either by short (2- to 4-week) periods of aerobic training at altitudes of 2,000 to 3,000 m or by equivalent exposure to hypoxic gas mixtures or chamber simulations of such altitudes, at least in subjects who were initially in good physical condition. However, the success of Kenyan distance runners when competing in international races, both at high altitude and at sea level, suggests that there may be some enhancement of endurance performance if an athlete undertakes more prolonged periods of aerobic training at high altitude. In a recent international event, 26 of the 32 successful distance runners had prepared themselves by prolonged residence at high altitudes (Dick, 1992).

The hemoglobin concentration is increased by residence at high altitudes, initially through hemoconcentration and subsequently by increased red cell synthesis. The threshold altitude for such a response is 2,200 to 2,500 m. But this potential advantage is often offset by the impact of the decreased plasma volume on maximal cardiac output (Shephard, 1974a). If aerobic training is undertaken at altitude and the individual subsequently returns to sea level, then hemolysis reverses any altitude-induced increase of hemoglobin level within a few days.

At very high altitudes, oxygen transport is further facilitated by the development of an increased muscle capillary density, an increase in myoglobin stores, and increased 2,3-diphosphoglycerate levels in the red cells (Sutton et al., 1992).

Psychological Influences

The aerobic training response of the average person depends very much on persistence with the prescribed regimen, in the face both of muscular discomforts and of other claims on leisure time. The psychological climate thus has a major impact on training responses. For example, if an elderly person is encouraged to "take life easy" and "enjoy a well-earned rest," then he or she is unlikely to make a substantial investment in training.

The exercise specialist can exert an important influence in modifying such inappropriate social norms, making moderate aerobic exercise a part of normal, adult behavior (Godin & Shephard, 1990). Currently, most patients have a substantial respect for the advice that they are given by their family physician, but too rarely does this advice include any specific exercise recommendation (Shephard, 1986c). A change in attitudes among the medical profession could have a major influence on both patient recruitment and adherence to training programs.

Pregnancy

During pregnancy, the circulation of the exerciser must be divided between the placenta and the skeletal muscles. However, there is growing evidence that moderate aerobic training is well tolerated, not only conserving the physical condition of the mother, but also contributing to a favorable outcome for the fetus (Brenner & Wolfe, in press).

Considerations in developing an appropriate exercise prescription for the pregnant woman (see chapter 5) include guarding the fetus against injury (from falls or collisions), hyperthermia, and hypoxia (the last being signalled by fetal bradycardia and a decrease of spontaneous fetal movements). The recommended activity should also make due allowance for alterations in the mother's circulation, respiratory mechanics, and body mass (McKenzie, 1992).

Youth

Some authors have suggested that preadolescent children have a diminished response to aerobic training, due to either inherently high levels of physical activity or immaturity of the responding systems (Bar-Or, 1983). Our data show that there is indeed little training response of any type before 8 years of age, mainly because the children lack the basic motor skills to engage in a vigorous program of physical activity (Shephard et al., 1977). However, our data also support a growing consensus (Rowland, 1985, 1992; Shephard, 1992a; Vaccaro & Mahon, 1987) that substantial gains of cardiorespiratory function and of muscle strength are possible among ordinary children aged 8 to 11 years (see Figure 4.6; also Shephard, 1992a). Earlier negative reports for the preadolescent (Bar-Or, 1983) can apparently be attributed

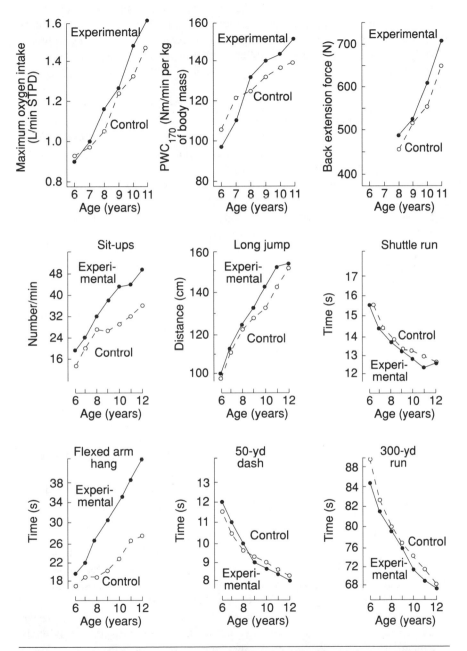

Figure 4.6 Development of fitness in schoolchildren. Experimental group received enhanced program of 5 hr physical education a week taught by a specialist; control group received standard program—one 40-min session a week. *Note*. Adapted from Shephard (1982b) by permission.

to such factors as the selection of children with too high an initial level of fitness, a training program that was inadequate in terms of its intensity, duration, or suitability to the age of the child, failure to allow for superimposed, seasonal changes in fitness (Shephard, Levallée, Jéquier, et al., 1978), and compensatory reductions of physical activity when the students were not engaged in the specified conditioning activities (Shephard, 1992a).

Provided that the nutritional intake is adequate, there is no evidence that vigorous aerobic training has any major influence on either normal growth patterns (Malina, in press; Shephard et al., 1984a) or other processes of maturation (e.g., increases in age at menarche or age at peak height velocity, or decreases the skeletal age; Shephard, 1991c; Shephard, Lavellée, Rajic, et al., 1978). Increases of aerobic power and its constituents develop in proportion to the normal increase of body size. Reports of delayed maturation and small body size in some categories of female athletes reflect selection by body build rather than a specific effect of regular physical activity on the growth process.

Participation in an aerobic training program sometimes (Pařízková, 1977) but not always (Shephard, 1982a) has at least a temporary effect in reducing obesity in children. However, this has only limited importance from the viewpoint of adult health, because unfortunately there is only a limited tracking of a favorable cardiac risk profile from childhood into adult life (Bar-Or, in press; Kemper, Storm-van Essen, & Verschuur, 1989; Montoye, 1985).

Old Age

Some studies that have attempted to gauge the trainability of elderly subjects have used unsatisfactory criteria of program response (Shephard, 1987a). For example, where estimates of conditioning have been based on changes in the directly measured maximal oxygen intake, initial test scores may have been biased downward by fears of overexertion on the part of the subject or the supervising physician, or by local muscle weakness. In such situations, the apparent aerobic training response would be exaggerated. Likewise, the initial physiological reaction to a submaximal test may be augmented by anxiety or a poor mechanical efficiency, so that the training-related change in submaximal performance may again have exaggerated the true improvement of maximal aerobic power (Shephard, 1987a). Despite these potential sources of bias, some early reports suggested a less-ready aerobic training of middle-aged and older subjects than those of who were younger (Benestad, 1965; DeVries, 1970).

More recent investigations have shown that, at least in terms of percentage gains, the aerobic training response is similar in young and older individuals (Shephard, 1987a, 1990b; Sidney & Shephard, 1978). But because of a slower rate of protein synthesis (Zackin & Meredith, 1989) and a lower intensity of exercise regimen, the speed of adaptation is commonly slower in the elderly than in younger people (Pollock et al., 1976; Seals, Hagberg, Hurley, Ehsani, & Hollosky, 1984; Sidney & Shephard, 1978).

The difference in maximal oxygen intake between continuing athletes and sedentary subjects remains much as in their younger years (Kavanagh, Lindley, et al., 1988a; Kavanagh & Shephard, 1977a; Shephard, 1988a), and 65-year-old subjects who themselves elect and persist in a high-intensity, high-frequency regimen may show gains of aerobic power as large as 7 to 8 μmol/(kg·s), or 10 ml/(kg·min), over a 3-month period (Sidney & Shephard, 1978). The response to aerobic training has enormous practical consequences for the maintenance of independence in the final years of life (Shephard & Montelpare, 1988), the sum of its benefits being equivalent to a 10- to 20-year difference in biological age.

Clinical Disorders

Most clinical conditions do not inhibit a typical training response, provided that the patient is able to undertake an adequate amount of exercise. A grossly obese person may be unwilling to comply with a standard exercise prescription, because of embarassment at clumsiness or an ungainly figure. Such reticence can sometimes be overcome by recommending unisex classes or private exercise sessions. In summer weather, such individuals also face problems caused by heavy sweating and an excessive elevation of core temperature; these difficulties can be resolved by using an air-conditioned gymnasium or by swimming in cool water. Finally, activity patterns may be restricted by a deterioration of major joints secondary to the increase of body mass; this problem is eased by the choice of weight-supported exercises (e.g., pool exercises, or Aquabics; Lawrence, 1981; Shephard, 1985c).

Some patients with myocardial ischemia have difficulty in following their exercise prescription because the required intensity of physical activity quickly induces severe anginal pain or dangerous cardiac arrhythmias. A modified interval-training program seems the best method of enabling such individuals to undertake an effective dose of exercise (Kavanagh & Shephard, 1975). The impact is more upon medical problems than discomfort. Problems are often reduced by the use of beta-blocking medication, although excessive doses can cause peripheral muscular fatigue and thus limit the training volume (Kullmer, Kindermann, & Singer, 1987; Tesch, 1985). The peripheral metabolic side-effects of beta-blocking drugs can be minimized by the use of cardio-selective agents.

Patients with extensive myocardial degeneration and compensated cardiac failure sometimes show a surprisingly good response to aerobic training (Kavanagh, Meyers, et al., 1992). Although we have seen an 8% to 10% increase in oxygen pulse over 12 weeks of conditioning, it seems likely that most of the observed gains reflect peripheral effects of training, possibly including a strengthening of muscles weakened by disuse.

Distressing dyspnea may limit attempts at aerobic exercise in patients with chronic obstructive lung disease. Here, the problem is commonly a vicious cycle of diminishing physical activity, loss of muscle strength, an increased accumulation of lactate during any exercise that is taken, a resultant exacerbation of dyspnea, and a further decrease of physical activity (Mertens et al., 1978). For such individuals, a prescription that includes specific muscle-strengthening exercises may help to break the vicious cycle. The administration of oxygen during aerobic training sessions may also enable the patient to progress to a point where compliance with the exercise prescription is encouraged by the internal reward of increasing self-efficacy.

Musculoskeletal lesions may preclude leg exercise. The specificity of training then becomes important, and the prescribed regimen should exercise as large a muscle mass as is practicable. In the frail elderly who are confined to their beds, a useful amount of training can still be accomplished from a sitting position (McNamara, Otto, & Smith, 1985).

Drug Therapy

The influence of beta-blocking drugs on the response to aerobic training has been discussed briefly. The increase of heart rate during a given bout of exercise is much smaller with such treatment, and perhaps for this reason, the aerobic training response of otherwise normal subjects is impaired. However, in cardiac patients (perhaps because of relief of angina), the response to aerobic training may be enhanced after the administration of beta-blocking drugs (Blood & Ades, 1988), unless compliance with the prescription is limited by local muscular fatigue (Kullmer et al., 1987; Tesch, 1985).

The blood-pressure-reducing action of regular aerobic exercise is enhanced if this is combined with a low-salt diet and the administration of diuretics. Conversely, addition of aerobic exercise to the treatment plan for a hypertensive patient reduces the requirement for antihypertensive medication (Tipton, 1984).

Anabolic steroids act mainly by increasing the rate of synthesis of skeletal muscle. They may induce a small increase of endurance performance, in part because of an increased synthesis of hemoglobin, though they also stimulate greater aggressiveness, which increases the subject's desire to participate in vigorous exercise.

Optimum Aerobic Training Recommendations

Based on the foregoing considerations, the American College of Sports Medicine (1990, 1991) now recommends that aerobic training be practiced 3 to 5 days/week at 50% to 85% of maximal oxygen intake. Because of the hazards of musculoskeletal injuries and possible cardiac emergencies, the lower end of the intensity range is recommended for subjects who have a low initial level of fitness. The suggested duration of training is 20 to 60 min a session, with longer sessions being adopted for the low-intensity programs. Further, if subjects are so unfit that they are unable to complete 60 min of exercise at a single session, then the training may be split into several segments with intervening rests.

The aerobic component of the prescription can be satisfied by vigorous participation in any sustained, large-muscle activity, such as walking, hiking, running, jogging, ergometer or road cycling, cross-country skiing, vigorous dancing, rope skipping, rowing, stair climbing, swimming, skating, or participation in endurance sports (Patton, Corey, Gettman, & Schovee, 1986).

Aerobic activities must be supplemented by sufficient strength training to maintain the individual's fat-free weight. The muscle-building component of the program requires at least two sessions a week, with participants making 8 to 12 repetitions of 8 to 10 exercises that involve the major muscle groups of the body.

Overtraining

Overtraining is more commonly a problem of international athletes than of the average exerciser. The overtrained subject shows a deterioration of physical performance and physiological scores relative to their peak attainments (Kuipers & Keizer, 1988; Milne, 1988; Verde, Thomas, Shek, et al., 1992a; Verde, Thomas, & Shephard, 1992). Associated phenomena include an intense psychological discouragement, sometimes with an increased vulnerability to infection (Nieman et al., 1990) and minor injuries.

The causes are probably multiple. Repeated, prolonged thermal stress may cause a substantial salt loss, a corresponding decrease of plasma volume, and reduction of peak cardiac output (Wyndham & Strydom, 1972). The cumulative alterations of mineral balance (Shephard, Kavanagh, & Moore, 1978) may exacerbate any abnormalities of cardiac rhythm, particularly in a patient with coronary atherosclerosis. Chronic hemorrhage and fecal blood loss (particularly if pain-relieving drugs have been prescribed; Robertson, Maughan, & Davidson, 1987), a poor absorption of iron, decreased red cell synthesis, and increased hemolysis (see chapter 2) may all contribute to anemia (Taunton, McKenzie, Clement, & Cook, 1986), so that less oxygen is carried by each unit volume of blood. The increased rate of metabolism leads to an increased production of free radicals, which can oxidize and peroxidize proteins, lipids, and DNA; such reactions can cause extensive cellular and tissue damage (Eichner, in press) with a potentially adverse effect on vascular disease, aging, and cancer. Catabolism is likely to exceed anabolic activity, causing an increased cortisol/testosterone ratio (Dressendorfer & Wade, 1991), myoglobinemia (R.B. Armstrong, 1984), myoglobinuria (Milne, 1988), and a substantial protein loss (Fisher, Baracos, Shnitka, Mendryk, & Reid, 1990). Energy intake may be insufficient to meet body needs, leading to progressive muscle wasting, loss of body fat, and a low blood-sugar level. In females, there may be associated amenorrhea and osteoporosis (Drinkwater et al., 1984, 1986; Prior, 1990). In both sexes, immune function may be suppressed, with a concurrent increase in the risk of minor infections (Mackinnon, 1992; Nieman et al., 1990; Shephard, Verde, et al., 1991). Leakage of Ca^{2+} ions activates proteolytic enzymes (R.B. Armstrong, Warren, & Warren, 1991). Repeated muscle soreness (Ebbeling & Clarkson, 1989; Jones, Newham, Round, & Tolfree, 1986; Kuipers & Janssen, 1985) and leakage of muscle enzymes (Noakes, 1987; Noakes, Kotzenburg, McArthur, & Dykman, 1983; Rogers, Stull, & Apple, 1985; Siegel, Silverman, & Evans, 1983; Stäubli, Roessler, Köchli, Peheim, & Straub, 1985) are strongly associated with the performance of eccentric exercise

(R.B. Armstrong, 1986; Sargeant & Dolan, 1987); such responses may progress to more serious musculoskeletal problems, including muscle tears and stress fractures of the bones. Finally, a suppression of testosterone levels may reduce the athlete's drive and aggressivenesss, compounding the negative psychological impact of boredom with repetitive training sessions that seem to be yielding ever smaller rewards. Measures such as the Profile of Mood States show adverse psychological changes, including an increase of state anxiety and a loss of vigor (Verde, Thomas, Shek, et al., 1992; Verde, Thomas, & Shephard, 1992).

Average subjects generally perform less than the prescribed amount of exercise, and thus they are unlikely to experience symptoms of overtraining. But occasional, obsessive individuals may undertake much more than the suggested training volume, with a corresponding potential of developing the various physiological and psychological problems seen in overtrained athletes.

Patients with anorexia nervosa often exhibit patterns of compulsive exercise, and it is controversial whether the compulsive exerciser is another manifestation of the same psychopathology. The distinction between compulsive exercise and anorexia nervosa is generally based on the nature of the primary obsession—exercise or food. The loss of body mass in the compulsive exerciser (5-10 kg) is much less dramatic than in the typical case of anorexia nervosa (e.g., many women with anorexia lose 20-30 kg of body mass, often showing a weight of only 35-40 kg at hospital admission; Garfinkel & Garner, 1982). Furthermore, if the patient with anorexia nervosa has resumed eating, the introduction of a moderate program of physical activity facilitates rather than hampers the rebuilding of lean tissue (C.T.M. Davies, von Döbeln, Fohlin, Freyschuss, & Thorén, 1978; Fohlin, 1978).

Nevertheless, the relentless pursuit of aerobic conditioning can lead to both cardiac and musculoskeletal problems, particularly in older adults. In the case of the runner, the likelihood of musculoskeletal injuries increases exponentially when the weekly training distance exceeds a certain threshold (Pollock et al., 1977, 1991). Prevention of over-use injuries requires moderation of an aerobic exercise prescription as soon as signs of musculoskeletal discomfort or myocardial irritability appear. Although eccentric movement is often the cause of musculoskeletal injury, progressive eccentric training also seems to make the muscles less vulnerable to soreness in subsequent bouts of physical activity (Ebbeling & Clarkson, 1990; Schwane, Williams, & Sloan, 1987). Finally, an adequate warmup before a session of aerobic training may help to avoid musculoskeletal injuries (DeVries, 1980; Safran, Seaber, & Garrett, 1989).

Maintenance and Loss of Training

If an exerciser progressively increases the dose of aerobic training, there may be a continuing, slow, upward progression of maximal oxygen intake. For example, following myocardial infarction, some middle-aged subjects who begin training at a very low aerobic power (19-20 μmol/[kg·s], 26-27 ml/[kg·min]—about 70%

of the age-related normal value) may reach final readings in excess of 45 μmol/(kg·s), or 60 ml/(kg·min), over the course of 3 to 4 years of progressive training (Shephard, 1981; see Figure 4.2, page 179). However, the average middle-aged adult is interested in defining the minimum dose of activity needed to sustain the gains in physical condition realized through a short course of training, rather than in making a belated attempt to match the characteristics of the superb, long-distance athlete.

Hickson et al. (1981, 1982, 1985) found that, once the desired level of aerobic training had been reached, the frequency or the duration of training sessions could be reduced by as much as two thirds without any adverse effect on physical condition. But if subjects decreased the intensity of training sessions, there was a substantial loss of aerobic power over the first 15 weeks of observation. Similarly, gains in strength could be sustained by one session of isotonic exercises a week, provided that the intensity of contractions was not reduced (Graves et al., 1988).

Certain aspects of bed rest have already been discussed. One of the distressing features of the average conditioning program is that many of its hard-won gains are dissipated very rapidly if training ceases. The deterioration of physical condition proceeds even faster if the subject loses normal gravitational stimulation, whether through space travel, bed rest or surgery (Coyle, 1988; Saltin et al., 1968). Thus, involvement in an exercise program can make little long-term contribution to health, unless participants are prepared to follow a maintenance regimen for the remainder of their lives.

A significant loss of cardiorespiratory condition occurs within 2 weeks of cessation of training (Coyle et al., 1984; Roskamm, 1967). The half-life of the loss in aerobic power is no more than 4 to 12 weeks (Fringer & Stull, 1974; Kendrick, Pollock, Hickman, & Miller, 1971; Roskamm, 1967). Thereafter, the rate of functional loss may slow down (Coyle et al., 1984; Klausen et al., 1981), but all effects of aerobic training are dissipated after 8 weeks (Orlander, Kiessling, Karlsson, & Ekblom, 1977) or 8 months (Knuttgen, Nordesjo, Ollander, & Saltin, 1973) of detraining.

Among the functional changes associated with detraining (Coyle et al., 1984) and bed rest (Saltin et al., 1968), we may note peripheral blood pooling (Blomqvist & Stone, 1982; Convertino, Hung, et al., 1982; Convertino, Sandler, 1982), a rapid loss of the trained person's 10%-advantage in plasma volume (Coyle, Hemmert, & Coggan, 1986; Cullinane, Sady, Vadeboncoeur, Burke, & Thompson, 1986), a somewhat slower decrease of stroke volume, a narrowing of the arteriovenous oxygen difference, and a decrease of maximal oxygen intake (Hoummard, 1992; Neufer, 1989; see Figure 4.7). W.H. Martin, Coyle, Bloomfield, and Ehsani (1986) pointed out the importance of venous tone to these various changes. In their study, the end diastolic volume and stroke volume were both diminished by detraining if tests were conducted in the sitting position, but were unchanged when the subject was tested supine. Similarly, the loss of aerobic power upon detraining could be largely countered by expansion of the plasma volume (Coyle et al., 1986).

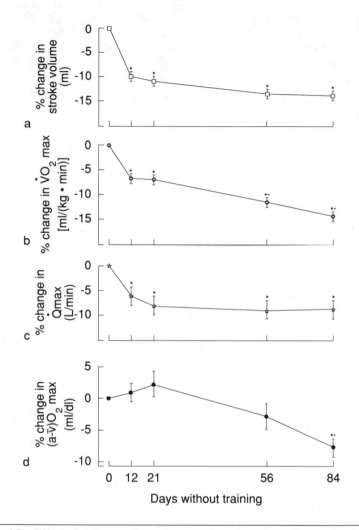

Figure 4.7   Effect of deliberate detraining on (a) stroke volume, (b) maximal oxygen intake, (c) plasma volume, and (d) arteriovenous oxygen. Subjects initially were aerobically trained. *Note*. Adapted from Coyle et al. (1984) by permission.

Detraining leads to a decrease of protein synthesis in skeletal muscle (Gibson et al., 1987). Muscle glycogen stores are diminished (Costill et al., 1985) and a decrease of muscle enzyme activity is visible after as little as 1 week of inactivity (Appell, 1990; Simoneau et al., 1987). The half-time of many of the enzymatic changes is about 12 days (see Figure 4.8), but values ultimately stabilize some 50% above the readings that would have been anticipated if the subjects had never trained.

Some authors have found a rapid loss of cardiac mass with detraining (Ehsani, Hagberg, & Hickson, 1978), but others have suggested on the basis of radiographic

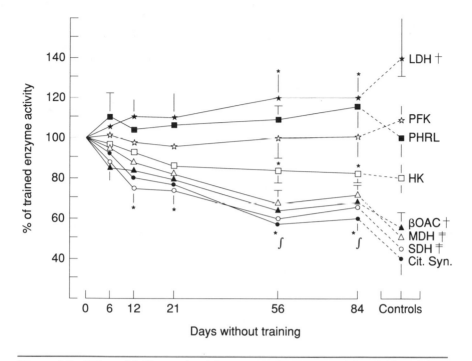

Figure 4.8   Effect of deliberate detraining on muscle enzyme activity. Subjects initially were aerobically trained. *Note.* Reprinted from Coyle et al. (1984) by permission. LDH = total lactate dehydrogenase; PFK = phosphofructokinase; PHRL = phosphorylase; HK = hexokinase; BOAC = beta-hydroxyacyl-CoA-dehydrogenase; MDH = malate dehydrogenase; SDH = succinate dehydrogenase; Cit. Syn. = citrate synthase.

measurements of cardiac volumes that the large heart of the endurance athlete persists through several years of detraining (Gallanti, Toncelli, Comeglio, Bisi, & Gallini, 1989; Saltin & Grimby, 1968). Dickuth et al. (1989) followed athletes for 24 years and observed only a 6% decrease of cardiac size during this period.

Lastly, with regard to prolonged bed rest, the loss of gravitational stimulation leads to a progressive demineralization of bone, with an increased risk of pathological fractures and renal calculi (Krølner & Toft, 1983; Wronski, Morey-Holton, Doty, Maese, & Walsh, 1987).

5
Chapter

The Goal of Improved Health

Improving personal health is a reason commonly cited both for undertaking regular physical activity and for maintaining aerobic fitness. In recent years, many reports have suggested that there are indeed associations between habitual physical activity, fitness, and health (Bouchard et al., 1990; see Figure 1.1, page 24). But the findings remain suggestive rather than conclusive, because they fail to satisfy the proof of a causal association demanded by statisticians.

Most commonly, observers have looked for an association between a high level of habitual aerobic activity and health, rather than between a good aerobic fitness score and health. This reflects in part the costs and the technical difficulties associated with accurately measuring health-related aspects of fitness on large population samples (Shephard, 1986c; see also chapter 3). There is also increasing recognition that a high aerobic fitness score does not necessarily mean that a person has maintained a high level of physical activity; the relationship between habitual physical activity and the attained level of fitness also varies with inherited, constitutional factors (Lortie et al., 1984; see also chapter 4). Finally, there are growing doubts that the types and intensities of physical activity most effective in boosting such traditional markers of aerobic fitness as maximal oxygen intake are necessary to improve long-term health. For example, S.N. Blair et al. (1989) noted in a prospective study of subjects who had completed a treadmill test at the Cooper Institute for Aerobics Research in Dallas, Texas, that although all-cause mortality decreased progressively in subjects with greater aerobic fitness, the biggest change was seen on moving from the most sedentary to the next fitness category (see Figure 5.1).

Because of the nature of the available data, this chapter will examine mainly the relationship between physical activity and health, noting that in studies where aerobic fitness has also been measured, habitually active individuals have generally had above-average fitness levels.

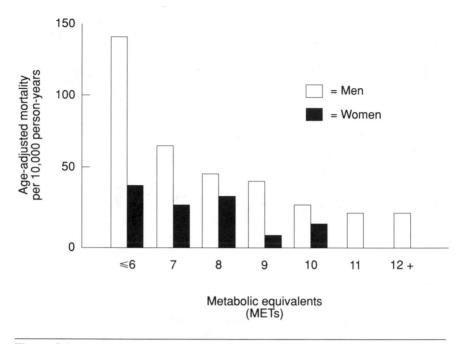

Figure 5.1 Relationship between initial fitness in METS and subsequent all-cause mortality. *Note.* Reprinted from Blair, Kohl, et al. (1989) by permission. Data for 3,129 women and 10,224 men initially tested at the Cooper Institute for Aerobics Research, Dallas, and then followed prospectively for an average of 8 years.

Aerobic Fitness and Lifestyle

The development of aerobic fitness may have a positive influence on health simply because it encourages the adoption of other positive health behaviors—for example, the regular use of a seat belt when driving or the cessation of cigarette smoking (S.N. Blair, D.R. Jacobs, & Powell, 1985; Marcus, Albrecht, Niaura, Abrams, & Thompson, 1991; Shephard, 1989b).

Investigators have approached the question of the fitness-lifestyle relationship by cross-sectional studies that compare various facets of personal lifestyle in physically active and sedentary subjects, by principal component analyses of health behaviors, and by prospective-controlled studies, particularly of the response to worksite fitness and health-promotional initiatives.

Cross-Sectional Studies

Regular physical activity shows statistically significant cross-sectional associations with good perceived health (Belloc & Breslow, 1972; Palmore, 1970), the control of obesity, and other favorable health behaviors, but correlations are quite weak (Shephard, 1986c; 1989b). Moreover, some categories of high-profile athletes are less cautious than their sedentary peers and thus have an increased likelihood of dying violent deaths, for example, in accidents caused by excessive driving speed or failure to observe traffic regulations (Polednak, 1978). On the other hand, Masters' athletes (who are primarily long-distance runners) tend to show a strong interest in health, and an above-average proportion of this group indicate regular use of a seat belt when in a moving vehicle (Kavanagh, Shephard, et al., 1992). A similar health consciousness is seen among active people in the general U.S. population (U.S. Dept. of Health & Human Services, 1981).

The proportion of smokers in sedentary and active samples of the general population is often quite similar (Shephard, 1986c). This may reflect a failure to distinguish the type of physical activity that is being undertaken (see Table 5.1). In particular, it is important to distinguish hedonistic, social types of activity from those pursuits that are undertaken with a deliberate intention of boosting personal fitness.

In studies where the active group has been restricted to those engaged in health-seeking forms of exercise, such as aerobics classes or distance running, the proportion of smokers has been substantially lower than in the general population (Perrier, 1979). Likewise, patients who stop smoking after coronary bypass graft surgery have substantially higher postoperative levels of aerobic activity than those who continue to smoke (Lapsley, Khuri, Patel, Strauss, & Sharma, 1991).

However, it remains uncertain from cross-sectional studies whether participation in aerobic activity has caused the favorable health behavior, or whether an underlying interest in good health has led to an increase of physical activity.

Principal Component Analyses

When a principal component analysis is applied to habitual physical activity and other health behaviors, the hypothesis is that the other behaviors will load on the same factor as physical activity. To date, the analyses undertaken suggest

Table 5.1
Association Between Active Lifestyle and Abstinence From Cigarettes

Percent smokers		
Active	Sedentary	Author
37%	42%	Canada Fitness Survey, 1983
37	39	US DHHR, 1981
31	37	Bradstock et al., 1984
44	56	Norwegian Confederation of Sport, 1984

Note. Cross-sectional studies collected by Shephard, 1986c; see source for details of references.

some association between the control of body mass and habitual aerobic activity (S.N. Blair et al., 1985; Shephard, 1989b). Regular, prolonged aerobic exercise is also linked to a substantial increase in blood concentrations of HDL-cholesterol, although the individual concerned must engage in a substantial weekly energy expenditure (equivalent to 18-20 km of jogging each week) before such an association is seen (Kavanagh et al., 1983; P.T. Williams et al., 1982; see Figure 5.3, page 234).

Longitudinal Studies on Smoking

P. Morgan, Gildiner, and Wright (1976) noted that an unusually high proportion of Masters' distance runners who had initially been smokers reported a later successful smoking withdrawal. It is tempting to explain this improvement of health behavior on the basis that exercise involvement demonstrated to the smokers some of the adverse effects of their addiction—for example, an impairment of ventilatory function or an exercise-induced anormality of their electrocardiogram such as ST segmental depression. Indeed we have heard patients make such comments at smoking withdrawal clinics (Rode et al., 1972).

But unfortunately for such a hypothesis, further questioning of Masters' runners (Kavanagh, Lindley, et al., 1988; Kavanagh, Shephard, et al., 1992) established that in most instances the decision to stop smoking antedated involvement in distance running. Kavanagh, Lindley, et al. (1988) thus argued that both successful smoking withdrawal and involvement in Masters' competition reflected an inherent interest in the adoption of a healthy lifestyle. Nevertheless, some athletes claimed that their participation in a regular aerobic training program was helpful in sustaining abstinence in the face of temptations to resume smoking (Kavanagh, Shephard, et al., 1992).

In a third study of exercise and smoking, we examined patients who had enrolled in a progressive-exercise rehabilitation program following myocardial infarction (Kavanagh et al., 1983). Before infarction, 80% of the group had been heavily addicted smokers. Immediately after infarction, the proportion of smokers dropped to 35%. No further change in the proportion of smokers was observed over 3 years of increasingly vigorous aerobic activity. But again, it remains arguable that exercise helped to avoid recidivism among the 45% who stopped smoking during their stay in hospital.

Longitudinal Studies of Overall Lifestyle

Prospective studies of worksite fitness and health-promotion initiatives have examined changes in various risk-taking behaviors of employees in the months following the implementation of such programs (S.N. Blair et al., 1986; Bly et al., 1986; Shephard, 1986b, 1986c; Shephard, Corey, & Cox, 1982). The current overall lifestyle of the individual employee is conveniently summarized using the Canadian Health Hazard Appraisal instrument (Spasoff, 1987; Spasoff et al., 1980). This is a simple questionnaire covering various aspects of personal lifestyle. On the basis of the subject's responses, the person's chance of dying from each of 12 major causes of death is estimated for the next 10 years of the person's life. Results are expressed as a composite risk score and a corresponding appraised age. Over the first 6 months of involvement in an employee fitness program, male recruits showed a substantial, 2-year decrease in appraised age (Shephard, Corey, & Cox, 1982). This was attributable largely to a reduction of cigarette and alcohol consumption, together with a decrease in body mass (see Table 5.2). However, there was no appreciable change of appraised age among female participants, perhaps because many of the women seemed to join the exercise classes more for social than for health reasons.

Prospective studies in the United States have likewise shown decreases of cigarette and alcohol consumption among participants in worksite fitness and lifestyle programs (S.N. Blair et al., 1986). It remains unclear whether the behavioral change is a consequence of exercise participation itself, or is due to other health-promotional efforts by those who are operating the fitness program.

Aerobic Fitness, Perceived Health, and Performance

When members of the general public indicate why they choose to participate in a program of regular aerobic exercise, they commonly voice an overall quest for improved health by a statement such as "I wish to feel better." Given our broad definition of health (see chapter 1), a positive change of mood state can make an important contribution to the wellness of an individual and thus to her or his performance at school or at work. However, it is less clearly established that a program of aerobic exercise is the most effective approach to an improvement of mood state.

Table 5.2
Change of Appraised Age Observed Over First 6 Months
of a Worksite Employee Fitness Program

Group	Change of appraised age (yr)	
	Men	Women
High adherents	−2.36	−0.13
Low adherents	−1.25	−0.12
Drop-outs	−1.19	−0.37
Nonadherents	+1.34	+2.46
Controls	−0.96	+1.41

Note. A decrease in appraised age implies a reduced risk of death from the 12 principal causes over the next 10 years. High adherents exercised two or more times per week. Nonadherents worked at the same location, but did not participate in the fitness program. Controls were drawn from a matched company, also in central Toronto. Reprinted from Shephard, Corey, and Cox (1982) by permission.

Improvement of Perceived Health

Many people claim that various types of exercise do indeed make them "feel better." In support of this contention, the amount of habitual activity that a person undertakes is inversely related to the number of disorders reported when completing the Cornell Medical Index, or CMI (Cheraskin & Ringsdorf, 1971). Similarly, participation in an aerobic training program leads to a decreased frequency of illnesses as assessed by the CMI (Sidney, 1975).

On the other hand, if psychometric tools, such as the Profile of Mood States, are used, it is surprisingly difficult to obtain objective evidence that a moderate program of aerobic exercise has induced an improvement of mood state in otherwise healthy individuals. In those with an initial disorder of affect, the beneficial response to such a program is more clear-cut.

Academic Performance

Many physical educators have apparently felt guilty about taking students' time from a heavily loaded curriculum to teach students what is widely regarded as a nonacademic subject. Early studies (Shaw & Cordts, 1960) failed to agree whether athletic involvement influenced academic achievement—favorably or not. Problems in interpreting the data of early investigations include their cross-sectional design, lack of an appropriate definition of exercise participation, and the difficulty of accurate measurement of academic achievement. Often, active students were defined on the basis of their winning an athletic letter. Such athletes are a highly selected group and inevitably differ from nonathletes in many characteristics, including the desire for high achievement, which may affect performance both on the track and in the examination hall. Often, athletes must also maintain a minimum of marks to retain a place in university, and sometimes they receive special coaching to compensate for travel off-campus. They may further gain various rewards—not only scholarship support, but also peer praise and heightened feelings of self-efficacy. Finally, if membership on a sports team is the basis of classification, a proportion of students who pursue vigorous individual activities, such as cycling, will be excluded from the active group.

Volle, Shephard, et al. (1982) and Volle, Tisal, et al. (1982) were able to conduct a controlled longitudinal experiment in which entire classes of primary-school students were switched from the standard physical education program (40 min/week, taught by a nonspecialist) to an enhanced regimen (60 min of daily exercise, taught by a physical education specialist and designed to enhance cardiorespiratory and muscular endurance); control classes in the same schools followed the standard physical education program. Over the 6-year study, the time that the experimental students allocated to academic work was necessarily reduced some 14% to accomodate the additional physical activity, but nevertheless, their academic performance was enhanced relative to that of control students.

There was apparently some linkage between the gains in academic performance and enhanced psychomotor performance (Volle, Tisal, et al., 1982). Other possible contributing factors may have been an enhanced mood state, an increase of arousal, and greater satisfaction with the overall school program. Moreover, the academic teachers may have taught their subjects better because they were free of teaching duties while the physical activity classes were proceeding, and thus had more time to prepare their instructional materials.

Perceived Health and Industrial Work

Several studies (see Table 5.3) have shown an improvement of health (measured by a reduction in the average number of medical insurance claims submitted) in the first few months after implementation of worksite programs of endurance exercise (Bowne, Russell, J.L. Morgan, Optenberg, & Clarke, 1984; Dedmon, 1988; Gibbs, Mulvaney, Henes, & Reed, 1985; Shephard, 1989d).

Initially, LaPorte (1966), Lindén (1969), and Massie and Shephard (1971) suggested that worksite fitness programs also lead to small gains of productivity and reductions in employee absenteeism. A possible explanation of these findings is that the physical activity itself, or some associated change of personal circumstance, leads to an improvement of mood state and optimization of cerebral arousal, with an enhancement of perceived health among those participating in the fitness program.

There may also be more specific benefits from physical training. For example, the gain in physical working capacity achieved during an aerobic training program may bring a worker's physique to a point where he or she can cope with both a day's employment and a minor ailment (e.g., a cold). Those unaccustomed to physical effort (Magora & Taustein, 1969) and those with weak trunk muscles (Alston, Carlson, Feldman, Grimm, & Gerontinos, 1966) seem particularly vulnerable to back injuries, and muscle-building programs apparently have reduced the

Table 5.3
Influence of Employee Fitness Program on Medical Costs

Author	Finding
Cox et al., 1981	Controlled study; costs reduced by equivalent of half-day hospital bed/year plus 3 medical consultations.
Bowne et al., 1984	46% reduction of medical costs for participants.
Gibbs et al., 1985	24% decrease in medical costs for participants.
Bly et al., 1986	Controlled study; 17% reduction of hospital costs Year I, 34% less in Year III relative to controls.
Patton et al., 1986	Costs $296/year less than nonparticipants.
Dedmon, 1988	$450/year health insurance savings.

Note. For details of references, see Shephard, 1992h.

incidence of back injuries among police and firefighters (Barnard & Anthony, 1980; Cady, P.C. Thomas, & Karwasky, 1985; Superko et al., 1983).

Unfortunately, many studies purporting to examine the health benefits of work-site fitness programs have been uncontrolled or poorly controlled (Shephard, in press-a). Thus, a part of the apparent response to exercise may have arisen because companies that provide fitness programs tend to recruit health-conscious employees (Baun et al., 1986), and the most health-conscious members of the labor force become the most enthusiastic participants in the fitness program.

Potential Causes of Well-Being and Enhanced Performance

Discussion continues on potential mechanisms whereby people might both feel better and perform better during and immediately following a bout of vigorous aerobic exercise. Successful performance of a sport or skilled activity can give a sense of self-efficacy and self-actualization. In a group setting, success may also win the praise of significant others (although conversely, a failure to meet the expectations of a coach or a fitness-class leader can have a negative impact upon mood state and self-image).

In some instances, physical activity (not necessarily aerobic in type) may provide a diversion from boring or unpleasant work. Participants may also find sensual pleasures associated with the exercise sessions (the excitement of competition, rapid body movement, physical danger) or they may enjoy the related social contacts (Kenyon, 1968). If a person is normally underaroused, the proprioceptive stimulation associated with vigorous movement may increase neuronal activity in the reticular formation of the brain, bringing the flow of impulses to what is an optimal level for job performance. On the other hand, if an individual normally faces a demanding job and is overaroused on leaving work, then gentle movement in a soothing environment may help reduce the activity of the reticular formation to a personally more acceptable level.

Biochemical factors may also contribute to the modulation of mood state—for instance, the secretion of arousing amines or relaxing beta-endorphins may be increased immediately following prolonged bouts of aerobic activity (Harber & Sutton, 1984).

Aerobic Exercise and Reproductive Function

Very heavy aerobic training apparently delays menarche in adolescents and may cause amenorrhea or irregular periods in young women who have already begun menstruating. Premenstrual breast tenderness, bloating, and mood changes are reduced by regular aerobic exercise. There is a decreased response to gonadotropin-releasing-hormone (D.C. Cumming, 1989), with a reduced frequency and amplitude of luteinizing hormone pulses, a shortening of the luteinizing phase of the menstrual cycle, and a decrease in the concentrations of circulating progesterone and estrogen. It is less clear whether exercise alone is responsible for these changes, or whether the cause is a metabolic or hormonal signal related to some combination of physical activity, emotional stress, and a negative energy balance (Beitins, McArthur, Turnbull, Skrinar, & Bullen, 1991; Feicht, T.C. Johnson, B.J. Martin, Sparkes, & Wagner, 1978; Myerson et al., 1991; Prior, 1990; Warren, 1985).

The reproductive systems of older women seem more resistant to an equivalent amount of training (Frisch et al., 1981), perhaps because older subjects usually have larger reserves of body fat. But amenorrhea can occasionally develop in quite obese older swimmers who are training hard (Frisch et al., 1984).

Normal menstrual cycles are usually resumed quite quickly once the training volume is reduced, but there is some medical concern, because the disorder is accompanied by calcium loss from trabecular bone. Prior (1990) has suggested that there may be compensating increases of cortical bone. In the absence of such compensation, the trabecular weakening could have long-term implications for health, increasing vulnerability to stress fractures and scoliosis (Cann, M.C. Martin, Genant, & Jeffe, 1984; Drinkwater et al., 1986; Warren et al., 1986).

Although the majority of studies of exercise and reproductive function have involved women, Prior (1990) has emphasized that very strenuous aerobic training induces analogous effects on the reproductive function of men. There are decreases in testosterone levels, decreased semen volume and quality, and decreased fertility—all reversible by a moderation of training.

Aerobic Exercise and Pregnancy

Over the past 2 decades, an increasing proportion of pregnant women have recognized the value of maintaining their aerobic fitness through a suitably adapted physical activity program (Lotgering & Longo, 1984; Wong & McKenzie, 1987). It has further been suggested that such activity has a favorable influence on the health of the mother both during and immediately following pregnancy.

Proponents of continued aerobic exercise for the pregnant woman have argued that aerobic conditioning shortens the duration of labor, reduces the frequency of perinatal complications, and improves the ultimate health of the newborn child (American College of Obstetricians & Gynecologists, 1985; Leaf, 1989; Paolone & Worthington, 1985; Wolfe, Ohtake, Mottola, & McGrath, 1989; Work, 1989). However, there is as yet only limited empirical support for the patterns of exercise currently being recommended to the pregnant woman (M.M. Gauthier, 1986; Kulpa, White, & Visscher, 1987).

Acute Effects on the Fetus

There can be little argument that an acute bout of vigorous aerobic activity redistributes maternal blood flow from the placenta toward the exercising muscles of the mother. But in normal pregnancy, it seems likely that compensatory mechanisms (an altered intrauterine distribution of flow, hemoconcentration, and a widening of the arteriovenous oxygen difference) protect the developing fetus from excessive exercise-induced hypoxia, unless the uterine circulation is already compromised by some preexisting pathology.

The response of the fetus to acute bouts of exercise has most commonly been evaluated by Doppler ultrasound recordings of its heart rate. Such studies show that in women with normal pregnancies, moderate dynamic exercise induces either no change or a moderate, 5- to 30-beats/min increase in fetal heart rate. Factors contributing to fetal tachycardia include an increase of arousal, a rise in core temperature, a placental transfer of catecholamines, and a reduction in maternal uterine blood flow (Collings, Curet, & Mullin, 1983). Maternal aerobic conditioning does not appear to alter the fetal response to a given intensity of exercise (Webb, Wolfe, Hall, Tranmer, & McGrath, 1989; Young, Bonen, Campagna, & Beresford, 1988). A very strenuous bout of aerobic exercise gives rise to the less favorable sign of fetal bradycardia in at least some pregnant women (Artal et al., 1986; Carpenter et al., 1988). Bradycardia and irregularities of fetal heart rhythm are particularly common in women with complicated pregnancies (e.g., those with a compromised uterine circulation or a preeclamptic state).

Other potential, exercise-induced changes in fetal health include alterations in the frequency of spontaneous limb movements and in patterns of breathing. Two studies found no change of fetal limb movements in response to moderate aerobic exercise (Katz, McMurray, Berry, & Cefalo, 1988; Platt, Artal, Semel, Sipos, & Kammula, 1983), but a third investigation noted some decrease of fetal movements in the first 7 min following treadmill exercise (Clapp et al., 1987). There have been some suggestions of a reduction in fetal breathing movements with vigorous aerobic exercise, although Platt et al. (1983) saw no change in such movements immediately following 15 min of mild treadmill exercise.

Effects on the Mother

Early investigators suggested that the involvement of women in vigorous athletic competition might strengthen the muscles of the pelvic floor and perineum, thus potentially hampering delivery, but might also strengthen the abdominal muscles, shortening the second stage of labor.

Evidence supporting either a positive or a negative impact of athletic involvement on the course of pregnancy (Zaharieva, 1972) is relatively weak. There is little correlation between maternal aerobic power and such factors as length of gestation, duration of labor, and obstetric complications (Clapp, 1989b; Kulpa et al., 1987; Pomerance et al., 1974). Berkowitz, Kelsey, Holford, and Berkowitz (1983) maintained that regular physical activity during pregnancy protected against preterm delivery, and Erkkola (1976) reported that women with a high physical working capacity had shorter spontaneous labors and gave birth to heavier infants than their sedentary peers. However, Clapp and Dickstein (1984) found that women who exercised beyond the 28th week of pregnancy gained an average of 4.6 kg less weight and delivered slightly lighter infants 8 days earlier than their inactive peers. Even so, D.C. Hall and Kaufmann (1987) noted that women who exercised regularly required delivery by Caesarian section less frequently.

Fetal Development

A number of animal studies have shown a negative long-term effect of habitual maternal exercise on fetal development. This has been attributed to a combination of hypoxia, hypoglycemia, and hyperthermia. The amounts of exercise involved have exceeded those generally undertaken by pregnant women (Clapp, 1989a, 1989b; McMurray & Katz, 1990). Hyperthermia during the first trimester apparently increases the risk of neural tube defects (N.L. Fisher & Smith, 1981), and hypoglycemia leads to a retardation of overall development (Clapp, Wesley, & Sleamaker, 1987).

Human data suggest that if the mother takes moderate aerobic exercise, there is little influence on infant birthweight or early measures of neonatal health, such as 1-min APGAR scores (Clapp, 1989b; D.C. Hall & Kaufmann, 1987; Kulpa et al., 1987). Clapp and Capeless (1990) commented that at birth, the infants of exercising mothers weighed 500 g less than those borne to sedentary mothers, but they argued that the lighter weight of the infants of the exercising mothers may have reflected merely a reduction in the body fat content of the fetus. A recent metaanalysis has confirmed that, on average, there is some reduction of fetal weight in mothers who exercise during pregnancy (Lokey, Tran, Wells, Meyers, & Tran, 1989).

The fitness and well-being of the mother are enhanced by continuing a program of moderate aerobic exercise during pregnancy (D.C. Hall and Kaufmann, 1987; Brenner, Monga, Webb, McGrath, & Wolfe, 1991). Such a regimen increases the probability of avoiding long-term adverse effects from the pregnancy. The infant may be a little smaller than that born to a sedentary mother, but this does not have an adverse effect on the infant's perinatal health. Women thus should be encouraged to maintain moderate physical activity throughout pregnancy.

Aerobic Exercise, Physical Working Capacity, and Quality of Life

The percentage of peak aerobic power that a subject can develop without experiencing excessive fatigue is greatly influenced by the nature and duration of the task that must be accomplished. An average person can use 100% of aerobic power for a few minutes, but depending on the volume of muscle that has been activated, the body posture that is adopted, and any adverse environmental circumstances such as an extreme of heat or cold, fatigue is likely if the activity demands more than 40% of aerobic power throughout a normal working day (I. Åstrand, 1967; I. Åstrand, Gahary, & Wahren, 1968; Hughes & Goldman, 1970; Shephard, 1992b, in press-a).

Bonjer (1968) has recommended even lower performance limits when aerobic activity is undertaken in industry—63% of maximal aerobic power for 1 hr, 53% for 2 hr, 47% for 4 hr, and 33% for 8 hr of work. The introduction of rest pauses to metabolize accumulated lactate improves tolerance to sustained aerobic exercise. On the other hand, a given rate of working is more poorly tolerated if the task is performed by a few specific muscle groups, particularly if the arms must be used above heart level (I. Åstrand, 1971; I. Åstrand et al., 1968). Likewise, a high environmental temperature reduces the safety margin, because a substantial fraction of the potential increase of cardiac output is then diverted from the working muscles to the blood vessels of the skin for cooling. Prolonged standing also reduces work tolerance, because fluid pools in the blood vessels and tissues of the legs. Awkward postures such as stooping or reaching are even more disadvantageous; a substantial effort is needed to maintain the posture, and it may no longer be possible to use many of the muscles that would otherwise be brought to bear on the primary external task. Finally, a long, tiring journey to and from work reduces tolerance of aerobic activity on the job.

In most circumstances, a young man with a peak oxygen consumption of 3 L/min, or 2.2 mmol/s, should tolerate 8 hr of work at an average intensity of 31 kJ/min, or 7.5 kcal/min. Effort of this level of severity is rarely required in modern industry. Peak oxygen-consumption figures for older men and women are typically 2.0 and 1.5 L/min, or 1.5 and 1.1 mmol/s, respectively. The industrial tolerance limits are correspondingly reduced to 21 and 15 kJ/min, respectively, figures that are exceeded in quite a number of jobs. Thus, one might anticipate that the older worker would show fatigue or a deterioration of productivity over an 8-hr shift. Equally, benefit might be anticipated from deliberate measures to increase the aerobic power of older employees: not only aerobic training, but also the correction of any obesity or anemia and the encouragement of smoking cessation.

In practice, the effects of aerobic fitness level on either productivity or absenteeism are generally small (Lindén, 1969; Shephard, 1989a) unless the work is arduous. Danielson and Danielson (1982) carried out a controlled study of people fighting forest fires in northern Ontario. An experimental group who received regular aerobic training were indeed more productive than the control group, but only under the most arduous conditions (e.g., hot and humid weather).

One possible reason why older people do not show greater evidence of fatigue in the workplace may be that as the safety limit is approached, they slow their pace of movement to a personally acceptable level. In some circumstances, a younger employee may also help an older worker who cannot bear the expected daily load. Experience may allow an older person to accomplish a given task with a smaller energy expenditure than a younger individual. Finally, some employees earn promotions that take them away from the shop floor.

Kilbom (1971a, 1971b) instituted a 7-week physical activity program for middle-aged female shop assistants. She noted that program recruits reported a greater feeling of physical well-being, particular comment being made regarding a reduction in swelling of the feet and calves at the end of the day.

Aging, Disability, and Handicap

A sedentary young adult usually has a fair margin between peak working capacity and the physical demands of normal daily life. However, as age advances, everyone experiences a progressive impairment of such components of physical fitness as aerobic power, muscle strength, and joint flexibility. The inevitable consequences of aging are often compounded by a progressive decrease in habitual physical activity and by the development of specific pathologies, such as osteoarthritis or stroke.

Physical ability decreases particularly rapidly in the senior citizen, and in the usual domestic environment faced by such individuals, disability becomes converted into handicap, as an increasing number of ordinary daily tasks such as climbing steps, bathing, and dressing become physically impossible. In Canada, the final period of life is typically marked by 8 to 10 years in which there is some limitation of physical activity, and 1 year of almost total dependency (Canada Health Survey, 1982). Moreover, perhaps because women have a longer overall life expectancy than men, on average they experience a longer period of disability.

The factors leading to dependency and institutionalization of the senior citizen are varied. Sometimes there is a medical explanation for the underlying impairment—the subject may suffer a progressive loss of intellect due to Alzheimer's disease or may experience a catastrophe, such as sudden stroke or blindness. In other cases, the factor precipitating dependence may be social or environmental. For instance, the death of a spouse or the removal of a near relative may cut off essential support and encouragement, converting disability into a handicap that precludes independent living. But in many instances, the primary problem is a progressive deterioration in some component of health-related fitness.

Loss of Health-Related Fitness and Dependency

In the present context, it is convenient to illustrate the interaction between the loss in various components of health-related fitness and the onset of dependence by reference to the age-related deterioration of aerobic power. The loss of oxygen transport in a sedentary person amounts to about 3 to 4 $\mu mol/(kg \cdot s)$, or 5 ml/(kg·min), during each decade of adult life—and deterioration occurs only a little more slowly in an endurance athlete (Shephard, 1988a). The peak aerobic power of a sedentary person thus drops from a value of 28 $\mu mol/(kg \cdot s)$, or 40 ml/(kg·min), as a young adult to only 14 $\mu mol/(kg \cdot s)$, or 20 ml/(kg·min), at the age of 65 years. By the time of retirement, the peak intensity of well-tolerated, steady aerobic activity is equivalent to an oxygen consumption of only 6 to 7 $\mu mol/(kg \cdot s)$ [8 to 10 ml/(kg·min)], or in a person weighing 70 kg, 9.6 to 14.7 kJ/min [2.3 to 3.5 kcal/min], no more than light work. As age advances, even a light task becomes fatiguing if it is sustained for 8 hr (Shephard, 1991c). Finally, around the age of 80 years, the peak aerobic power has dropped to a critical threshold (probably 9 to 10 $\mu mol/[kg \cdot s]$, or 12 to 14 ml/[kg·min]) where many of the ordinary tasks of daily living can no longer be accomplished unaided, even with frequent rest breaks.

The threshold of aerobic power below which physiological impairment is translated into an overt handicap depends very much on the individual's environment. Independence can be maintained for much longer if a senior citizen lives in a barrier-free environment or a small, labor-saving apartment with some domestic help than if they are trying, unaided, to maintain, a large, multistoreyed house with a garden.

Influence of Habitual Physical Activity on Independence

Participation in a regular aerobic training program can increase maximal oxygen intake by 4 to 8 μmol/(kg·s), or 5 to 10 ml/(kg·min), even in a senior citizen (Sidney & Shephard, 1978; Shephard, 1987a). Relating this gain to the normally anticipated, age-related loss of aerobic power, we may note that a conditioning program can yield the equivalent of a 10- to 20-year reduction in biological age (Shephard, 1991c).

It follows that if a low aerobic power is the prime cause of dependency, then regular aerobic training should set back the age at which overt handicap and institutionalization result by a corresponding margin of 10 to 20 years. Empirical evidence that active living has such an effect was obtained by Shephard and Montelpare (1988) in a survey of senior citizens. Relative to their independently living peers, those who had suffered disability or were institutionalized had engaged in much less physical activity at the age of 50 years (see Table 1.5).

Disability and Quality-Adjusted Lifespan

Investigators are just beginning to develop methods of measuring quality-adjusted lifespans (Kaplan, 1985). However, we can see intuitively that if a person has preserved sufficient health-related fitness to maintain independence during the later years of retirement, then their quality of life will be much higher than that of someone who has been obliged to enter an institution or who has become heavily dependent on daily nursing care. Ten years of dependent survival might be equivalent to no more than 5 disability-free years. Thus, even if the average age of death is relatively similar for active and inactive seniors (Paffenbarger, 1988; Pekkanen et al., 1987), the active senior could still gain a 5-year advantage of quality-adjusted life expectancy.

Paraplegia and Quadriplegia

Arguments about the contribution of a well-maintained level of aerobic fitness to productivity, independence, and quality of life have particular importance to people having paraplegia or quadriplegia The aerobic power of such individuals is typically low, because of such factors as blood pooling in paralyzed muscles, loss of normal means to increase heart rate and myocardial contractility, an increased afterloading as the heart endeavors to perfuse small, vigorously contracting arm muscles, and, in many instances, an inactive overall lifestyle (Shephard, 1989e). At the same time, the energy cost of wheelchair ambulation can be quite high, particularly when the subject is ascending a ramp or crossing a carpeted surface, and the oxygen cost of such activity is further exacerbated because the mechanical efficiency of rim propulsion is relatively low.

Both the aerobic power and the muscle strength of a person with spinal injury can be increased by appropriate training programs (G. Davis & Shephard, 1990; G. Davis, Plyley, & Shephard, 1991). Noreau and Shephard (1992) found that the productive activity of such individuals correlated to their peak aerobic power, the relationship persisting even after the data had been controlled for leisure-time aerobic activity. They postulated that a large aerobic power might be serving as surrogate for muscle strength, and they argued that strength sufficient to surmount architectural barriers was a critical factor when such individuals attempted to undertake productive activity in the community.

Acute Disease, Immune Function, and Aerobic Exercise

Aerobic activity has both immediate and more prolonged effects upon the risks of acute disease, because it modifies exposure to infection and alters immune function. It may also influence the course of a preexisting disease process.

Altered Exposure Patterns

If aerobic exercise is taken outdoors, there is a likelihood of increased exposure to many air contaminants (Silverman, Urch, Corey, & Shephard, 1990). In particular, peak concentrations of particulate matter and absorbed vapors are commonly two to three times higher outdoors than indoors (Phair, Carey, & Shephard, 1958).

The biological effects of any given concentration of an air contaminant are also likely to be increased during vigorous aerobic exercise, because nasal breathing is supplemented by oral breathing at respiratory minute volumes of more than 30 to 40 L/min (Niinimaa, Cole, Mintz, & Shephard, 1980). Under resting conditions, a substantial fraction of large, airborne particles, and as much as 90% of soluble vapors, are absorbed as the inspirate passes through the nose (Ainsworth & Shephard, 1961; Oberst, 1961). During aerobic exercise, oral breathing exposes the trachea more directly to both pollutants and cold, dry air. The mucus becomes thicker, and ciliary movement is slowed (Rylander, 1968). Both of these responses hamper the elimination of particles (including bacteria and viruses) from the respiratory tract. Similarly, if a person exercises vigorously while suffering from a sinus infection, mucus may be aspirated into the chest, spreading infection into the smaller air passages.

On the other hand, the concentration of virus and bacterial particles per unit volume of respired air is likely to be much lower outdoors than at places of passive, indoor entertainment. Furthermore, the concentrations of some major air contaminants of importance to health (e.g., environmental tobacco smoke; Surgeon General, 1986) are much higher indoors than outdoors.

In a number of instances, swimming in infected water has been incriminated as the cause of epidemics of anterior poliomyelitis and of *Salmonella typhi* or *Giardia lamblia* infections (Jokl, 1977). Improved sanitation now has reduced such hazards to more acceptable levels, at least in developed countries; but crowded public swimming pools are still responsible for a troubling incidence of conjunctival and middle-ear infections (Crone & Tee, 1974), and some reports still link gastrointestinal infections to swimming in seawater contaminated by untreated sewage.

The macerated skin of the athlete who competes in a hot environment is also less resistant to staphylococcal lesions (e.g., boils and carbuncles), whereas wet surfaces in changing areas provide an increased opportunity for the transmission of fungal infections, such as tinea pedis, or athlete's foot, and tinea cruris, a related infection of the groin).

Finally, endurance activities, such as cross-country running, may take the participant into regions where there is risk of infection from insect vectors (e.g., mosquito-borne malaria or meningitis) and contaminated soil (e.g., that harboring tetanus).

Immune Function

A single bout of vigorous aerobic exercise suppresses various aspects of cellular and humoral immune function, such as the ratio of helper to suppressor T cells and serum immunoglobulin levels (Mackinnon, 1992; Shephard, 1991a; Shinkai, Shore, Shek, & Shephard, 1992). The maximum response is seen about 30 min following the exercise session, and the normal resting values of most immune parameters are restored 30 to 60 min later (see Figure 5.2). Because the disturbance of immune function is quite transient, it is unlikely that it has any substantial impact on clinical variables, such as resistance to acute infections, HIV, or cancer.

Moderate aerobic training apparently boosts resting immune function and diminishes the impact of even a single bout of exercise on immune parameters (Shephard, Verde, et al., 1991). However, the evidence concerning strenuous aerobic training is somewhat less favorable. Several weeks of excessively heavy training is associated with a persistent depression of resting immune function (Shephard, Verde, et al., 1991). Moreover, various authors have commented that athletes have a surprisingly high incidence of upper respiratory infections (Berglund & Hemmingson, 1990), and episodes of overtraining apparently increase the susceptibility of the trainee to acute infections. For example, during the final 2 months of preparation for the Los Angeles marathon run, Nieman et al. (1990) noted a twofold increase in the incidence of respiratory infections among those who ran more than 97 km/week. Furthermore, in the week following the run, there was a 5.9-fold increase in the risk of infectious episodes among participants relative to similarly experienced runners who had not participated in the event.

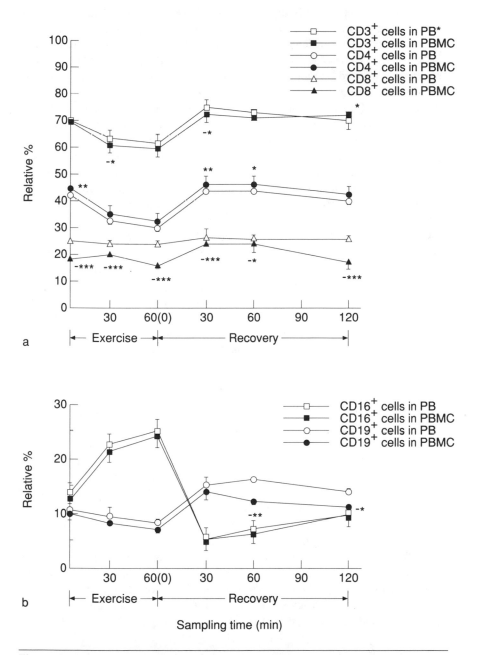

Figure 5.2   Acute effects of exercise on various categories of immunocompetent cells including (a) CD3, CD4 (helper T cells) and CD8 (suppressor cells), and (b) CD16 (NK cells) and CD 19 lymphocytes. *Note*. Reprinted from Shinaki et al. (1992) by permission. *PB, peripheral blood; PBMC, washed peripheral blood mononuclear cells. Subjects performed 60 min exercise at 60% to 70% of maximal oxygen intake.

Patients in the chronic phase of rheumatoid arthritis respond favorably to a program of moderate aerobic exercise. It remains unclear whether benefit is attributable to a direct influence of training on this immune disorder, whether pain relief comes from an increased production of neuropeptides, or whether function is improved by mobilization of the affected joints and strengthening of the surrounding muscles. At least one report has claimed that regular exercise is also beneficial in systemic lupus erythematosus (Robb-Nicholson et al., 1989).

There is growing evidence that the response to moderate aerobic exercise has a beneficial influence on the course of HIV infection (Antoni et al., 1990; LaPerriere, Schneiderman, Antoni, & Fletcher, 1990; Liesen & Uhlenbruck, 1992). However, the mechanism may be indirect (e.g., a decrease of anxiety and depression, with an enhanced release of endogenous opioids or a reduced secretion of corticosteroids), rather than a specific boost of immune function or an attack on the virus itself.

Well-trained individuals have a decreased risk of gastrointestinal and reproductive system cancers (Bartram & Wynder, 1989; Kohl, LaPorte, & S.N. Blair, 1988; Shephard, 1990e), although it is unclear whether this benefit arises from such factors as a reduction of body fat and a speeding of gastrointestinal transit, or whether it can be linked to an influence of aerobic training on cytokines and natural killer-cell function. Aerobic exercise increases blood levels of a number of cytokines, but it may also reduce the numbers and activity of natural killer-cells, in part by the action of prostaglandins (Mackinnon, 1992).

Course of Acute Infections

Vigorous aerobic exercise may modify the course of acute infections by increasing core temperature (the multiplication rates of some microorganisms are highly susceptible to local environmental temperatures; Roberts, 1979). Regional effects may also arise from a redistribution of blood flow to the active tissues. For instance, if a person is infected with the virus of anterior poliomyelitis, then the microorganism tends to localize in the anterior horn cells that are linked to the muscles that have been engaged in vigorous aerobic activity (Jokl, 1977).

Viral myocarditis (e.g., an infection of the myocardium by a strain of influenza virus) is aggravated by acute bouts of exercise, with a risk of provoking sudden death. The contribution of viral myocarditis to cardiac catastrophes is smaller than was once believed (Bouhour & Borgat, 1985), but our own data include one postcoronary patient from the Toronto Rehabilitation Centre who entered a marathon run with an undisclosed influenzal infection and died after covering 8 km of the course (Shephard, 1981).

Cardiac Disease

Exercise has long been considered a useful antidote to ischemic heart disease, but more recently it has also been prescribed for children with various forms of congenital heart disease, adults with hypertension, peripheral atherosclerosis, or congestive failure, and patients of all ages who have undergone coronary bypass and cardiac transplant operations.

Primary Prevention

Epidemiologists (Mausner & Bahn, 1974) distinguish between the primary, secondary, and tertiary prevention of disease. Primary prevention is implemented before the subject has developed any subclinical pathology. Secondary prevention is begun after the onset of pathological changes. For example, a patient may have some atheromatous streaking of the major arteries, but this has not yet been translated into a clinical manifestation of ischemic heart disease (IHD), such as angina or intermittent claudication. Tertiary prevention, or rehabilitation, follows the onset of clinical disease. Thus, a tertiary program for the patient with ischemic heart disease will seek to prevent a recurrence of myocardial infarction.

The distinction between primary and secondary prevention has particular importance in conditions with a long time course. For example, the intraarterial deposition of atherosclerotic lipids begins in early childhood (McGill, 1980; Ylä-Herttula, 1985). Many people in developed societies have quite advanced atherosclerosis by the time they reach early adulthood (Enos, Holmes, & Bayer, 1953). Thus, to be successful, primary prevention of IHD must begin in early childhood.

Prospective studies on high-risk adult populations—for example, those living in Finland (Frick et al., 1987) and in North America (Lipid Research Clinics Program, 1984)—have shown that serum cholesterol can be reduced by a combination of a low-fat diet and cholesterol-sequestrating drugs. There are fewer cardiac events following such treatment, but the evidence regarding a decrease of overall mortality is less convincing, particularly after the therapeutic intervention has ceased. An increase of physical activity, likewise, has beneficial metabolic effects in high-risk populations. It improves the lipid profile, increases insulin sensitivity, and reduces the systemic blood pressure (Després, Bouchard, & Malina, 1990). However, perhaps because youngsters have a better initial cardiac-risk status, the benefits of increased aerobic activity and a reduced intake of saturated (i.e., animal) fat (Keys, Anderson, & Grande, 1957) are less readily demonstrated in school-age children than in adults, particularly if the evidence is sought from longitudinal studies rather than cross-sectional comparisons between athletic and sedentary individuals (Després et al., 1990).

Secondary Prevention

Sustained aerobic exercise likely benefits the secondary prevention of ischemic heart disease. An increase of aerobic activity is effective in controling several important cardiac risk factors, including obesity (Brownell & Kaye, 1982; Pařízková, 1982); a high serum-cholesterol concentration (here, the benefit of exercise is more easily demonstrated in adults—Kavanagh et al., 1983 [see Figure 5.3];

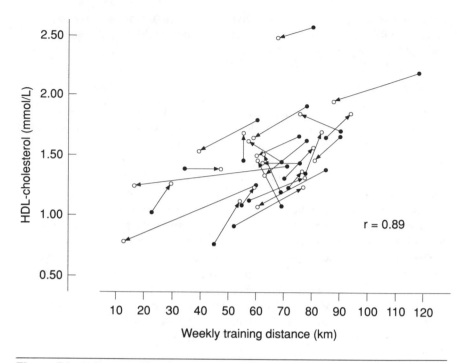

Figure 5.3 Influence of jogging distance on plasma levels of HDL-cholesterol. Each line represents two observations at 1-yr interval on a single postcoronary patient. The overall correlation between HDL-cholesterol concentration and weekly training distance is r = 0.89. *Note.* Adapted from Kavanagh et al. (1983) by permission.

P.T. Williams et al., 1982—than in children—Després et al., 1990); glucose tolerance (Björntorp, 1981; Vranic & Berger, 1979; Vranic & Wasserman, 1990); and hypertension (Hagberg et al., 1983; Tipton, 1991; Ylitalo, 1981). In animals, an increase of physical activity can actually cause a regression of atherosclerotic lesions (Kramsch, Aspen, Abramowitz, Kreimendahl, & Hood, 1981), but in humans, epidemiological evidence can do no more than prove that the progression of vascular lesions is slowed if aerobic exercise is used as a means of secondary prevention.

Studies from both North America and Europe (Berenson, 1980; Clarke, Schrott, Leaverton, Connor, & Lauer, 1978; Després et al., 1990; Gilliam, Katch, Thorland, Weltman, 1977; Montoye, 1985; Verschuur, 1987; Wilmore & McNamara, 1974) have shown that, largely as a consequence of low levels of aerobic activity, many young children already manifest several of the accepted, major risk factors for future ischemic heart disease, including hypertension, obesity, a high serum cholesterol, and a low HDL- to LDL-cholesterol ratio. From the viewpoint of secondary prevention, it is less certain how far such risk factors track from childhood into adult life (Kemper et al., 1989; Orchard, Donahue, Kuller, Hodge, & Drash, 1983; Verschuur, 1987; Webber, Cresanta, Voors, & Berenson,

1983). For example, the correlation between the extent of obesity seen in young adolescents and their subsequent levels of obesity diminishes progressively as observations are extended through the teen years into early adulthood (Kemper et al., 1989; also see Table 5.4).

The impact of aerobic activity on the incidence of ischemic heart disease in adults was originally explored in terms of cross-sectional comparisons between athletes and sedentary individuals, between workers in physically demanding jobs and those in sedentary occupations, and between ethnic groups with varying levels of habitual physical activity (Shephard, 1981, 1985b). In general, such data suggested an association between regular, vigorous aerobic activity and a low risk of ischemic heart disease. Moreover, the risk gradient was largest in the best-controlled studies (Powell et al., 1987). However, problems of interpretation remain, due to self-selection of the exercise regimen and a possible linkage between exercise participation and other favorable health behaviors. For example, Karvonen et al. (1974) showed that cross-country skiers lived some 4 years longer than their sedentary peers, but much of the apparent benefit of prolonged aerobic exercise may have occurred because the majority of the skiers were lifelong nonsmokers. Likewise, J.N. Morris, Heady, and Raffle (1956) demonstrated that a sedentary group of workers (bus drivers) were fatter than a supposedly similar, but physically active group (bus conductors) upon hiring, when their Transit Authority uniforms were first issued. The drivers started their careers with a greater risk of coronary heart disease than the conductors. In other studies, there have been differences of income, education, diet, and race between physically active and sedentary groups. Cross-sectional studies cannot, by definition, establish a causal relationship between either physical activity or aerobic fitness and subsequent health experience.

Many potentially confounding factors can be eliminated by means of a prospective study. J.N. Morris, Kagan, Pattison, Gardner, and Raffle (1966) chose 667 bus crew without initial evidence of heart disease and followed their cardiovascular health over a 5-year period. During this time, 7% developed clinical or

Table 5.4
Cardiac Risk Factors From Adolescence (13 yr) to Early Adult (21 yr)

Variable	Correlation, 21- vs. 13-yr value	
	Males	Females
Total cholesterol	0.70	0.65
HDL-cholesterol	0.42	0.52
% Fat	0.59	0.62
Systolic pressure	0.49	0.35
Diastolic pressure	0.35	0.32

Note. Data from Kemper et al. (1989, p. 237).

electrocardiographic signs of coronary artery disease. Cardiac incidents were more common in obese than in thin subjects, and drivers were also at a disadvantage relative to conductors; but the two factors that contributed most to the risk of coronary attack were a high systolic blood pressure and a high serum cholesterol.

More recently, several other prospective studies (see Tables 5.5 and 5.6) have followed subjects who were initially characterized in terms of either their activity patterns (Leon et al., 1987; J.N. Morris, Everitt, Pollard, Chave, & Semmence, 1980; J.N. Morris, Clayton, et al., 1990; Paffenbarger, 1988; Scragg, Stewart, Jackson, & Beaglehole, 1987) or their initial levels of aerobic fitness (S.N. Blair et al., 1989; Ekelund et al., 1988; Leon et al., 1987; Lie, Mundal, & Erikssen, 1985; Peters, Cady, Bischoff, Bernstein, & Pike, 1983; Slattery & Jacobs, 1988). In all cases, regular physical activity or an above-average level of aerobic fitness was associated with a subsequent advantage in terms of ischemic heart disease morbidity and mortality. Moreover, the protection gained from a high level of physical activity was enhanced in subjects with other risk factors, such as a high systolic blood pressure, a high serum cholesterol, or continued cigarette smoking (Paffenbarger, 1988; Peters et al., 1983). S.N. Blair et al. (1989) stressed that the association between initial aerobic fitness and protection against ischemic heart disease persisted after adjustment of the data for the impact of potentially associated risk factors, including smoking habits, blood cholesterol, blood pressure, blood glucose levels, and a parental history of ischemic heart disease. It remains arguable from such studies that, for some reason, those with an inherently low risk of ischemic heart disease choose to exercise. In partial answer to the criticism of self-selection of an active lifestyle, Paffenbarger, Hyde, Wing, Jung, and Kampert (1991) demonstrated that benefit was enhanced if subjects increased their physical activity over the period of observation, but protection was lost if initially active subjects became sedentary. Nevertheless, there remains the difficulty that those who develop manifestations of ischemic heart disease subsequently may move from an active to a sedentary form of employment or reduce their leisure activity.

Originally, it was recommended that, in order to optimize cardiovascular benefit, subjects should undertake 30 min of vigorous activity at 70% of maximal oxygen intake three to five times a week (American College of Sports Medicine, 1991; also chapter 4). However, further analysis of the data linking fitness with subsequent prognoses suggested that much of the cardiovascular benefit was associated with quite small increments of physical activity and aerobic fitness (e.g., progression from a sedentary state, with a peak oxygen intake of 6 METS, to mild activity with a peak oxygen intake of 7 METS; S.N. Blair et al., 1989; see Figure 5.1, page 216); in some studies, prognosis actually worsened in subjects taking the highest levels of physical activity (Leon et al., 1987; Paffenbarger, 1988). Most adults can realize the 7-METs standard of peak performance through a regimen that involves such activities as rapid walking, gardening, and deliberate stair climbing, without participating in more vigorous forms of aerobic training. From the psychological point of view, it has been argued that it is much easier to shape sedentary behavior toward a modest initial exercise involvement than

Table 5.5
Relationship Between Habitual Physical Activity and Subsequent Risk of Ischemic Heart Disease

	Habitual activity level					
	1 (low)	2	3	4 (high)		Author
Fatal	1.0	.54	.38	.27		Morris et al., 1980
Nonfatal	1.0	1.0	.68	.35		
Total	1.0	.81	.57	.32		
Total	1.0	.88	.81			Leon et al., 1987
Fatal[a]	1.0	1.9	.50	.10	(male)	Scragg et al., 1987
	1.0			.20	(female)	
Nonfatal	1.0	1.2	.50	.20	(male)	
	1.0	.90	.70	.20	(female)	
Total	1.0		.61			Paffenbarger, 1988

Note. Data presented as relative risk. All studies adjusted for age differences. Data of Paffenbarger (1988) also adjusted for differences in cigarette habit and blood pressure status.
[a]Fatal attacks = all sudden deaths within 24 hr; data for men and for women shown separately.

attempt to induce a sudden, drastic increase in physical activity patterns. Such an approach is also attractive from the medical viewpoint, because it much less likely that a small increase in the intensity of physical activity will cause either musculoskeletal or cardiac problems.

Tertiary Prevention

There has been much discussion concerning the optimal design of programs for the tertiary prevention of ischemic heart disease, the evidence that benefit is gained from such programs, and the possible mechanisms involved in any therapeutic response (Shephard, 1981, 1989d).

PROGRAM DESIGN.   Gottheiner (1960) was the first person to advocate a systematic exercise rehabilitation of postcoronary patients. At first, programs were very cautious in nature, and training did not begin for 6 months or longer postinfarction, in order to ensure complete scarring of the affected area of the ventricular wall. Such a delay in treatment allowed considerable detraining to occur, and the patient's interest in adopting a better lifestyle kindled by the acute

Table 5.6
Relationship Between Physical Fitness and Subsequent
Incidence of Ischemic Heart Disease

	Physical fitness level				
	1 (low)	2	3	4 (high)	Author
T	1.0		.20	(high blood pressure)	Peters et al., 1983
	1.0		.23	(high cholesterol)	
	1.0		.29	(smoker)	
	1.0		.15	(two of above)	
F	1.0	.42	.39	.19	Lie et al., 1985
F	1.0	.54	.54	.15	Ekelund et al., 1988
F[a]	1.0	.41	.44	.35	Blair et al., 1989

Note. Risk of fatal (F) and total (T) attack shown relative to sedentary comparison group.
[a]All-cause death rate.

cardiac incident had often waned by the time exercise was permitted. Thus, very light, *Phase I* exercise now commences within 24 hr of infarction, unless the patient shows signs of heart failure, ominous aneurysmal bulging of the cardiac shadow at radiography, shock, intractable anginal pain, or abnormalities of cardiac rhythm that cannot be controlled by appropriate medication.

Beginning with movements of individual muscles (at an energy cost <10 kJ/min), the patient progresses to walking distances of 1 km at a stretch by the end of 4 weeks. Enrollment in a formal, supervised, outpatient program of progressive aerobic exercise begins about 8 weeks after infarction (Kavanagh, 1992). The exercise prescription is increased as rapidly as is judged safe based on regular laboratory exercise tests, physical observation of performance in the gymnasium, and (in some laboratories) individualized cardiac monitoring by telemetry. Current consensus holds that unless the patient falls into a high-risk category (with electrocardiographic evidence of continuing myocardial ischemia, abnormalities of heart rhythm not controlled by medication, or evidence of congestive failure), telemetric monitoring of training sessions is a costly and unnecessary luxury (Van Camp & Peterson, 1986).

The Toronto Rehabilitation Centre program (Kavanagh, 1992) offers an appropriate model for rehabilitation of the patient who is living in a large city. During the first 8 weeks, the patient attends *Phase II* classes two to three times a week. Staff monitor physiological and psychological responses to a program of carefully graded aerobic exercise throughout the 8 weeks. The patient is instructed in techniques of walking, jogging, and pulse counting, any symptoms are discussed, and light home activities are prescribed for 3 of the remaining days in each week. If there is evidence of exercise-induced angina, the patient is advised to reduce activity to a slow walk whenever such a symptom occurs and not to resume more intense activity until the discomfort has passed. Exercise should not be pushed to the point of provoking frequent bouts of severe pain, which cause the patient unnecessary anxiety; there is also a risk that cardiac failure may develop while the myocardium is hypoxic (Parker, diGiorgi, & West, 1966). The typical, symptom-free patient progresses from walking 1.6 km in 30 min to covering 4 km in 57 min over the 8-week observation period. He or she then graduates to the *Phase III* program, attending the rehabilitation center once a week for 9 months, and once a month for a further 6 months.

Phase III participants also receive a personal exercise prescription specifying activities that are to be followed for at least 4 other days a week. Given the heavy opportunity cost of traveling to and from the rehabilitation center, this plan yields a much higher compliance rate (Shephard, Corey, & Kavanagh, 1981) than do programs that require the patient to attend a fixed location for 3 sessions of supervised activity each week.

Supervised activity sessions comprise a group discussion with the program director, 10 min of calisthenics for warm-up, 25 to 30 min of an individually prescribed walk-jog, 15 min of an enjoyable game, such as volleyball, and a final, extended cool-down. The home prescription notes the distance to be covered each day, the duration of exercise, the permitted pulse-rate ceiling, and any special indications for stopping exercise, such as the appearance of anginal pain or the development of an irregular heart rhythm. Adherence to the prescription is checked by having the patient complete a diary sheet each week and by then checking this report against the individual's progress as observed during monitored exercise sessions. Whereas some patients may undertake less than the recommended dose of exercise, there is also a danger that those with Type A personalities will attempt to progress faster than suggested, hoping to show a better training response than others enrolled in the same program.

Upward adjustment of the exercise prescription follows the typical, long-distance training plan. First, the time specified for covering a given distance is reduced. When the patient can accomplish the faster speed without problem, the distance is lengthened to restore the initial duration of the training session. The time for covering the new distance is then shortened, and the entire process is repeated. Using this type of plan, some patients have advanced from an aerobic power that was only 70% of the sedentary norm immediately postinfarction to as much as 112% of normal 3 to 4 years later (Shephard & Kavanagh, 1975).

Cardiac rehabilitation programs originally avoided muscle building, on the grounds that resistance exercise would cause a dangerous elevation of blood pressure and a depression of the cardiac ejection fraction during exercise sessions (Painter & Hanson, 1984). However, recent data have suggested such programs are safe (DeBusk, Valdez, Houston, & Haskell, 1978; Kelemen et al., 1986; Vander, Franklin, Wrisley, & Rubenfire, 1986), and with an appropriately graded program of brief contractions at less than 60% of maximal voluntary force, the rise of systolic pressure is no greater than would be seen during a sustained bout of aerobic exercise (Haslam, McCartney, McElvie, & McDougall, 1988). Further, by restoring lost muscle strength, a well-planned program of muscle building may increase the individual's sense of self-efficacy (K.J. Stewart, Mason, & Kelemen, 1988) and help to avoid a recurrence of infarction while performing unsupervised physical activities (Faigenbaum, Skrinar, Cesare, Kraemer, & Thomas, 1990; McKelvey & McCartney, 1990).

EVIDENCE OF BENEFIT.   Some investigators have argued that the pathological changes seen in atherosclerotic vessels are irreversible. There have been reports of exercise-induced regression of fatty streaking of vessels in animals (Kramsch et al., 1981), but postmortem studies of human adults do not reveal any fewer fatty, atherosclerotic plaques in the coronary vessels of normally active subjects than in the vessels of sedentary individuals. On the other hand, postmortem examination does show less fibrous scarring of the myocardium in active than in sedentary subjects (J.N. Morris & Crawford, 1958).

A variety of cross-sectional studies suggest that exercised patients fare much better than sedentary groups following myocardial infarction, the likelihood of a fatal recurrence being two to three times greater in those who do not exercise (Shephard, 1981). However, the supposed control groups in such studies have commonly comprised those who were living far from the treatment center, those unwilling to exercise, or those excluded from the exercise program by their medical adviser. It is thus arguable that much if not all of the apparent benefit seen in such studies is an artifact of patient selection.

During the past decade, about a dozen laboratories have attempted to assign postcoronary patients on a randomized or a stratified randomized fashion to aerobic exercise and control programs. Individual trials have been marred by difficulty in recruiting a sufficient number of subjects, a high drop-out rate, poor compliance with both experimental and control programs, and a relatively short follow-up period. Moreover, because of advances in medical treatment, the recurrence rate has proved to be much lower than was anticipated when the experiments were originally designed. Thus, with one exception, results have been statistically inconclusive. Individual laboratories have adopted different subject recruitment criteria and exercise protocols. The extent of advice offered on other aspects of personal lifestyle has also varied from one study to another. But accepting that all experiments were attempting to test the value of progressive aerobic exercise in tertiary prevention, a number of metaanalyses have now been completed (May, Furberg, Eberlin, & Geraci, 1983; Oldridge, Guyatt, Fischer, & Rimm, 1988; Shephard, 1989c). All of these analyses suggest that exercise leads to a statistically significant 20% to 30% reduction in the incidence of fatal recurrences of myocardial infarction (see Table 5.7). On the other hand, the incidence of nonfatal infarctions is similar in exercised and control groups. The inference from the metaanalyses is thus that progressive aerobic exercise adds 2-3 years to the lifespan of the average postcoronary patient.

Table 5.7
Endurance Exercise in Tertiary Prevention of Ischemic Heart Disease

Author	Sample size	Entry	Follow-up	Treatment	Exercise group			Control group		Therapeutic benefit	
					N	Deaths	Annual%	N	Deaths	Annual%	Ex/control
Kentala, 1972	298 (165)**	6-8 week	1 yr	Individually supervised, 2-3 times per week	152 77^x	26 11	17.1 7.2	146 81^x	32 11	21.9 6.9	0.81 1.04
Kallio, 1981	375 (74F,301M)	Hospital discharge (2 week)	3 yr	Exercise + health education	188	41	7.3	187	56	9.9	0.73
*Kallio et al., 1988	375 (74F,301M)	Hospital discharge (2 week)	10 yr (3-yr program)	Exercise + health education	188^x	82	8.2	187^x	97	9.7	0.85
*Hamalainen et al., 1988	456	Hospital discharge (2 week)	6 yr (3-month program)	Exercise + health education; controls received community-based program	228	45*	7.5	228	55*	9.2	0.82
Palatsi, 1976	380	2-3 months	29 months (1-yr program)	Daily home program (nonrandomized allocation based on time of recruitment)	180	18	4.1	200	28	5.8	0.64

(continued)

Table 5.7 (*continued*)

Author	Sample size	Entry	Follow-up	Treatment	Exercise group			Control group			Therapeutic benefit	
					N	Deaths	Annual%	N	Deaths	Annual%	Annual%	Ex/control
Wilhelmsen et al., 1975	315 (35F,280M)	3 months	4 yr	Individually supervised, 3 times per week, hospital-based	158	28	4.4	157	35	5.6	0.80
Shaw, 1981	651	2-36 months	3 yr	Individually supervised, 3 times per week	323	15	1.3	328	24	2.1	0.63
Rechnitzer et al., 1975	751 733 retained	2-12 months	3-4 yr	Partially supervised 2-4 times per week; controls received homeopathic exercise	379	15*	0.98	354	13*	0.91	1.08
Vermuelen et al, 1983	98	—	5 yr	—	47	2	0.85	51	5	1.90	0.45
Marra et al., 1985	161	2 months	4-1/2 yr	Individually supervised, increasing to 4 times per wk; controls received homeopathic exercise	81	6	1.35	80	5	1.90	0.45

(continued)

Table 5.7 (*continued*)

Author	Sample size	Entry	Follow-up	Treatment	Exercise group			Control group			Therapeutic benefit	
					N	Deaths	Annual%	N	Deaths	Annual%	Annual%	Ex/control
Roman, 1985	193	2 months	up to 9 yr	Individually supervised, 2-4 times per week	93	16	3.6	100	27	5.8		0.59
Carson et al., 1982	303	6 weeks	25 months (12-week program)	Individually supervised, 3 times per week	151	12	3.9	152	21	7.9		0.57
Lamm et al., 1982	1360	4-12 weeks	3 yr (6-week-3-yr program)	Individually supervised, 3 times per week	705	105	5.0	655	105	5.3		0.93
TOTAL	5325				(370)			(447)				(0.83)

Note. Reprinted from Shephard (1989d) by permission.
*Coronary deaths + assuming 4-yr follow-up of all subjects.
**Numbers suitable for long-term follow-up
xSame subjects as previous sample.

The issue of enhanced functional capability is at least as important as any exercise-induced extension of lifespan. When first seen a few months following myocardial infarction, the average patient has a maximal oxygen intake that is only about 70% of that of an age-matched peer. However, 3 years of progressive aerobic training can restore the maximal oxygen intake of the average patient to near the age-related, normal value (Kavanagh et al., 1979). Indeed, some of the postcoronary patients attending the Toronto Rehabilitation Centre have progressed to a maximal oxygen intake of over 45 μmol/(kg·s), or 60 ml/(kg·min), and after 3 years of training, one previously sedentary man was able to run a marathon race in as short a time as 3 hours 17 minutes (Kavanagh, Shephard, & Pandit, 1974; Shephard, Kavanagh, Tuck, & Kennedy, 1983a).

Psychosocial factors, such as the degree of spousal support and the extent of disability benefits, have a marked influence on the patient's return to the labor force following myocardial infarction (Shephard, 1981). Nevertheless, an improvement of health-related fitness generally shortens the period of absence from work and increases the likelihood of ultimate return to paid employment. An early analysis of patients attending the Toronto Rehabilitation Centre found that 71% returned to full-time work at their previous jobs, 12% found new full-time jobs, 6% accepted part-time jobs, and only 10% remained unemployed. More recent studies have shown an employment differential of 10% to 30% favoring the exercised groups (Shephard, 1989c).

POSSIBLE MECHANISMS OF BENEFIT FROM EXERCISE.   How could regular aerobic exercise help a person to live with damaged coronary vessels? The original hypothesis was that an exercise-induced oxygen lack stimulated both a general enlargement of the arterial tree (Stevenson, 1967) and the development of a collateral blood supply to parts of the myocardium beyond a locus of vascular narrowing or occlusion. Some animal experiments tended to support this explanation (Eckstein, 1957, but not Schaper, 1982), although benefit was not seen if occlusion occurred after aerobic training had been completed (Burt & Jackson, 1965). Attempts to demonstrate that moderate aerobic exercise stimulates the development of collateral vessels in human subjects have also been unconvincing (Kattus & Grollman, 1972; Kavanagh, 1989). Possibly, the person with myocardial ischemia has difficulty in exercising hard enough to stimulate collateral formation.

Plainly, prolonged, moderate, aerobic exercise helps to establish a better balance between the intake and usage of energy, due to both the immediate metabolic demands of the exercise session and a small continuing increase of metabolism after the activity has ceased. Body fat is metabolized, the total serum cholesterol is reduced, and there may be an increase in absolute HDL-cholesterol concentration, or the ratio of HDL- to LDL-cholesterol (Kavanagh et al., 1983). All of these changes favor a slower accumulation of atherogenic lipids in the coronary vessels. Physical activity also decreases the clotting tendency of the blood (Drygas, 1988), further reducing the likelihood that existing atherosclerotic plaques will expand to cause a critical (i.e., >70%) narrowing of the coronary vessels.

Exercise-induced gains of aerobic power and muscle strength, together with a reduction of body mass, reduce the stress imposed on the heart for a given external rate of working, whether assessed in terms of the rise in systemic blood pressure or the secretion of adrenaline. A lower blood pressure and a lower heart rate reduce the work rate of the heart, and thus the myocardial oxygen demand, to the point where ischemia can be avoided despite an unaltered narrowing of the coronary vessels. The slower exercise heart rate leads to a relative lengthening of the diastolic phase of the cardiac cycle, when most of the perfusion of the left ventricle occurs (Scott, 1967). There may also be an increase of myocardial contractility. In itself, this last change tends to increase the myocardial oxygen demand, but because the end diastolic dimensions are also reduced, the ventricular wall tension associated with a given blood pressure is decreased. The lower wall tension in turn facilitates blood flow through the perforating coronary vessels, arteries that traverse the ventricular wall to supply the vulnerable sub-endocardial areas of the myocardium.

Finally, exercise offers psychological benefits. Light physical activity offers pleasurable relaxation, camaraderie, and joie de vivre, whereas more vigorous physical activity may provide an outlet for the dangerous, hostile component of Type A behavior (Friedman & Rosenman, 1974).

Exercise and Beta-Blockade

Many patients with ischemic heart disease are now treated with beta-blocking drugs in order to control hypertension and to reduce the incidence of arrhythmias. After beta-blockade, the heart rate fails to show the anticipated increase during vigorous aerobic exercise, and thus the heart rate cannot be used to regulate the intensity of an exercise prescription. Because peripheral metabolic actions of the sympathetic-adrenergic system are inhibited, the patient may complain of muscular fatigue (Kullmer et al., 1987), and the relative metabolism of fat, carbohydrate, and protein may be affected (P.E. Hall, S.R. Smith, & Kendall, 1987). Such changes limit the possibility of using either the rating of perceived exertion or the respiratory gas exchange ratio to monitor the intensity of physical activity in patients who are receiving beta-blocking medication (Tesch, 1985).

After beta-blockade, the heart rate shows little increase during bouts of aerobic exercise, but there is only a small diminution of peak oxygen intake, at least in normal subjects (Hughson, 1989; Tesch, 1985). Presumably, the heart is able to compensate at least partially for the therapeutic bradycardia by an increase of stroke volume at the expense of an increase of end diastolic volume and thus a diminution of cardiac reserve. Equally, current consensus holds that aerobic training induces a relatively normal increase of maximal oxygen intake in post-coronary patients who are taking beta-blocking drugs. Presumably, the exercise sessions impose at least a normal (and usually a greater than normal) load on the ventricles (Blood & Ades, 1988; Wilmore et al., 1990), and patients whose angina is relieved are able to train harder.

Exercise as a Precipitant of Heart Attacks

A review of clinical histories of patients who had sustained nonfatal myocardial infarctions suggested that a higher-than-expected proportion of such incidents occurred while the person was engaged in some type of physical activity (Shephard, 1974b). It was estimated that physical activity increased the immediate risk of a heart attack by a factor of at least 5. A similar analysis of recurrent infarctions suggested that postcoronary patients had a sixfold increase in the risk of a cardiac emergency while they were exercising (Shephard, 1979b). Vuori, Suurnakki, and Suurnakki (1982) analyzed fatal episodes of exercise that were subjected to autopsy in Finland (see Table 5.8). The risk of such incidents varied somewhat with age and with the type and intensity of the activity that was being undertaken, but the overall danger was of a similar order to that found in Canada: The relative risk of dying was increased 2- to 13-fold while the individual was exercising.

Does such evidence negate the preventive value of regular aerobic activity? A substantial proportion of exercise-induced cardiac incidents involved unaccustomed types of physical activity, for which the person was ill conditioned. In other instances, intense physical activity was combined with a strong emotional stimulus (Shephard, 1974b; 1981). It is thus possible that if there were better guidelines for exercise, the immediate hazards of an active lifestyle could be reduced. However, even if this hope is not realized, exercise will remain of practical value to the participant, because there is a substantial reduction of cardiac risk during the intervening hours of rest (Siscovick, Weiss, Fletcher, & Lasky, 1984). Taking an appropriately weighted account of the average risks applicable to both physically active and inactive periods of the day, the exerciser gains a substantial overall advantage of prognosis relative to a sedentary peer (Shephard, 1974b, 1981; Siscovick, 1990; Siscovick et al., 1984).

Congenital Heart Disease

Aerobic training has considerable value in enhancing the effort tolerance of children with many forms of congenital heart disease. Often, the children have

Table 5.8
Relative Risk of Sudden Death During Exercise vs. Sedentary Conditions

Activity	20-39 yrs	40-49 yrs	50-69 yrs
Nonstrenuous exercise	2.5	3.6	2.5
Strenuous exercise	10.0	13.1	5.3
Walking	0.0	0.2	0.5
Jogging	9.3	4.7	0.7
Cross-country skiing	9.3	9.0	6.1

Note. Based on data covering all autopsied sudden deaths (74,694) over 11 years in a Finnish population of 4.5 million. Reprinted from Vuori et al. (1982) by permission.

been unnecessarily restricted by either their physicians or their parents, and in consequence they perform at substantially less than their potential (G.R. Cumming, 1989; Mocellin, 1985). The main indications for a cautious approach to exercise for such individuals are diagnoses of aortic stenosis, aortic dilatation (Marfan's syndrome, Ehlers-Danlos syndrome), abnormal coronary vascular supply, abnormalities of heart rhythm associated with congenital septal lesions, syncope associated with pulmonary hypertension, and severe congestive failure.

Hypertension

Many patients with a high resting blood pressure exhibit an exaggerated blood pressure response to a single bout of aerobic exercise (Tipton, 1984), for example, a systolic reading greater than 230 mm Hg and a diastolic reading greater than 110 mm Hg (Attina, Guiliano, Arcangeli, Musante, & Cupelli, 1986). There have been suggestions that this exaggerated exercise response might offer a means of diagnosing individuals at risk of future hypertension (Jetté et al., 1988). Possible factors contributing to the hypertensive response include enhanced central and peripheral responses to catecholamines, autonomic dysfunction, impaired muscle vasodilatory capacity, reduced myocardial compliance, and increased baroreceptor sensitivity (Tipton, 1984).

In contrast, there is growing evidence that regularly repeated aerobic activity leads to a small but therapeutically useful decrease in systemic blood pressure (Tipton, 1984, 1991). Early studies of athletes (Kral, Chrastek, & Adamirova, 1966) and of active Michigan residents (Montoye, Metzner, & Keller, 1972) suggested an association between regular physical activity and a reduced risk of hypertension. Animal experiments have also demonstrated that the progressive rise of resting blood pressure in hypertensive rats is slowed by regular aerobic exercise (Hagberg, 1990). A multiplicity of human longitudinal experiments, reviewed by Tipton (1984, 1991) have shown a 5 to 25 mm Hg reduction of systolic readings and a 3 to 15 mm Hg reduction of diastolic readings following aerobic training. Hagberg (1990) concluded that the average response in patients with essential hypertension was a 10.8 mm Hg reduction of systolic and a 8.2 mm Hg reduction of diastolic pressures. This compares favorably with what is achieved by many pharmacological interventions, whereas complications of drug therapy, such as postural hypotension, are avoided. Regular aerobic exercise alone may suffice to control mild hypertension, and in more severe cases, exercise may reduce the dose of hypotensive medication that is required.

The optimum regimen emphasizes regular exercise in the range of 40% to 70% of maximal oxygen intake. Early fears that hypertensive individuals might develop a dangerous response to resistance training were probably exaggerated (Tipton, 1991). Indeed, carefully planned resistance exercises are tolerated quite well both by hypertensive and by coronary patients (Fleck, 1988; A.P. Goldberg, 1989; K.A. Harris & Holly, 1987; Kelemen, 1989). The patients who fail to respond favorably to an exercise program include those with a resting blood pressures in excess of 230/110 mm Hg, a significantly elevated, resting plasma-catecholamine concentration, or cardiac enlargement (Tipton, 1991).

To date, the possible contributions of alterations in autonomic function, baroreceptor sensitivity, and plasma volume to the changes in blood pressure induced by aerobic training remain unclear. Likewise, researchers do not agree as to whether the main hypotensive mechanism is a peripheral vasodilatation or a decrease of cardiac output (Hagberg, 1990).

Peripheral Arterial Disease

From the mid-1960s, there have been persistent reports that patients with peripheral manifestations of atherosclerosis, such as intermittent claudication, derived benefit from a program of progressive aerobic exercise (Jonason, Jonzon, Rinqvist, & Oman-Rydberg, 1979). The time to onset of pain in the calf muscles of a claudicant patient can be substantially extended by a program of progressively increasing physical activity, although the mechanism of benefit remains unclear.

There is no evidence that training improves function simply through a reduction of body mass or an improvement in the mechanical efficiency of walking. Possibly, conditioning of the heart may allow it to develop a higher systemic pressure against the afterloading imposed by the sclerosed arteries, thus improving muscle perfusion. But the typical claudicant patient is unlikely to reach an intensity of effort at which much cardiovascular training can occur. There may also be peripheral changes facilitating aerobic metabolism, such as an increased capillarization of the muscle and a resultant shortening of the diffusion distance, or an increase of local enzyme activity in the active muscles.

Congestive Failure

Conventional wisdom held that physical activity should be minimized in the patient who had developed congestive cardiac failure. It was reasoned that even if heart failure was initially well compensated, any increase of cardiac demand would quickly lead to a dangerous episode of congestive failure.

However, similarly to many other clinical disorders, it appears that the traditional treatment of congestive failure led to overprotection with adverse functional consequences. Our recent experiments (Kavanagh, Myers, et al., 1992) have indicated that despite an average age of 62 years, patients with compensated congestive heart failure could progress to walking 17 km/week over a 12-week period. Such activity had a substantial, favorable effect on the quality of life and led to useful 10% gains in peak power output and peak maximal oxygen intake.

In the short term (i.e., 4 weeks of training), the training response may be traced to a reversal of excessive peripheral vasoconstriction (Jetté, Heller, Landry, & Blümchen, 1991). But in the longer-term study of Kavanagh et al. (1992b), an increase of myocardial contractility seemed a significant mechanism, because training was accompanied by a roughly equal increase in oxygen pulse, and at the end of the program, the subjects were able to exercise to a higher systemic blood pressure.

Coronary Bypass Surgery

The plan of training for the patient who has undergone coronary bypass surgery is generally similar to that adopted for the patient who has sustained a myocardial infarction. However, because the underlying pathology has been largely corrected by surgery, the rate of progression of training can usually be more rapid for the patient who has received a bypass graft or angioplasty than for the individual who has uncorrected, coronary vascular narrowing (Goodman, 1989).

Range-of-motion exercises may be begun as soon as 12 hr after surgery, and indeed, early mobilization reduces the likelihood of pain at the site of the sternal incision, which can otherwise hamper the training plan. Because of persistent sternal discomfort, it is generally wise to avoid swimming as a source of aerobic exercise, at least in the early phases of rehabilitation.

Progression of atherosclerosis and recurrence of coronary narrowing are common problems in this group of patients. A comprehensive, exercise stress test is desirable at least once a year, both to monitor the state of the coronary vessels and to provide ongoing motivation for continued tertiary prevention.

Cardiac Transplantation

Patients who have undergone orthotopic cardiac transplants have a considerable disadvantage when attempting to perform any type of aerobic activity, because they lack the increases of myocardial contractility and heart rate that would normally be mediated via the sympathetic nervous system (Shephard, 1991d). Physiological abnormalities are compounded by a combination of rejection episodes, intercurrent infections, and adverse effects of immunosuppressant therapy that lead to both a loss of skeletal muscle mass and a further weakening of cardiorespiratory condition. An aerobic training program can do much to enhance quality of life and (probably) to avert the accelerated atherosclerosis that complicates the postoperative course of these patients.

Because of the lack of sympathetic innervation, the patient must use breathlessness, the rating of perceived exertion, or the type of exercise to be performed as a guide to an appropriate intensity of exercise. Muscle weakness may modify both exertional perceptions and breathlessness, and a set walking pace may provide the most reliable indicator of an appropriate intensity of effort.

The Toronto Rehabilitation Centre has now completed a 16-month training study of a group of 36 patients who had received an orthotopic cardiac transplant. The functional response was apparently very favorable (Kavanagh, Yacoub, Mertens, Kennedy, & Campbell, 1988). Unfortunately, it was not possible to include a control group, although it was argued that the improvement of performance over the period of aerobic training did not represent spontaneous postoperative recovery, because the benefit seen was independent of when treatment was begun relative to the date of surgery.

Respiratory Diseases

Aerobic exercise has been recommended for patients with a variety of respiratory disorders, including asthma, cystic fibrosis, and chronic obstructive lung disease.

Asthma

In patients with hypersensitive airways, the acute response to vigorous aerobic exercise is a bronchospasm (Morton & Fitch, 1989; Neijens, Duiverman, & Kerrebijn, 1985; Shephard, 1977b). In rare cases, the response may even progress to a life-threatening allergic reaction. Factors exacerbating the bronchospasm include oral breathing and the inspiration of cold, dry, or polluted air. Patients who are severely affected can take prophylactic medication (e.g., cromolyn sodium), or they can exercise in a warm, humid environment (e.g., swimming in a heated pool that is not too heavily chlorinated).

A diagnosis of asthma is no contraindication to rigorous endurance training. Indeed, a number of world-class swimmers have suffered from asthma (Morton & Fitch, 1989). On the other hand, many parents and some physicians are overprotective of children with bronchospasm. Substantial gains of aerobic power can be realized by a period of residence at a camp where a progressive regimen of aerobic exercise can be implemented without parental protection (Shephard, 1979a). Such a regimen can do much for the child's functional capacity, although there are usually no important changes of pulmonary function, and the liability to exercise-induced attacks of bronchospasm is not reduced by such training (Neijens et al., 1985).

Cystic Fibrosis

Exercise intolerance and exertional dyspnea are common complaints of the patient with cystic fibrosis. The limiting link in the oxygen transport chain becomes alveolar ventilation. There is a major decrease of ventilatory efficiency due to enlargement of the respiratory dead space, and patients commonly attempt to use their entire maximal voluntary ventilation during vigorous aerobic exercise (Orenstein & Nixon, 1989). In the later stages of the disease, the respiratory problems are often compounded by right ventricular dysfunction.

Involvement in an aerobic training program can be helpful to such patients, providing a means of increasing the endurance of their ventilatory muscles (Keens et al., 1977). The conditioning program increases peak oxygen transport (Orenstein et al., 1981) and possibly facilitates the clearance of mucus from the airways (Zach, Oberwaldner, & Hausler, 1982). Because their sweat has a high salt concentration, patients with cystic fibrosis should be encouraged to take additional salt when they exercise in warm weather.

Chronic Obstructive Lung Disease

The patient with advanced chronic obstructive lung disease often faces a most unpleasant bout of dyspnea if he or she attempts to undertake aerobic exercise (N.L. Jones & Killian, 1990; Kearon, Summers, Jones, Campbell, & Killian, 1991). Fear of breathlessness leads to a vicious circle of declining physical activity, loss of cardiovascular condition and muscle strength, increased dyspnea, and further reductions of habitual activity (N.L. Jones, 1989; Mertens et al., 1978).

The onset of the disorder is gradual. There is no critical incident, comparable to a heart attack, that can trigger a radical change of personal lifestyle. However, if the patient with chronic obstructive lung disease can be persuaded to begin an aerobic exercise program, the vicious cycle of dyspnea and inactivity can be reversed, with substantial functional improvement (Shephard, 1976). Even if the electrocardiogram shows evidence of right ventricular strain, there is no evidence that an increase of habitual physical activity will worsen prognosis or precipitate right ventricular failure (Bass, Whitcomb, & Forman, 1970).

The design of an appropriate training regimen must take into account the severity of the illness, the nutritional status of the patient, any coexisting cardiovascular disease, and any bronchial hyperreactivity (Rebuck, D'Urzo, & Chapman, 1985). If there is substantial arterial unsaturation, it may be helpful to begin the training process by walking on the treadmill while breathing oxygen (Woolf & Suero, 1969). The functional improvement seen with any program of aerobic activity tends to be task specific. This is a strong argument in favor of adopting treadmill exercise as the training mode, because an increased ability to walk will add much to quality of life for the COLD patient.

There is no evidence that aerobic training improves any of the usual indices of pulmonary function in chronic obstructive lung disease (Niederman et al., 1991). Indeed, it would be surprising if mere physical activity could restore pulmonary tissue that has been destroyed by disease. Nevertheless, exercises designed to strengthen the respiratory muscles sometimes help to counter airflow obstruction (Hanel & Secher, 1991; Pardy & Leith, 1985). Part of the reported improvement in condition following any training program is undoubtedly psychological, a placebo response to a new pattern of treatment or greater medical support, a lessening of fears about a given intensity of breathlessness, or a reaction to a greater sense of self-efficacy (Rebuck et al., 1985). The deterioration of cardiovascular condition resulting from years of physical inactivity may also be slowly corrected, although many patients have difficulty in reaching the intensity of effort at which a cardiovascular training response would be anticipated. There may be some useful biomechanical changes; initially, the COLD patient tends to be very nervous, walking with small, halting steps, but a longer-paced and more efficient walk is adopted as confidence of movement is regained. Finally, the leg muscles are strengthened, so that they are more easily perfused. There is thus a reduced production of lactate at any given fraction of aerobic power (Mertens et al., 1978; Schols et al., 1991). This in turn reduces the drive to the ventilatory center and thus the extent of dyspnea at a given intensity of exercise (Casaburi et al., 1991).

Metabolic Disorders

Aerobic exercise is helpful in correcting obesity, in normalizing the lipid profile, and in controlling maturity-onset diabetes.

Obesity

Obesity is well recognized to be a risk factor for ischemic heart disease. It is less clear whether this risk persists after allowance for associations of obesity with high blood pressure and an adverse lipid profile (Keys et al., 1972). The question seems unimportant from the therapeutic point of view, because a reduction of excess weight modifies the other risk factors and thus diminishes the chances of heart attack (Ashley & Kannel, 1974). The Society of Actuaries (1959) has long accepted that an excessive body mass in relation to height is associated with an increased risk of death from a number of important clinical disorders, but it is worth emphasizing (1) that mass must be 20 to 30 kg above the actuarial ideal to have a large effect on mortality, and (2) that an unusually low body mass relative to height also carries an adverse prognosis.

METHODS OF ASSESSMENT. In epidemiological surveys, obesity is commonly approximated by use of the ponderal index (body mass/height^2). A value greater than 25 kg/m^2 is regarded as a signal of increased risk of ischemic heart disease. Ratios of mass to height, such as the ponderal index, take no account of the nature of the excess body mass, whether fat, muscle, or bone. In a population sense, this is usually unimportant, because the main cause of excess mass is accumulation of fat. But mass-to-height ratios can be very misleading when advising the individual patient. The reason why an individual has an excess body mass relative to actuarial norms may be unusually well-developed muscles or a heavy skeletal frame, rather than an accumulation of fat. It is unclear whether a heavy muscle or bone mass also worsens life expectancy. Certainly, the work load imposed on the heart depends on the total weight to be displaced rather than the relative proportions of muscle and fat that make up the body weight. Furthermore, there is a link between body build and personality: An aggressive, muscular mesomorph is the type of person who is most likely to undertake a dangerous burst of physical activity, thus precipitating a heart attack. The Metropolitan Life Assurance Company (1983) provided a partial answer to the problem of body build by adding some skeletal dimensions (bi-acromial diameters) to their tables of actuarial norms. But if the objective is to assess obesity, it seems logical to estimate body composition more directly, using such techniques as skinfold measurement, whole-body impedance determinations, or hydrostatic weighing.

Skinfold data allow the observer to assess not only the total burden of body fat but also its distribution. There is growing evidence that a masculine, abdominal pattern of fat distribution has a particularly strong association with atherosclerosis, diabetes, and insulin resistance. It is thus useful to record the ratio of waist- to hip-skinfold readings (S.N. Blair, Ludwig, & Goodyear, 1988; Bouchard & Després, 1989; Joos, Mueller, Hanis, & Schull, 1984).

CAUSES OF OBESITY. Many obese people claim that they do not overeat. Nevertheless, the basic cause of their obesity must be an imbalance between the intake of food and daily energy expenditures (Bray, 1990). Several factors may explain denial of overeating. For example, account must be taken, not only of the size of meals, but also of the number and nature of intervening snacks such as candy, cookies, heavily sugared coffee, soft drinks, and alcohol. This is not to imply that frequent meals are intrinsically bad. Indeed, by curbing peaks and troughs of blood sugar levels, they can help to reduce overeating (Leveille & Romsos, 1974). However, care must be taken to count the energy equivalent of all such snacks when estimating the daily intake of food energy.

The obese person may absorb food a little more efficiently than a thinner individual, but such differences are small. A taste for sweet foods may encourage the obese person to use carbohydrate rather than fat as a metabolic fuel, with a correspondingly greater yield of external work per joule of food energy that is consumed. Gross disturbances of hormonal function are unlikely, but if thyroid secretion is below average, there will be less uncoupling of the linkage between food breakdown and the generation of high-energy phosphate bonds. Further, a solid layer of subcutaneous fat conserves body heat, so that less energy must be dissipated in order to keep the obese person warm.

Finally, many observers look for evidence of gross overeating. But the excess of food intake relative to energy expenditure is generally small, even in a person who is quite obese. If 10 kg of fat has been accumulated over 10 years of adult life, the metabolic error averages less than 40 MJ a year, or about 1% of normal food intake. The problem could be something as simple as adding a little extra sugar to the daily coffee or avoiding a 10-min walk each morning. Brownell, Stundard, and Albaum (1980) noted that when there was a choice between use of the stairs or an escalator, obese subjects were substantially more likely to choose the escalator than were their leaner peers. When a person has become obese, habitual activity is further restricted (Bullen, Reed, & Mayer, 1964; Chirico & Stunkard, 1960; Durnin, 1966; Ishiko, Ikeda, & Enomoto, 1968; Stefanik, Heald, & Mayer, 1959). The energy cost of most tasks is increased, and aerobic fitness is usually poor, so that any exercise leaves the overweight member of the group hot, tired, and breathless. The person who is overweight may also be embarrassed by his or her ungainly figure.

TREATMENT.   If the affected individual is prepared to take a long-term view of treatment, moderate obesity can be corrected through a small adjustment of diet or physical activity schedules to create a negative energy balance. Wilmore (1983) reviewed 55 studies of exercise programs in lean and moderately obese subjects. All except five showed a reduction of body fat in as little as 7 to 22 weeks, the average loss being 1.6%. The response is greater and is more readily demonstrated in those who are moderately obese than in individuals who are initially close to their ideal weight (Kukkonen, Rauramaa, Siitonen, & Hanninen, 1982). However, those who are moderately obese rapidly regain their initial excess weight if they leave the exercise program.

It is difficult to reduce body fat in the person with massive obesity (Krotkiewski et al., 1979), partly because they have difficulty undertaking substantial amounts of exercise and partly because they have a larger-than-average total number of fat cells. The majority of studies have found that obese individuals are habitually somewhat less active than thinner subjects, but because the cost of any given movement is increased by the greater body mass, the difference of daily energy expenditure between fat and thinner people is often quite small (Bray, 1990).

Many physicians use dietary restrictions or appetite-suppressing drugs rather than exercise to treat obesity. This is partly because doctors have been taught more about medications than about exercise, and partly because the obese person seems a high-risk candidate for an exercise regimen. However, diet plans have an abysmally low, long-term success rate (Innes, Campbell, Campbell, Needle, & Munroe, 1974; Sohar & Sneh, 1973). An increase of aerobic activity has several therapeutic advantages relative to dieting alone: (1) A positive change of mood state is induced by exercise, in contrast to the depression and reduction of habitual activity that typically accompanies dietary restriction (Behnke & Wilmore, 1974); (2) a temporary, appetite-suppressing, increase of blood sugar is seen immediately following vigorous exercise (Katch, Martin, & Martin, 1979; Mayer, 1960); (3) there is a reduced loss of lean tissue as overall body mass diminishes (Babirack, Dowell, & Oscai, 1974; Keys, Brozek, Henschel, Mickelson, & Taylor, 1950; Pavlou, Steffe, Lerman, & Burrows, 1985; Walberg, 1986; but not Van Dale, Saris, Schoffelen, & ten Hoor, 1987); and (4) there is possibly a lesser reduction of resting metabolism in response to a given negative daily energy balance, a benefit observed by Göranzon and Forsum (1985), and Tremblay, Després, & Bouchard (1985), but not by Henson, Poole, Donahoe, & Heber (1987).

The obese person generally begins an exercise regimen at a low level of physical condition and is thus faced by several handicaps, including an above-average vulnerability to cardiac catastrophe, musculoskeletal problems, and heat stress. Moderate, weight-supported, aerobic activity (e.g., swimming, pool exercises, or cycling) is recommended, rather than very intense workouts that could place a load that is too heavy on the knees, hips, and spine. Not only is a moderate regimen much safer for such individuals, but it also assures a greater relative metabolism of fat than would be seen with more intensive aerobic exercise (Christensen & Hansen, 1939). Moreover, an obese person can sustain a moderate energy expenditure for a substantial period but would be quickly exhausted by more intensive aerobic exercise. Thus, a program based on moderate intensity exercise is likely to increase the daily energy expenditure much more than would a prescription recommending bouts of very vigorous aerobic activity.

Optimization of Lipid Profile

The risk of ischemic heart disease is increased by a high, total serum cholesterol and a deficiency of the scavenging HDL-cholesterol with a low HDL- to LDL-cholesterol ratio (Goldbourt & Medalie, 1979; Lipid Research Clinics Program, 1984; G.J. Miller & Miller, 1975; N.E. Miller, Forde, Thelle, & Mjos, 1977). Particular importance is attached to blood levels of HDL-2-cholesterol (P.D. Wood & Stefanik, 1990). Some families show very high serum-cholesterol concentrations, with a related propensity for heart attacks at an early age. Such families may suffer from an inherited defect of hepatic lipase. This enzyme converts HDL-2 to HDL-3 by removal of cholesterol and phospholipid from the lipid particles. Thus, if the activity of the enzyme is low, cholesterol accumulates to a much greater extent than would be predicted from the subject's habitual physical activity and dietary intake of animal fat. However, population levels of cholesterol are also much higher in North America than in many less privileged societies, and it seems plain that much of the current epidemic of hypercholesterolemia arises from an excessive overall intake of food energy, a diet that is rich in saturated (animal) fat, and an inadequate level of daily physical activity.

The therapeutic options when treating a patient with a high serum cholesterol are similar to those for the control of obesity, including the administration of drugs, stringent dieting, and an increase of physical activity. Trials such as the Lipid Research Clinics Program (1984) have demonstrated the feasibility of inducing clinically significant reductions of serum cholesterol using a combination of cholesterol-sequestrating resins and radical changes of diet. However, the benefit resulting from a reduced intake of saturated fat alone is small unless the daily energy balance becomes negative, because a substantial fraction of the total cholesterol pool of the body is synthesized in the liver, using excess energy derived from foodstuffs other than animal fat. A further disadvantage of attempting to adopt a very low intake of animal fat is that such a radical change of diet is disrupting both for patients and their families. The prospect of consuming therapeutic resins for the remainder of their lives may be extremely daunting.

The response of the serum lipid profile to short periods of aerobic training is equivocal, but an aerobic exercise regimen of 12 weeks or longer seems quite effective in augmenting levels of HDL-cholesterol, particularly the important HDL-2 component (Haskell, 1984; Kavanagh et al., 1983; P.T. Williams et al., 1982; see Figure 5.3, page 234). Nevertheless, a threshold, weekly dose of physical activity (18-20 km of walking or jogging a week) is still required for benefit. Some authors have suggested that strength training can also augment HDL-cholesterol. Such reports are hard to interpret, because sometimes a control group was lacking, body mass decreased, inadequate care was taken to establish the initial cholesterol level, or sampling was not repeated to ensure that any apparent effects of the exercise program were other than transient (Kokkinos & Hurley, 1990). In fact, 20 weeks of vigorous strength training seems to have little impact on either HDL-cholesterol or lipoprotein lipase activity in subjects with initial high-cholesterol levels (Kokkinos et al., 1991).

Kiens et al. (1980) found that 12 weeks of aerobic training induced a 10% increase of apolipoprotein A-I, the apoprotein associated with HDL-cholesterol. On the other hand, Wood et al. (1983) saw no change in either A-I or A-II apolipoproteins in those participating in an endurance training regimen, although they did find a decrease in serum concentrations of apoprotein B, the principal apolipoprotein of LDL-cholesterol.

Diabetes

Young patients with Type I, insulin-dependent diabetes mellitus are well able to participate in aerobic activities, provided that the underlying endocrine disorder is well controlled. Medical clearance should exclude hyperglycemia, ketosis, and neural or vascular complications, such as a peripheral neuropathy, hypertension, or a proliferative retinal angiopathy. When exercising, the diabetic should keep an appropriate reserve of readily assimilable energy at hand (Berger & Kemmer, 1990). Regular participation in an aerobic training regimen is particularly important to such individuals, because they have an increased risk of atherosclerosis.

Insulin sensitivity is improved by aerobic training, but there is no evidence that blood glucose levels are better regulated, even if the subject shows a substantial increase of maximal oxygen intake (Landt, Campaigne, James, & Sperling, 1985; Wallberg-Henriksson, Gunnarsson, Henriksson, Ostman, & Wahren, 1984; Wasserman, Lickley, & Vranic, 1985).

If treatment is based on an intramuscular injection of insulin, care must be taken that the exercise session does not induce a sudden, local increase of muscle blood flow, with a corresponding surge in insulin level and the development of acute hypoglycemia. An increased intake of carbohydrate may be an appropriate precaution when undertaking a single bout of aerobic exercise, but if the patient is committed to a systematic increase of daily activity, then a reduction of insulin dosage is usually required.

Type II diabetes typically develops in association with the obesity of late middle-age or early old-age (at about 60 years). In such individuals, hyperglycemia is associated with insulin resistance and often with other cardiovascular risk factors, such as hypertension and hyperlipoproteinemia (Panzram, 1987; Reaven, 1980). Type II diabetes has become particularly prevalent among many indigenous populations such as North American Indians and Pacific Islanders (H. King, Zimmet, Raper, & Balkau, 1984; Szathmary & Holt, 1983), because of the substantial decrease of habitual physical activity in such communities over the years.

It has been hypothesized that an increase of aerobic activity increases the sensitivity of the insulin receptors in Type II diabetes. In consequence, mild cases may no longer require insulin (Bogardus et al., 1984; Reitman, Vasquez, Klimes, & Nagulesparan, 1984; Schneider, Amorosa, Khachadurian, & Ruderman, 1984). Perhaps because of poor motivation and limited compliance with the prescribed exercise regimen (Berger & Kemmer, 1990), the impact of an aerobic training program on glucose tolerance has yet to be categorically demonstrated in older, Type II diabetics (National Institutes of Health, 1987). Any exercise prescription for this population must be approached cautiously, because many of the affected individuals have advanced cardiac and peripheral vascular atherosclerotic disease. Nevertheless, many such individuals would find daily physical activity a pleasant alternative to adoption of a complicated diet and regular insulin injections for the remainder of their lives.

Osteoporosis, Osteoarthritis, and Rheumatic Arthritis

A progressive age-related loss of bone mineral begins around 30 years of age, and in women the process is greatly accelerated in the 5 perimenopausal years

(E.L. Smith, Rabb, et al., 1989; E.L. Smith et al., 1990). Young adults may also face a loss of bone minerals during the conditions of weightlessness encountered in space exploration. Moderate weight-bearing aerobic exercise is usually a helpful preventive measure, but in middle-aged adults with weakened bone structures, attempts at too rapid progression of an exercise prescription may lead to stress fractures, particularly of the metatarsal bones. The osteoporotic process attains more general clinical importance in the later years of retirement. At this stage, the main bones of the body have been sufficiently weakened that even mild trauma can be enough to cause a fracture. Unfortunately, conditions such as a fractured hip can cause a substantial morbidity and mortality at this age.

A number of cross-sectional comparisons suggest that athletes have a greater total body calcium, or a greater density of the lumbar vertebrae, than their sedentary peers (Aloia et al., 1978; Dalen & Olsson, 1974; R. Marcus & Carter, 1988; Nilsson & Westlin, 1971). But if the athletes have performed exercise mainly with their legs, they may show no difference in the mineral density of the radius relative to that of sedentary individuals, and if the sedentary subjects are heavier than the active group, the calcaneal density may also show no intergroup difference (Brewer, Meyer, Keele, Upton, & Hagan, 1983).

In many studies, the stimulus to an increase of bone density has apparently come from weight-bearing activity, but in some cases, bone density is most closely correlated with an index of muscle strength such as lean body mass and thus the local forces applied internally to the bones (Doyle, Brown, & Jachance, 1970). The apparent correlation between bone density and maximal oxygen intake (Chow, Harrison, Brown, & Hajek, 1986) may come, not from the direct relationship of maximal oxygen intake to aerobic activity, but rather from its association with lean body mass (Aloia et al., 1978).

A regular exercise program slows or arrests the age-related loss of bone calcium (Chow, Harrison, & Notarius, 1987; Sidney et al., 1977; Talmage et al., 1986). Huddlestone, Rockwell, Kulund, and Harrison (1980) found a 13% advantage in local calcium content in the playing arm of tennis competitors. However, many training experiments (Krølner et al., 1983; E.L. Smith, Smith, Ensign, & Shea, 1984; M.K. White, Martin, Yeater, Butcher, & Radin, 1984) have shown less dramatic benefits than those inferred from cross-sectional surveys. Problems in longitudinal studies include nonrandom allocation of subjects between exercised and control groups, an inadequate daily intake of calcium, measurements on a limited number of bone sites, and a negative effect of the physical activity program on overall energy balance. At best, bone density has been 1% to 2% higher in the active groups. In the first year of the study by E.L. Smith et al. (1984), there was a 3.8% decrease of radial density in physically active individuals (perhaps because calcium was being shifted from the arms to other parts of the skeleton), although density increased relative to controls in Years 2 and 3 of the same study. Possibly, cross-sectional studies exaggerate the beneficial influence of exercise on bone density, because subjects are more likely to participate in active sports if their muscles and bones are initially strong enough to allow prolonged aerobic training without injury (R. Marcus & Carter, 1988).

One clinical concern is that whereas moderate aerobic exercise increases bone mineral content, overvigorous physical activity may have a converse effect on bone health, particularly in young women (Cann et al., 1984; Drinkwater et al., 1984; Nelson et al., 1986). If a training regimen is pursued to the point of amenorrhea, then the density the trabecular bone in the lumbar spine may be reduced by at least 10%, although there may be no change in the density of the cortical bone of the radius (R. Marcus & Carter, 1988). Investigators have generally claimed that body fat stores were approximately equal in amenorrheic women who lost bone calcium and eumenorrheic individuals who did not, although in many of the distance competitors who showed a decrease of bone density, food intake was inadequate, the overall energy balance was negative, and calcium intake was grossly inadequate for the amenorrheic state. There is thus a need to test whether the very heavy aerobic training has an adverse effect on the bone density of young women who are in energy balance and have an adequate calcium intake.

Osteoarthritis

The precise etiology of osteoarthritis, a painful, degenerative condition of the bone articulations, is unknown. The frequent discrepancy between the deterioration of joints visible on radiographs and the severity of symptoms is particularly puzzling. Genetic factors (e.g., limb malalignment) may predispose to osteoarthritis, but injuries incurred in sport or at work are often regarded as the main cause. If there is a history of major trauma (Chantraine, 1985; Panush & Brown, 1987) or repeated overloading of the cartilaginous surface, then the blame placed on sport or occupation may be appropriate. To cite one example, some (but not all) observers have found a high incidence of osteoarthritic lesions in the shoulders and elbows of those who operate pneumatic drills (E.L. Smith et al., 1990).

On the other hand, Soh and Micheli (1985) found that 25 years after leaving a university, those who had been track stars had a lower incidence of osteoarthritis of the knee and hip than those who had represented their college as swimmers. Likewise, middle-aged adults who continue to participate in such physical activities as distance running do not have a higher incidence of osteoarthritis than their sedentary peers (Lane et al., 1986; Panush et al., 1986). But it remains arguable that in such studies, those vulnerable to musculoskeletal problems have been selectively eliminated from the active group.

Thus, present data do not offer convincing evidence that aerobic activity provokes osteoarthritis, unless a joint surface is injured by trauma. However, controlled longitudinal studies are needed to confirm this viewpoint.

Rheumatic Diseases

Rheumatoid arthritis is one expression of an immune disorder that can affect many parts of the body, including the cardiovascular system (pericarditis, peripheral arteritis), the lungs (pleuritis and fibrosis), the peripheral nerves (neuropathy, neuritis), the tendons, and the muscles. All of these manifestations potentially have an adverse impact on physical performance.

During the acute phase of the disease, the best treatment is rest of the inflamed area. During the chronic phase, function can be greatly improved by adopting a progressive regimen of aerobic exercise (Ekblom, 1985). Cycling and rowing are well tolerated in the early phases of the disease, but if there is extensive degeneration of the joints, water-supported sports such as swimming and pool exercises are preferred activity options. Relative to inactive controls, an exercise program not only improves subjective and functional status, but also slows deterioration of the affected joints (Ekblom, 1985).

Cancer

Early studies suggested that relative to the general population, athletes had a somewhat above-average, overall death rate from cancer (Polednak, 1978). Possible contributing factors to an adverse outcome include an increased exposure to ultraviolet radiation (particularly in swimmers and sailors), athletic trauma and associated x-irradiation, a high intake of animal protein and thus of nitrites, an exercise-induced increase in free-radical formation, abuse of anabolic steroids, a high consumption of cigarettes and/or alcohol after retiring from certain types of sport, and sport-specific risks, such as exposure to toxic agents through the use of tanned leather equipment (Shephard, 1990e).

More recently, animal experiments, occupational studies, and long-term follow-up of individuals with active leisure pursuits have all suggested that regular aerobic exercise can protect athletes against cancer of the colon, and (in women, at least) against cancer of the reproductive system (Bartram & Wynder, 1989; H.W. Kohl et al., 1988; Shephard, 1990e, 1992f). It remains unclear whether such physical activity stimulates host defenses, or merely alters other risk factors for the cancer in question, perhaps by increasing gastrointestinal motility, controlling obesity, reducing blood levels of reproductive hormones, or encouraging adoption of a healthy overall lifestyle.

Suitably adapted aerobic training programs can also be helpful in alleviating some of the effects of established disease and in restoring physical condition after successful treatment of the cancer (Shephard, 1990e).

Animal Studies

Animal experiments (almost without exception) have linked physical activity with a retardation of growth in such tumors as sarcomas, adenocarcinomas, and mammary carcinomas (Mackinnon, 1992; Shephard, 1990e). Benefit apparently persists only while the exercise program is sustained (Rashkis, 1952). The single negative experiment (Thompson, Ronan, Ritacco, & Tagliafero, 1989) began enforced running 14 days after tumor induction. In this study, tumor growth was greater for animals performing what was described as a moderate exercise program than for those that were asssigned to a lower intensity regimen.

It is somewhat easier to control diet and physical activity patterns in animal than in human experiments. Longitudinal experiments can also be completed more quickly in small mammals than in humans. On the other hand, there are obvious difficulties in extrapolating from animal data to human responses. The neoplasm induced in the animal model is experimental rather than spontaneous in type, the pattern of physical activity and the diet differ widely from that of the typical human subject, and there are problems in matching either the age at tumor induction or the duration of exercise treatment between small mammals and much longer-lived humans.

Occupational Studies

In most occupational surveys, the classification of physical activity at work is relatively crude. Serious problems arise from job transfers, because those who become sick tend to move from physically active to sedentary employment even before a diagnosis of cancer has been established. Moreover, a physically active job category is commonly linked with a low socioeconomic status, a poor overall lifestyle, occupational exposure to known carcinogens, and membership of a particular race or ethnic group. With one exception (Gerhardsson, Norell, Kiviranta, Pedersen, & Ahlboom, 1984), occupational studies have made no allowance for the important factor of compensating differences of leisure activity between active and inactive job categories. Increasingly, a higher overall weekly energy expenditure is observed among those engaged in office work than in those employed in heavy industry.

H.L. Taylor et al. (1962) found all-cancer rates were 52% higher among railway workers with sedentary jobs (office clerks) than in those with a more active job classification (track section men), although data were not controlled for possible differences in smoking habits between the two samples. Persky et al. (1981) linked a high resting heart rate (presumably, an overall measure of current sedentary living less vulnerable to problems of recent job transfer) with a high incidence of colonic cancer, after controlling their data for age, systolic blood pressure, relative body weight, serum cholesterol, and smoking habits. Garabrant, Peters, Mack, and Bernstein (1984); Gerhardsson et al. (1986); Huseman, Neubauer, & Duhme (1980); Vena et al. (1985); and Vena, Graham, Zielezny, Brasure, and Swanson (1987) all noted positive associations between their classifications of the intensity of occupational activity and the risk of colon cancer. Data were controlled for age and socioeconomic status but not for smoking habits. Vena et al. (1987) further commented that the less active female employees had an increased risk of breast cancer. In contrast, Paffenbarger, Hyde, and Wing (1987) found no significant effect of occupation upon the overall risk of cancer in Californian longshore workers when data were controlled for the individual's cigarette smoking, age, and blood pressure.

Studies of Leisure Activity

Studies of leisure activity are generally based on questionnaires (see chapter 3), although in a few instances (e.g., S.N. Blair et al., 1989), there have been initial measurements of aerobic fitness. Physically active leisure is a self-selected behavior, and currently it tends to be associated with a high socioeconomic status and other favorable habits of lifestyle that might reduce the risk of various types of cancer.

Paffenbarger et al. (1986, 1987) classified male university alumni on the basis of their reported patterns of physical activity as students. Involvement in university athletic programs was associated with a reduced incidence of rectal cancer (risk ratio 0.46) but an increased vulnerability to prostatic cancer (risk ratio 1.66). A prospective study followed a medically screened cohort of the same population for up to 16 years. A sedentary lifestyle was associated with a 47% increase in the incidence of all forms of cancer relative to those individuals with a weekly energy expenditure greater than 8MJ. The one weakness in this study was the possibility that vague ill health may have restricted the initial activity patterns of those who later developed cancer.

Frisch et al. (1985, 1989) carried out a similar analysis of female university alumnae. Those who reported a history of vigorous physical activity as students had a below-average prevalence of breast cancers (1:1.86) and cancers of the reproductive system (ovary, uterus, cervix, and vagina, 1:2.53). Women who had been physically active as students also had a lower-than-expected incidence of benign tumors of the reproductive system (Wyshak, Frisch, Albright, Albright, & Schiff, 1986). These studies were well controlled for potential interfering variables, but one important weakness was the use of prevalence data. Thus, women who had already died of cancer were excluded from the analyses. It is also likely that many subjects changed their activity patterns after they had left university.

Several other recent reports, including an analysis of data from the Framingham study (Ballard-Barbash et al., 1990), the U.S. National Health and Nutrition Examination Survey (Albanes, A. Blair, & Taylor, 1989), and a prospective study of subjects attending the Cooper Institute for Aerobics Research (S.N. Blair et al., 1989; Shephard, in press-b) suggest that all-cancer death rates are lower in subjects with physically active leisure pursuits. The NHANES study, while showing an association between an active lifestyle and a reduced likelihood of reproductive cancers, found no association between reported physical activity patterns and all-cancer death rates. On the other hand, the follow-up of patients attending the Cooper Institute for Aerobics Research suggested that even after allowing for the likely effect of smoking, the risk of death from all types of cancer was halved on moving from the lowest quintile of aerobic fitness to the next two quintiles, and that there was a further reduction of risk among those who were initially in the highest two fitness quintiles (Shephard, 1992f).

Possible Mechanisms of Protection Against Cancer

There is no agreement on potential mechanisms whereby regular physical activity could protect the individual against either all forms of cancer or specific types of tumor (Bartram & Wynder, 1989; H.W. Kohl et al., 1988).

A vigorous bout of aerobic exercise influences the blood level of many hormones, some of which (such as estrogen) influence the course of reproductive cancers. Physically active individuals are also less fat, and adipose tissue is the site where aromatization converts sex hormones to more potent analogs (Pearson, 1978; Simopoulos, 1987; Siiteri, 1987). Moreover, physical activity increases gastrointestinal motility (Cordain, Latin, & Behnke, 1986; Holdstock, Misiewicz, Smith, & Rowlands, 1970). The exerciser thus has less exposure to nitrosamines (which are formed from dietary nitrites by the action of intestinal bacteria), and to other carcinogens formed from bile acids and resins. Finally, intergroup differences in the consumption of dietary fat may be an important determinant of the risk of cancer (Nauss, Jacobs, & Newperne, 1987).

At the cellular level, an appropriate dose of aerobic exercise may have a favorable effect on the function of the immune system, including changes in the numbers and proportions of T and B lymphocytes and an increase in the number or the activity of natural killer cells (Mackinnon, 1992; Shephard et al., 1991). Further, though aerobic activity tends to increase the production of mutagenic free radicals, there is a more than compensatory increase in the activity of the enzymes that break down these same mutagens (Jenkins, 1988).

In most human studies, it is difficult to reach a final conclusion because of the problem of self-selection. Those who elect a vigorous occupation or choose to engage in vigorous leisure pursuits may differ genetically from more sedentary members of the population, and those who are physically active in their leisure time may also have adopted a range of other healthy behavior patterns that offer protection against carcinogenesis.

Exercise in Therapy

Exercise has an immediate mood-elevating effect, which can be of considerable help to the cancer patient. It also stimulates appetite and encourages the conservation of lean tissue, thereby tending to slow the clinical course of the disease (Pearson, 1978).

Following clinically successful radiation treatment and chemotherapy, physical condition is usually poor. A program of progressive aerobic training can thus help to normalize function, increasing the quality of the remaining period of life (Whittaker et al., 1991).

Disorders of Affect

Studies of postcoronary patients (Kavanagh, Shephard, Tuck, & Qureshi, 1977) demonstrated that many of this group suffered severe depression in the first few months following myocardial infarction. However, the abnormal mood state was apparently corrected as these same individuals became involved in an aerobic training program and they sensed an improvement of their functional capacity.

Paivio (1967) argued that whereas exercise reduced anxiety and corrected depression in patients who showed an initial abnormality of mood state, changes were minimal in those patients who began their program with normal psychometric scores.

A recent metaanalysis by North, McCullagh, and Z.V. Tran (1990) confirmed that although exercise decreased depression in a variety of patient-categories, both immediately and in the longer term, the response was greatest in those individuals who were initially sufficiently disturbed to require medical or psychological care. Both state and trait depression scores diminished with training, and the exercise regimen proved more effective therapy than relaxation techniques or participation in other enjoyable activities. Indeed, the benefit resulting from the exercise regimen matched that obtained from psychotherapy, although in seriously depressed individuals a combination of exercise and psychotherapy was judged the best treatment plan.

Mechanisms That Improve Disorders of Affect

The mechanisms responsible for the improvement of affect with participation in an exercise program remain unclear. Contributing psychological factors probably include (1) an increase in the sense of self-efficacy and restoration of an internal locus of control when a difficult physical skill is mastered, (2) the social rewards associated with group interaction and personal attention from the leader of the exercise class, (3) an interruption of the downward spiral of negative thoughts by new, positive experiences, and (4) distraction from the worries and stresses of daily life. Favorable physiological influences include an increase of working capacity, so that daily tasks are more readily accomplished, an increased secretion of monoamine neurotransmitters (particularly noradrenaline), and the possible release of beta-endorphins.

Potential for Exercise Addiction

Several authors have commented on the potential for addiction to the trance-like "high" that develops during endurance running (Sachs, 1982; Shephard, 1992h). It is uncertain whether this is a pharmacological addiction—for example, to the beta-endorphins secreted during the exercise—or a psychological addiction to various other aspects of the running experience. The evidence of addiction that has been adduced includes a strong desire to continue exercising when this is manifestly bad for health (e.g., when there is an unhealed fracture), and withdrawal symptoms, such as anxiety, restlessness, and depression that persist for several days when opportunity for exercise is denied.

A moderate level of exercise addiction may have positive features—for example, it may sustain compliance with an exercise training program in the face of external barriers that would otherwise provide an excuse for inactivity. However, a major exercise addiction has adverse consequences for physical, social, and psychological health. Moreover, the associated trance-like state gives the distance runner a sense of personal invulnerability, which can contribute to collisions with motor vehicles (Shephard, 1992h).

Bed Rest and Surgery

The loss of physical condition associated with a period of local immobilization or general bed rest is a matter of common experience. Parallel effects have been noted during space missions, when normal gravitational stimuli are lacking. It also seems logical that if the body is placed under added stress, whether from a severe illness or a combination of anesthesia and surgical intervention, the person with a high level of health-related fitness will have an added initial margin of functional capacity that will increase the likelihood of a favorable treatment outcome.

Bed Rest

Bed rest forces adoption of a horizontal posture for most of the day. There is a substantial reduction in overall energy expenditure, a reduction of the local stresses imposed on muscles and bones, and possible psychological responses to confinement and moderate isolation (Greenleaf et al., 1977; Greenleaf & Kozlowski, 1982).

Perhaps the most widely publicized and detailed study of bed rest was conducted by Saltin and associates (1968). They tested three sedentary and two athletic young men, demonstrating a negative water balance, with a progressive loss of plasma, red cell, and extracellular fluid volumes, a deterioration of cardiovascular function and maximal oxygen intake, and a progressive decrease of tissue enzyme activity over 20 days of bed rest. Recovery was equally rapid once normal activity patterns were resumed, and because training continued, the sedentary subjects surpassed their initial baselines of aerobic fitness (see Table 5.9). Other observers (Greenleaf et al., 1977; P.C. Johnson, Driscoll, & Carpentier, 1971; Morse, 1968; H.L. Taylor, Henschel, Brozek, & Keys, 1949; Zager, Melada, Goldman, Gonzales, & Luetscher, 1974) have generally confirmed these observations.

Additional effects of prolonged bed rest include an increase of the alveolar-arterial pressure gradient, perhaps due to a progressive atelectasis of lung tissue (Cardus, 1967), a loss of balance related as much to a loss of neural coding as to muscle weakness (Haines, 1974), and a loss of bone calcium (Issekutz, Blizzard, Birkhead, & Rodahl, 1966; Krølner & Toft, 1983; Krølner, Toft, Pors-Nielsen, & Tondevold, 1983). The loss of overall body mass and tissue nitrogen is surprisingly small over the usual short-term laboratory experiment (Dietrik, Whedon, & Shore, 1948; Fuller, Bernauer, & Adams, 1970; Greenleaf et al., 1977; Saltin et al., 1968), although it is likely to become a more significant problem if bed rest is continued for several months.

The deterioration in aerobic fitness reflects a deterioration of overall blood volume, an increase of the peripheral at the expense of the central blood volume, and possibly a decrease of myocardial contractility (Bergman, Hoffler, Johnson, & Wolthuis, 1976). The functional loss is proportional to the duration of bed rest and is similar in sedentary and in trained individuals (Greenleaf & Kozlowski,

Table 5.9
Effects of Bed Rest and Subsequent Reconditioning on Cardiovascular Function

Variable	Initial	After bed rest	After reconditioning
Maximum oxygen intake			
(μmol/[kg·s])	32.0	23.7	38.0
(ml/[kg·min])	43.0	31.8	51.1
Maximum heart rate			
(beats/min)	193	197	191
Maximum stroke volume			
(ml)	104	74	120
Maximum cardiac output			
(L/min)	20.0	14.8	22.8
Maximum a-v difference			
(ml/L)	162	165	171
Heart volume			
(ml)	860	770	895

Note. Reprinted from Saltin et al. (1968) by permission.

1982). Among 22 young men, there was a 6% loss of PWC_{170} at 7 days (Friman, 1976), and 12 middle-aged men showed a 15% decrease of maximal oxygen intake after 10 days (Convertino, Hung, et al., 1982; Convertino, Sandler, et al., 1982). Other reports show losses of 9% (Sullivan et al., 1985) and 27% (Saltin et al., 1968) at 3 weeks.

Fluid losses during bed rest can be minimized if subjects undertake isometric or resisted muscle contractions while they are confined to bed (Greenleaf et al., 1977). Once activity is resumed, aerobic power is apparently normalized somewhat more rapidly in sedentary than in physically active individuals (Saltin et al., 1968).

General Surgery

Blood loss may impair aerobic performance for a few days following major surgery. Carswell (1975) found a 20% reduction of predicted aerobic power 4 days after gastric surgery. Other studies (Adolfsson, 1969; C.D. Wood et al., 1985) have noted an 8% to 13% decrease of PWC_{170} one week after such procedures. There is some suggestion that the absolute loss of function may be larger in those who have a high initial state of aerobic training (Adolfsson, 1969), but nevertheless, trained individuals had a better postoperative condition than would have been the case if they had been sedentary (Carswell et al., 1978).

Muscle wasting is not responsible for the loss of functional capacity, because the postoperative reduction of working capacity is equally marked if the loss of muscle nitrogen is halved by amino-acid infusion (C.D. Wood et al., 1985).

Likewise, there are only minimal changes in the aerobic enzyme activity of the limb muscles following surgery (Sullivan, Merola, Timmerman, Unverferth, & Leier, 1986).

A recumbency-induced decrease of plasma volume is the most probable explanation of the decrease in aerobic power of surgical patients, although there is also some evidence that transfusions that maintain total body hemoglobin avert the postoperative decrease of functional capacity (A. Young, 1990).

Local Immobilization

The immobilization consequent to musculoskeletal injury causes a local loss of muscle strength and a more general deterioration of physical condition. The limited evidence available suggests that both local resistance exercises and more general programs of aerobic conditioning can speed the recovery of function following injury (Fried & Shephard, 1969, 1970; Oldridge, 1990). However, more information is needed on the optimal type and dose of training at various points during recovery.

Acute Infection

Acute infection, like general surgery or local immobilization, causes immediate decrements of muscle strength and aerobic power, with an enhanced tendency to fatigue. The onset of the functional loss is rapid, but the effects can last for some weeks and the mechanisms involved are at present unclear (A. Young, 1990).

It is difficult to assess the precise impact of acute infections on aerobic fitness, because preinfection data are usually lacking. Two studies have suggested that the immediate postfebrile PWC_{150} is reduced by about 14% relative to recovery values (Bengtsson, 1956; Friman, 1976).

Some viral infections seem to reduce the activity of muscle enzymes (Aström, Friman, & Pilström, 1976). However, a loss of blood volume due to sweating and recumbency, plus other unidentified factors, contribute to the overall deterioration in condition (Hedin & Friman, 1982).

Aerobic Fitness and Clinical Outcome of Surgical and Medical Treatment

Because modern surgery is well controlled and most patients have a substantial reserve of cardiorespiratory function while resting, initial aerobic fitness has only a marginal impact on the outcome of surgery. Bagg (1984) found the 12-min walking distance to be a poor predictor of postoperative respiratory complications, and Schilling and Molen (1984) noted that whereas the patients' Canadian Home Fitness Test scores were inversely related to their lengths of stay in surgical wards, the test data failed to predict the likelihood of postoperative cardiac or respiratory complications. Possibly, measures of aerobic fitness might give a better guide to the outcome of surgical procedures if the analysis were restricted to senior citizens, who have a much smaller initial margin of cardiorespiratory function.

There have been no human studies of the value of aerobic training in countering infection, other than the investigations of the immune system discussed previously. However, in animals, training on exercise wheels apparently increases resistance to *Salmonella typhi*, tularemia, and pneumococcal infections (Cannon & Kluger, 1984; Ilbäck, Friman, Beisel, A.L. Johnson, & Berendt, 1984).

Space Travel

Given that most of the changes observed with bed rest, surgery, and acute infection seem due to a temporary loss of normal gravitational stimulation, there has been considerable interest in the physical condition of healthy adults following periods of weightlessness in space.

The effects of prolonged weightlessness include a progressive loss of lean tissue, body fat, hemoglobin, and bone calcium, with a decrease of cardiac stroke volume, poor orthostatic tolerance, a lowered physical working capacity, a fall of systemic blood pressure both in rest and exercise, and a decrease of blood volume (Buderer, Rummel, Michel, Mauldin, & Sawin, 1976; P.C. Johnson, Leach, & Rambaut, 1973; P.C. Johnson, Nicogossian, Bergman, & Hoffler, 1976; Rummel, Michel, & Berry, 1973; Rummel, Sawin, Buderer, Mauldin, & Michel, 1975; Vogel & Whittle, 1976; Wronski & Morey, 1983).

Originally, it was anticipated that prior, rigorous aerobic training would prevent many of these complications and would facilitate adaptation to the space environment. But in practice, perhaps because of lower circulating levels of catecholamines, endurance athletes have sometimes shown a poorer adaptation to weightlessness than those with an average level of aerobic fitness (Klein, Wegmann, & Kuklinski, 1977). The performance of physical work during the flight reduces the loss of aerobic power while the subject is weightless (Sawin, Rummel, & Michel, 1975), and repeated local application of negative counterpressure ("suction") to the legs helps to avert the loss of orthostatic tolerance (P.C. Johnson et al., 1976).

Musculoskeletal Injuries

If health benefit is to be derived from an increase of physical activity, it is important that this not be outweighed by the adverse effects of musculoskeletal injuries incurred during the performance of sport.

A recent study from Holland (Reijnen & Velthuijsen, 1989) suggested that, at least in young adults, the social costs of medical services and injury-related work loss were actually greater in active than in sedentary individuals. The majority of the musculoskeletal injuries responsible for this finding arose during soccer games. Likewise, Nicholl, Coleman, and Williams (1991) found that participation in several vigorous sports (including soccer and rugby football) was associated with increased medical costs, the cumulative effect of all vigorous activities matching the estimated economic impact of diabetes. We found that more than a half of Masters' competitors (predominantly distance runners) had had an injury of sufficient severity to stop training for 1 week or more during the course of a typical year (Kavanagh, Lindley, et al., 1988). In a younger sample of distance runners, Koplan, Powell, Sikes, Shirley, and Campbell (1982) found that 35% of subjects needed to reduce their running distance because of injury during the year following a distance road race; 13% of men and 17% of women sought medical attention during this same period. Some 44% of participants in aerobic dance classes noted one or more musculoskeletal complaints over a 16-week period (Garrick et al., 1986), and about a quarter of these injuries were severe enough to modify participation.

The average, well-run aerobic fitness program has a somewhat lower incidence of musculoskeletal injuries. S.N. Blair, Kohl, and Goodyear (1987) noted that 24% of participants at the Cooper Institute for Aerobics Research experienced an injury that caused them to stop running for at least 7 days over the course of a year. Shephard, Corey, Renzland, and Cox (1982) analyzed health care costs over the first year of an employee fitness program and found no increase in the demand for orthopedic services among participants relative to nonparticipants.

Plainly, the likelihood of injury depends on the type and intensity of exercise. MacIntosh et al. (1972) demonstrated that in university-level athletes, the annual toll of injuries increased tenfold on moving from intramural to intercollegiate programs, whereas Pollock et al. (1977; 1991) suggested that the incidence of injuries in a jogging program rose steeply as the duration of activity was extended from 15 through 30 to 45 min a session. Further, some sports are much more hazardous than others, and indeed there is evidence that the excitement of a dangerous activity sometimes encourages participation (Shephard, Godin, & Valois, 1989).

Adverse factors that increase the incidence of injuries in aerobic dance classes (Garrick et al., 1986) include a history of prior orthopedic problems and a minimal commitment to aerobic dance (attending only one session a week). In other activities, the main determinant of injury is the total volume of training that is undertaken each week, for example, the weekly training distance of the jogger (S.N. Blair et al., 1987; S.J. Jacobs & Berson, 1986; Koplan, Powell, Sikes, Shirley & Campbell, 1982; Powell, Kohl, Caspersen, & Blair, 1986) or the swimmer (Rovere & Nichols, 1985). Perhaps because individuals with a high level of aerobic fitness exercise more and at a higher intensity than subjects who are less fit, there is little relationship between the predicted maximal oxygen intake of the individual and susceptibility to injury (e.g., among soccer players; Eriksson, Jorfeldt, & Ekstrand, 1986).

Conclusion

Although there is some evidence that overvigorous physical activity can precipitate both musculoskeletal injuries and heart attacks, this is generally a response to excessive enthusiasm. With the moderate conditioning regimen currently recommended to the average person (American College of Sports Medicine, 1990, 1991), the impact on health is more likely to be positive than negative.

The observations of Paffenbarger (1988) suggest that middle-aged adults who embark on a program of aerobic training may extend their life expectancy by as much as 2 years. However, this is contingent on the participant continuing the exercise program for the remainder of their lives. Cynics have pointed out rightly that a large part of the added 2 years of lifespan must be spent in exercising and traveling to and from exercise facilities. Thus, it could be argued that if the person does not enjoy the recommended program of physical activity, there is very little to be gained from it. Plainly, if fitness professionals are to motivate sedentary people to increase their habitual activity, the proposed program must be enjoyable in itself, and it must leave the participant feeling better rather than worse at the end of the day. This is a very strong reason for promoting moderate rather than very intensive forms of aerobic exercise.

It is difficult to excite a young adult about the prospect of living to 80 rather than 78 years of age, and immediate gains in the quality of life may be a much stronger reason to become physically active. If an exercise program makes a 35-year-old man feel 50% better, this represents a 15- to 20-year extension of the quality-adjusted lifespan, a major benefit that would be difficult to assure through some alternative form of therapeutic intervention. More importantly from the motivational standpoint, the benefit begins immediately, although it will continue into later life.

Even for the senior citizen, the prospects of independence and a higher quality of life during the retirement years are likely to be more attractive goals than a mere prolongation of existence. The active senior citizen who is still able to maintain an independent lifestyle at 95 or 100 years of age has succeeded in turning back the biological clock by 15 to 20 years. Again, this is a benefit that cannot be matched by any dietary or pharmacological intervention.

The gains in well-being and our broad definition of health that result from the regular practice of aerobic exercise have major implications for both the happiness and the economic security of an aging population. It is to be hoped that governments will continue their efforts to modify attitudes and social norms, so that an ever-growing proportion of people accept and experience such benefits.

Appendix

Units of Fitness Measurement, Abbreviations, and Body Size Standardization

This appendix offers details of the currently accepted units and abbreviations appropriate to the study of fitness, together with a discussion of possible methods of standardizing data for interindividual differences of body size.

Standard International Units

At one time, fitness and nutritional data were expressed in a wide variety of physical units, including imperial (feet, pounds), metric (meters, kilograms), mechanical (foot-pounds, horsepower), thermal (calories), and electrical (watts) systems of measurement. Confusion has been greatly reduced and the comparison of studies facilitated by the introduction and gradual acceptance of standard international (SI) units for physical and chemical measurements (Ellis, 1971). Features of the SI system are (1) the use of interlinked, metric, gravity-independent units, and (2) the adoption of an approved system of abbreviations for each variable.

mass—Mass expresses the quantity of matter present in a given object. In an earlier era, investigators spoke of body weight. However, weight varies with the acceleration due to gravity, and thus with the individual's distance from the center of the earth. At an altitude of 4,000 meters, gravitational acceleration is diminished by about 0.13%, and because the earth is not completely spherical, the gravitational force is also about 0.53% greater at the poles than at the equator.
   The commonly used unit of mass is the kilogram (kg); 1 pound = 0.454 kg.

distance—The fundamental unit of distance is the meter (m), although because of the speed of the human competitor, endurance events are commonly measured in kilometers (km); 1 mile = 1.609 km, 1 foot = .305 m.

time—The standard SI unit of time is the second (s). Again, those interested in endurance fitness tends to think in terms of minutes rather than seconds, although if SI units are to be multiplied together as intended, it is necessary to convert data from minutes to seconds; 1 min = 60 s.

force—Force is that which changes the state of rest or motion of an object, and it is measured as the product of mass and gravitational acceleration, expressed in newtons (N). In a normal gravitational field, a mass of 1 kg exerts a force of 9.81 newtons. Another unit of force found in some older literature is the kilopond (kp), the force exerted by 1 kg in unit gravitational field. Under standard conditions, 1 kp = 1 kg = 9.81 N.

work—Work is performed when a force acts against an opposing resistance to produce motion. The quantity of work undertaken is given by the product of force and distance. The basic unit is the joule (J), developed when a force of 1 N is exerted over a distance of 1 m. The exercise scientist finds it convenient to think in terms of kilojoules (kJ, or 1,000 joules) and megajoules (MJ, or 1,000 kJ).

Much of the older literature on nutrition is expressed in calories (the amount of energy required to heat 1 g of water from 15° to 16°C). The calorie and kilocalorie are not accepted international units. Under standard conditions, 1 calorie = 4.186 joules.

power—Power is the rate of performing work (that is, work divided by time). The unit is the watt, equivalent to a power output of 1 J/s, or 60 J/min. Under standard conditions, 1,000 kg·m/min = 1,000 kp·m/min = 163.5 W; 1,000 ft lb = 22.6 W; 1 kcal/min = 69.8 W; 1 horsepower = 736 W.

pressure—Pressure is the force developed per unit area. The standard unit is the pascal, observed when a force of 1 N is applied to an area of 1 m^2. Ambient pressures are expressed in kilopascals (kPa). Older generations of respiratory physiologists are accustomed to stating pressures in mm Hg, or Torr (the corresponding height of a column of mercury that is supported in a closed tube in unit gravitational field); 100 mm Hg = 13.3 kPa. Formerly, osmotic pressures were expressed in mm Hg, but they are now more commonly reported as milliosmoles. In dilute solutions, solutes exert a characteristic pressure proportional to their molar concentration. At a concentration of 1 μmol/L, and a temperature of 37°C, the pressure is .701 kPa.

Clinicians are even more closely wedded to use of the mercury column when reporting blood pressures, and kilopascals are only now beginning to be used for this purpose.

temperature—Temperatures are expressed in degrees Celsius (°C) or as an absolute temperature in degrees Kelvin (°K), 273 degrees higher than the temperature in degrees Celsius.

oxygen consumption, carbon dioxide output, and lung volumes—The SI system has proposed that all chemical reactions, including those involving gases, be expressed in molar terms. A gram molecule of any dry gas, measured under standard conditions of pressure (P) and temperature (T) (STPD—101.2 kPa, or 760 mm Hg at 0°C, or 273°K), occupies a volume (V) of 22.4 liters; 1 liter of oxygen at STPD thus contains 44.6 millimoles (mmol). In practice, volumes of oxygen and carbon dioxide are measured experimentally at ambient pressure and temperature, saturated with water vapor at the prevailing temperature (ATPS), but data can be converted to STPD volumes by application of Boyle's and Charles' Laws:

$$P_A V_A / T_A = P_S V_S / T_S$$

where the subscripts, A and S, refer to ambient and standard conditions, respectively.

Measurements of ventilatory capacity and power are commonly expressed as perceived by the body (i.e., as the equivalent volume at body temperature and pressure, saturated with water vapor at body temperature, BTPS); 1 L STPD = approximately 1.1 L ATPS = 1.21 L BTPS.

The SI units for gas exchange are, theoretically, micromoles per second (μmol/s). For example, an oxygen consumption of 1 L/min should be written 44.6 mmol/min or 744 μmol/s. The advantage of expressing oxygen intake and carbon dioxide output in molar units is that data can then be related directly to changes in other body metabolites. However, the use of molar gas volumes is at present a new practice.

Rates of oxygen consumption are also sometimes expressed as METS (i.e., ratios to resting metabolic rate). 1 MET = 3.5 ml/(kg·min) = 156 μmol/(kg·min) = 2.60 μmol/(kg·s).

chemical compounds—Concentrations of other chemical compounds should also be expressed in molar units (mol/L), although in many older reports concentrations are expressed in milligrams per deciliter (mg/dl) of blood. Conversion factors for some compounds commonly encountered by the exercise scientist are given in Table A.1.

Standard Abbreviations for the Cardiorespiratory System

The standard symbols used to represent gas transfer (Cotes, 1965; Pappenheimer, 1950) were originally developed by respiratory physiologists, and they are now widely accepted. They look complicated at first inspection, but there is a simple underlying logic.

The dot above a symbol indicates a time derivative. Thus, V is a static volume, but $\dot{V}$ represents the same volume displaced in unit time. The subscript specifies the site of measurement; thus $\dot{V}_E$ is the volume of gas expired in unit time (usually expressed per minute rather than per second) and $\dot{V}_A$ is the corresponding rate of alveolar ventilation. Capital subscripts refer to the gas phase, and lower case subscripts indicate the blood phase. Thus $\dot{Q}$ is the total cardiac output in unit time, and $\dot{Q}_c$ is the slightly smaller volume of blood flowing through the pulmonary capillaries during the same interval. The solubility coefficient lambda (λ) is introduced to accommodate the change from the gas to the blood phase at the alveolar-capillary interface. Lambda is a dimensionless number reflecting the

Table A.1

Molar Equivalents of Some Compounds of Interest in Exercise and Fitness Research

Compound	Older units	Molar equivalent
Glycogen[a] (resting muscle)	15g/kg	343 mmol/kg
Glucose (resting blood)	80 mg/dl	4.44 mmol/L
Cholesterol (resting serum)	200 mg/dl	5.2 mmol/L
Triglyceride[b] (resting)	120 mg/dl	1.4 mmol/L
Lactic acid (peak blood)	100 mg/dl	11.1 mmol/L
ATP[c] (resting muscle)	2.5 g/kg	4.75 mmol/kg
CP[d] (resting muscle)	3.0 g/kg	14.1 mmol/kg

[a]Older units were for wet tissue; newer units are expressed relative to dry tissue mass, about 27% of the wet-tissue mass, assuming also that the molar equivalent of a glycogen-derived glucosyl unit is 162.
[b]Precise value depends on structure of fatty acid; example is for triacylglycerol with molecular mass of 864.
[c]Adenosine triphosphate.
[d]Creatine phosphate.

ability of unit volume of blood to carry a specific quantity of a given gas under standard conditions of pressure.

Standardization of Fitness Data for Body Size

When comparing fitness variables or the resulting performance of physical tasks between populations (e.g., between children and adults, women and men, or short and tall people), the method that is chosen to standardize data for interpopulation differences of body size can have an important influence on conclusions. For example, as adolescent children mature, it may appear that they maintain a constant level of aerobic fitness (the inference from a height^2 adjustment of maximal oxygen intake data; Bailey, 1974) or that they are showing a progressive deterioration of physical condition (the inference from a height^3, or body mass, adjustment of findings; Shephard, 1982a). The choice of standardization procedure may be based on dimensional theories, or it may be derived from empirical considerations.

Dimensional Theories

The search for appropriate dimensional models can be traced back to Archimedes, who proposed laws for geometrically similar bodies, and Borelli, who observed that geometrically similar animals could jump to approximately the same height, whereas the maximum velocity of running was relatively independent of an animal's size. Such theories were developed further by Von Döbeln (1966) and Asmussen and Christensen (1967). The Scandinavian authors argued that unidimensional variables such as leverage and stride length were proportional to height (H), that bidimensional variables such as muscle force (a function of cross-sectional area of the active fibers) could be related to H^2, and that volumetric measurements such as body mass, heart volume, and lung volumes were proportional to H^3. Von Döbeln (1966) attempted to include time in his schema by equating it with height. He reasoned that from Newton's laws of motion, acceleration = force/mass, or $H^2/H^3 = 1/H$. Further, by definition, acceleration = distance/time^2. Making the somewhat debatable assumption that distance was a function of H, he suggested that acceleration = H/time^2. Equating the two formulae, H/time^2 = 1/H, so that H^2 = time^2, and thus time could be considered a function of H.

By an extension of this same reasoning, work = force × distance, a function of $H^2 \cdot H^1$, or H^3, and power (i.e., the rate of working, or the corresponding oxygen intake) was a function of work/time, H^3/H, or H^2.

We may immediately note one substantial limitation of the Scandinavian approach, in that all body parts are presumed to grow in proportion to overall stature. This is a somewhat inappropriate assumption when comparing young and older children, women and men, or different racial groups (Shephard, 1982a). It is thus not surprising that in practice, experimental data do not always conform to the suggested power functions of standing height. In a cross-sectional study of Danish boys, Asmussen (1973) found that muscle force varied as height$^{2.89}$ and that aerobic power increased as height$^{2.90}$. Shephard et al. (1980) had similar findings in a semilongitudinal study of children living in the Trois Rivières region of Québec (see Table A.2). Some authors have attributed discrepancies between

Table A.2
Power Functions Relating Standing Height to Various Physiological Measurements

Variable	All students	Enhanced activity* Boys	Girls	Control program Boys	Girls
Vital capacity	2.68	2.68	2.76	2.68	2.71
Maximal oxygen intake	2.78	3.21	2.76	3.21	2.66
Peak power output	3.37	3.58	3.60	3.37	2.94
Handgrip force	3.23	3.12	3.34	3.29	3.16
Back extension	2.72	2.62	2.91	2.69	2.76
Leg extension	2.88	2.40	3.42	2.80	2.96

Note. Data from Shephard et al. (1980).
*Students in enhanced program performed 1 hr of aerobic activity a day, whereas students in control program followed the normal primary-school physical education program.

the Scandinavian dimensional theory and their experimental data to the use of cross-sectional results or to interference from the pubertal growth spurt. However, such explanations cannot explain the lack of conformity in the Trois Rivières data; these measurements were semilongitudinal in type and were obtained when the students were 6 to 11 years of age.

Empirical Standardization

Because the theoretical basis of any proposed height standardization remains controversial, it seems preferable to adopt an empirical approach, using the size variable that shows the strongest correlation with the physiological measurements that require standardization. On this basis, body mass is as good as any simple, alternative method of standardizing maximal oxygen intake, peak power output, and the maximal voluntary force of selected muscle groups. Thus, oxygen consumption is expressed in $\mu mol/(kg \cdot min)$, or $ml/(kg \cdot min)$. The body mass standardization penalizes the person with a high percent body fat, although from a performance perspective the penalty is often fair, because the oxygen cost of most activities varies with the individual's weight.

Another empirical possibility, sometimes used for such variables as respiratory minute volume, cardiac output, and resting metabolism, is to express data per unit of body surface area, which is usually estimated from a function of both height and body mass. Because the rate of resting heat loss depends on the body surface that is available for convection, radiation, and evaporation of sweat, such an approach has some logic under resting conditions, but it is less appropriate when standardizing exercise data.

References

Aaron, E.A., Henke, K.G., Pegelow, D.F., & Dempsey, J.A. (1985). Effects of mechanical unloading of the respiratory system on exercise and respiratory muscle endurance. *Medicine and Science in Sports and Exercise*, **17**, 290.

Aaron, E.A., Johnson, B., Pegelow, D., & Dempsey, J. (1990). The oxygen cost of exercise hyperpnea: A limiting factor? *American Review of Respiratory Diseases*, **141**, A122.

Adams, A. (1966). Effect of exercise upon ligament strength. *Research Quarterly*, **37**, 163-167.

Adams, L., Chronos, N., & Guz, A. (1982). Dependence of the intensity of breathlessness on $F_{I,O2}$ during heavy exercise in normals. *Journal of Physiology*, **327**, 51P-52P.

Adams, L., Chronos, N., Lane, R., & Guz, A. (1986). The measurement of breathlessness induced in normal subjects: Individual differences. *Clinical Science* **70**, 131-140.

Adams, T.D., Yanowitz, F.G., Fisher, A.G., Ridges, J.D., Nelson, A.G., Hagan, A.D., Williams, R.R., & Hunt, S.C. (1985). Heritability of cardiac size: An echocardiographic study of monozygotic and dizygotic twins. *Circulation*, **71**, 39-44.

Adolfsson, G. (1969). Rehabilitation and convalescence after surgery. *Scandinavian Journal of Rehabilitation Medicine*, **1**, 14-15.

Ahlborg, G., & Felig, P. (1982). Lactate and glucose exchange across the forearm, legs, and splanchnic bed during and after prolonged exercise. *Journal of Clinical Investigation*, **69**, 45-54.

Ahn, B., Nishibayashi, Y., Okita, S., Masuda, A., Takaishi, S., Paulev, P.E., & Honda, Y. (1989). Heart rate responses to breath-holding during supramaximal exercise. *European Journal of Applied Physiology*, **59**, 146-151.

Ainsworth, M., & Shephard, R.J. (1961). The intrabronchial distribution of soluble vapours at selected rates of gas flow. In C.N. Davies (Ed.), *Inhaled particles and vapours* (pp. 233-248). Oxford: Pergamon Press.

Albanes, D., Blair, A., & Taylor, P.R. (1989). Physical activity and risk of cancer in the NHANES I population. *American Journal of Public Health*, **79**, 744-750.

Alderson, J., & Crutchley, D. (1990). Physical education and the national curriculum. In N. Armstrong (Ed.), *New directions in physical education* (Vol. 1, pp. 37-62). Champaign, IL: Human Kinetics.

Alekseev, V.P. (1991). Coronary atherosclerosis and ischemic heart disease in aboriginal and newcomer populations of Yakutia. In B. Postl, P. Gilbert, J. Goodwill, M.E.K. Moffatt, J.D. O'Neil, P.A. Sarsfield, & T.K. Young (Eds.), *Circumpolar health 90* (pp. 406-407). Winnipeg: Canadian Society for Circumpolar Health.

Allen, J.G. (1966). Aerobic capacity and physiological fitness of Australian men. *Ergonomics*, **9**, 485-494.

Aloia, J.F., Cohn, S.H., Babu, T., Abesamis, C., Kalici, N., & Ellis, K. (1978). Skeletal mass and body composition in marathon runners. *Metabolism*, **27**, 1793-1796.

Alston, W., Carlson, K.E., Feldman, D.J., Grimm, Z., & Gerontinos, L. (1966). A quantitative study of muscle factors in the chronic low-back syndrome. *Journal of the American Geriatric Society*, **14** 1041-1047.

American Alliance for Health, Physical Education, Recreation and Dance. (1980). *Health related fitness test*. Washington, DC: Author.

American College of Obstetricians and Gynecologists. (1990). *Planning for pregnancy, birth, and beyond* (pp. 1-260). Washington, DC: Author.

American College of Sports Medicine. (1978). The recommended quantity and quality of exercise for developing and maintaining fitness in healthy adults. *Medicine and Science in Sports*, **10**, 7-10.

American College of Sports Medicine. (1990). The recommended quantity and quality of exercise for developing and maintaining cardiorespiratory and muscular fitness in healthy adults. *Medicine and Science in Sports and Exercise*, **22**, 265-274.

American College of Sports Medicine. (1991). *Guidelines for graded exercise testing and exercise prescription* (4th ed.). Philadelphia: Lea & Febiger.

American Heart Association. (1981). *The exercise standards book*. Dallas: Author.

American Medical Association. (1966). *Report of committee on exercise and physical fitness*. Chicago: Author.

Andersen, K.L. (1967). Work capacity of selected populations. In P.T. Baker & J.S. Weiner (Eds.), *The biology of human adaptability* (pp. 67-90). Oxford: Clarendon Press.

Andersen, K.L., & Hart, J.S. (1963). Aerobic working capacity of Eskimos. *Journal of Applied Physiology*, **18**, 764-768.

Andersen, K.L., & Magel, J.R. (1970). Physiological adaptation to a high level of habitual activity during adolescence. *Internationale Zeitschrift für Angewandte Physiologie*, **28**, 209-227.

Andersen, K.L., Masironi, R., Rutenfranz, J., & Seliger, V. (1978). *Habitual physical activity and health*. Copenhagen: World Health Organization Regional Office for Europe.

Andersen, P., & Saltin, B. (1985). Maximal perfusion of skeletal muscle in man. *Journal of Physiology*, **366**, 233-249.

Anderson, T.W., & Shephard, R.J. (1968a). The effects of hyperventilation and exercise upon the pulmonary diffusing capacity. *Respiration*, **25**, 465-484.

Anderson, T.W., & Shephard, R.J. (1968b). Physical training and exercise diffusing capacity. *Internationale Zeitschrift für Angewandte Physiologie*, **25**, 198-209.

Andres, R. (1985). Mortality and obesity: The rationale for age-specific height-weight tables. In R. Andres, E.L. Bierman, & W.R. Hazzard (Eds.), *Principles of geriatric medicine*, (pp. 311-318). New York: McGraw Hill.

Andres, R. (1990). Assessment of health status. In C. Bouchard, R.J. Shephard, T. Stephens, J. Sutton, & B. McPherson (Eds.), *Exercise, fitness and health*, (pp. 133-136). Champaign, IL: Human Kinetics.

Andrew, G.M., Brooker, B., & Brawley, L. (1974). Effects of adult fitness classes on heart and lung functions at rest and exercise. *Canadian Association for Health, Physical Education and Recreation Journal*, **41**(2), 33-37.

Anholm, J.D., Stray-Gunderson, J., Ramanathan, M., & Johnson, R.L. (1989). Sustained maximal ventilation after endurance exercise in athletes. *Journal of Applied Physiology*, **67**, 1759-1763.

Antoni, M.H., Schneiderman, N., Fletcher, M.A., Goldstein, D.A., Ironson, G., & LaPerriere, A. (1990). Psychoneuroimmunology and HIV-1. *Journal of Consulting and Clinical Psychology*, **58**, 38-49.

Appell, H-J. (1990). Muscle atrophy following immobilisation: A review. *Sports Medicine*, **10**, 42-58.

Apthorp, G.H., Bates, D.V., Marshall, R., & Mendel, D. (1958). Effects of acute carbon monoxide poisoning on work capacity. *British Medical Journal*, (ii), 476-478.

Arbesu, N. (1991). Aerobic and anaerobic physical capacity of Cuban schoolchildren subjected to different motor regimens. In R.J. Shephard & J. Pařízková (Eds.), *Human growth, physical fitness and nutrition* (pp. 99-108). Basel: S. Karger.

Armstrong, L.E., & Maresh, C.M. (1991). The induction and decay of heat acclimatisation in trained athletes. *Sports Medicine*, **12**, 302-312.

Armstrong, R.B. (1984). Mechanisms of exercise-induced delayed onset muscular soreness: A brief review. *Medicine and Science in Sports and Exercise*, **16**, 529-538.

Armstrong, R.B. (1986). Muscle damage and endurance events. *Sports Medicine*, **3**, 370-381.

Armstrong, R.B. (1987). Cardiac output distribution during prolonged exercise in animals. *Canadian Journal of Sport Sciences*, **12**(Suppl.), 71S-76S.

Armstrong, R.B., Warren, G.I., & Warren, J.W. (1991). Mechanisms of exercise-induced muscle fibre injury. *Sports Medicine*, **12**, 184-207.

Artal, R., Rutherford, S., Romem, Y., Kammula, R.K., Dorey, F.J., & Wiswell, R.A. (1986). Fetal heart rate responses to maternal exercise. *American Journal of Obstetrics and Gynecology*, **155**, 729-733.

Asahina, K. (1975). Relationship between growth and fitness. In K. Asahina & R. Shigiya (Eds.), *JIBP synthesis* (pp. 23-39). Tokyo: University of Tokyo Press.

Ashley, F.W., & Kannel, W.B. (1974). Relation of weight change to changes in atherogenic traits: The Framingham study. *Journal of Chronic Diseases*, **27**, 103-114.

Asmussen, E. (1973). Ventilation at transition from rest to exercise. *Acta Physiologica Scandinavica*, **89**, 68-78.

Asmussen, E., & Christensen, E.H. (1939). Einfluss der Blütverteilung auf den Kreislauf bei körperlicher Arbeit [Influence of blood volume on circulation during body work]. *Skandinavisches Archiv für Physiologie*, **82**, 185-192.

Asmussen, E., & Christensen, E.H. (1967). *Kompendium: Legem sölvelsernes Specielle Teori.* Copenhagen: Kobenhavns Universitets Fond til Tilverbringelse of Läremidler.

Asmussen, E., & Nielsen, M. (1960). Alveolar-arterial gas exchange at rest and during work at different O_2 tensions. *Acta Physiologica Scandinavica*, **50**, 153-166.

Astakhova, T., Rjabikov, A., Astakhov, V., Bondareva, Z., Lutova, F., & Bulgakov, Y. (1991). Risk factors and chronic non-communicable diseases in native residents and newcoming population of Chukotka. In B. Postl, P. Gilbert, J. Goodwill, M.E.K. Moffatt, J.D. O'Neil, P.A. Sarsfield, & T.K. Young (Eds.), *Circumpolar health 90* (pp. 408-409). Winnipeg: Canadian Society for Circumpolar Health.

Åstrand, I. (1960). Aerobic work capacity in men and women with special reference to age. *Acta Physiologica Scandinavica*, **49**(Suppl. 169), 1-92.

Åstrand, I. (1967). Degree of strain during building work as related to individual aerobic work capacity. *Ergonomics*, **10**, 293-303.

Åstrand, I. (1971). Circulatory responses to arm exercise in different work positions. *Scandinavian Journal of Clinical and Laboratory Investigation*, **27**, 293-297.

Åstrand, I., Åstrand, P.O., Christensen, E.H., & Hedman, R. (1960). Myohemoglobin as an oxygen store in man. *Acta Physiologica Scandinavica*, **48**, 454-460.

Åstrand, I., Gahary, A., & Wahren, J. (1968). Circulatory responses to arm exercise with different arm positions. *Journal of Applied Physiology*, **25**, 528-532.

Åstrand, P.O. (1952). *Experimental studies of physical working capacity in relation to age and sex.* Copenhagen: Munksgaard.

Åstrand, P.O. (1961). *Fysiologiska synpunkter pa skolungsdomens fysika fostran. Preliminär rapport till folksam.* Stockholm: Central Gymnastic Institute.

Åstrand, P.O., & Rodahl, K. (1986). *Textbook of work physiology* (3rd ed.) New York: McGraw Hill.

Åstrand, P.O., & Saltin, B. (1961a). Maximal oxygen uptake and heart rate in various types of muscular activity. *Journal of Applied Physiology*, **16**, 977-981.

Åstrand, P.O., & Saltin, B. (1961b). Oxygen uptake during the first minutes of heavy muscular exercise. *Journal of Applied Physiology*, **16**, 971-976.

Åstrand, P.O., Ekblöm, B., & Goldberg, A.N. (1971). Effects of blocking the autonomic nervous system during exercise. *Acta Physiologica Scandinavica*, **82**, 18A.

Åstrand, P.O., Engström, L., Eriksson, B., Karlberg, P., Nylander, I., Saltin, B., & Thorén, C. (1963). Girl swimmers, with particular reference to respiratory and circulatory adaptation and gynaecological and psychiatric aspects. *Acta Paediatrica Scandinavica*, **147**(Suppl.), 1-75.

Åström, E., Friman, G., & Pilström, L. (1976). Effects of viral and mycoplasma infections on ultrastructural and enzyme activities in human skeletal muscle. *Acta Pathologica Microbiologica Scandinavica*, **84**(A), 113-122.

Attina, D.A., Guiliano, G., Arcangeli, G., Musante, R., & Cupelli, V. (1986). Effects of one year of physical training on borderline hypertension: An evaluation by bicycle ergometer exercise testing. *Journal of Cardiovascular Pharmacology*, **8**(Suppl. 5), S145-S147.

Avellini, B.A., Shapiro, Y., & Pandolf, K.B. (1983). Cardio-respiratory physical training in water and on land. *European Journal of Applied Physiology*, **50**, 255-263.

Babb, T.G., Viggiano, R., Hurley, B., Staats, B., & Rodarte, J. (1991). Effect of mild to moderate airflow limitation on exercise capacity. *Journal of Applied Physiology*, **70**, 223-230.

Babirack, S.P., Dowell, R.T., & Oscai, L.B. (1974). Total fasting and total fasting plus exercise: Effects on body composition of the rat. *Journal of Nutrition*, **104**, 452-457.

Bagg, L.R. (1984). The 12-min walking distance: Its use in the pre-operative assessment of patients with bronchial carcinoma before lung resection. *Respiration*, **46**, 342-345.

Bagley, M., Berg, K.E., Latin, R., & LaVoie, J. (1991). Energy expenditure of short-term exercise recovery in trained runners. *Journal of Applied Sports Science Research*, **5**, 182-188.

Bahr, R., & Sejersted, O.M. (1991). Effect of feeding and fasting on exercise post-exercise oxygen consumption. *Journal of Applied Physiology*, **71**, 2088-2093.

Bailey, D.A. (1974). Exercise, fitness, and physical education for the growing child. In W.A.R. Orban (Ed.), *Proceedings of national conference on fitness and health* (pp. 13-22). Ottawa: Health & Welfare Canada.

Bailey, D.A., Ross, W.D., Weese, C., & Mirwald, R.L. (1978). Size dissociation of maximal aerobic power during growth in boys. In J. Borms & M. Hebbelinck (Eds.), *Pediatric work physiology* (pp. 140-151). Basel, Switzerland: Karger.

Bailey, D.A., Shephard, R.J., & Mirwald, R.L. (1976). Validation of a self-administered home test of cardio-respiratory fitness. *Canadian Journal of Applied Sport Sciences*, **1**, 67-78.

Bailey, D.A., Shephard, R.J., Mirwald, R.L., & McBride, G.A. (1974). Current levels of Canadian cardio-respiratory fitness. *Canadian Medical Association Journal*, **111**, 25-30.

Bake, B., Bjure, J., & Widimsky, J. (1968). The effect of sitting and graded exercises on the distribution of pulmonary blood flow in healthy subjects studied with the ^{133}Xenon technique. *Scandinavian Journal of Clinical and Laboratory Investigation*, **22**, 99-106.

Baker, J.A., Humphrey, S.J.E., & Wolff, H.S. (1967). Socially acceptable monitoring instruments (SAMI). *Journal of Physiology*, **188**, 4P.

Baker, L.G., Ultman, J.S., & Rhoades, R.A. (1974). Simultaneous gas flow and diffusion in a symmetric airway system: A mathematical model. *Respiratory Physiology*, **21**, 119-138.

Bakers, J.H., & Tenney, S.M. (1970). The perception of some sensations associated with breathing. *Respiratory Physiology*, **10**, 85-89.

Balke, B. (1954). Optimale korperliche Leistungsfahigkeit, ihre Messung und Veränderung infolge Arbeitsmüdung [Optimal body training activity, its measurement, and its variation as a result of conditioning]. *Internationale Zeitschrift für Angewandte Physiologie*, **15**, 311-323.

Ballard-Barbash, R., Schatzkin, A., Albanes, D., Schiffman, M.H., Kreger, B.E., Andersen, K.M., & Helsel, W.E. (1990). Physical activity and the risk of large bowel cancer in the Framingham study. *Cancer Research*, **50**, 3610-3613.

Bangsbo, J., Gollnick, D., Graham, T.E., Juel, C., Kiens, B., Mizuno, M., & Saltin, B. (1990). Anaerobic energy production and O_2 deficit-debt relationship during exhaustive exercise in humans. *Journal of Physiology*, **422**, 539-559.

Banks, T.P. (1943). Army physical conditioning program. *Journal of Health and Physical Education*, **14**, 195.

Barnard, R.J., & Anthony, D.F. (1980). Effect of health maintenance programs on Los Angeles City firefighters. *Journal of Occupational Medicine*, **22**, 667-669.

Bar-Or, O. (1983). *Pediatric sports medicine*. New York: Springer-Verlag.

Bar-Or, O. (in press). Childhood and adolescent physical activity and fitness and adult profile. In C. Bouchard, R.J. Shephard, & T. Stephens (Eds.), *Physical activity, fitness, and health*. Champaign, IL: Human Kinetics.

Bartram, H.P., & Wynder, E.L. (1989). Physical activity and colon cancer risk? Physiological considerations. *Journal of Gastroenterology*, **84**, 109-112.

Bass, H., Whitcomb, J.F., & Forman, R. (1970). Exercise training: Therapy for patients with chronic obstructive pulmonary diseases. *Diseases of the Chest*, **57**, 116-121.

Bassey, E.J., Fentem, P.H., MacDonald, I.C., & Scriven, P.M. (1976). Self-paced walking as a method for exercise testing in elderly and young men. *Clinical Science*, **51**, 609-612.

Bassey, E.J., Patrick, J.M., Irving, J.M., Blecher, A., & Fentem, P.H. (1983). An unsupervised "aerobics" physical training programme in middle-aged factory workers: Feasibility, validation, and response. *European Journal of Applied Physiology*, **52**, 120-125.

Bassey, E.J., Morgan, K., Dalloso, H.M., & Ebrahim, S.B. (1989). Flexibility of the shoulder joint measured as range of abduction in a large representative sample of men and women over 65 years of age. *European Journal of Applied Physiology*, **58**, 353-360.

Baun, W.B., Bernacki, E.J., & Tsai, S.P. (1986). A preliminary investigation of the effect of a corporate fitness program on absenteeism and health care cost. *Journal of Occupational Medicine*, **28**, 18-22.

Beaudry, P. (1968). Pulmonary function of the Canadian Eastern Arctic Eskimo. *Archives of Environmental Health*, **17**, 524-528.

Beaver, W.L., & Wasserman, K. (1970). Tidal volume and respiratory rate changes at start and end of exercise. *Journal of Applied Physiology*, **29**, 872-876.

Bechbache, R.R., Chow, H.K.K., Duffin, J., & Orsini, E.C. (1979). The effects of hypercapnia, hypoxia, exercise, and anxiety on the patterns of breathing in man. *Journal of Physiology*, **293**, 285-300.

Bedingfield, E.W., & Wronko, C.J. (1981). *Biomechanical analysis of ice versus roller skating*. Report to the Canadian Amateur Speed Skating Association, cited by Quinney (1990).

Beeckmans, J., & Shephard, R.J. (1971). Computer calculations of exercise dead space: The role of laminar flow and development of a clinical prediction formula. *Respiration*, **28**, 232-252.

Behnke, A.R., & Wilmore, J.H. (1974). *Evaluation and regulation of body build and composition*. Englewood Cliffs, NJ: Prentice Hall.

Beitins, I.Z., McArthur, J.W., Turnbull, B.A., Skrinar, G.S., & Bullen, B.A. (1991). Exercise induces two types of human luteal dysfunction: Confirmation by urinary free progesterone. *Journal of Clinical Endocrinology*, **72**, 1350-1358.

Belloc, N.B., & Breslow, L. (1972). Relationship of physical health status and health practices. *Preventive Medicine*, **1**, 409-421.

Bender, P.R., & Martin, J. (1985). Maximal ventilation after exhausting exercise. *Medicine and Science in Sports and Exercise*, **17**, 164-167.

Benestad, A.M. (1965). Trainability of old men. *Acta Medica Scandinavica*, **178**, 321-327.

Bengtsson, E. (1956). Working capacity and exercise electrocardiogram in convalescents after acute infectious diseases without cardiac complications. *Acta Medica Scandinavica*, **154**, 359-373.

Berenson, G.S. (1980). *Cardiovascular risk factors in children*. New York: Oxford University Press.

Berg, K.W., LaVoie, J.C., & Latin, R.W. (1985). Physiological training effects of playing youth soccer. *Medicine and Science in Sports and Exercise*, **17**, 656-660.

Berger, M., & Kemmer, F.W. (1990). Discussion: Exercise, fitness, and diabetes. In C. Bouchard, R.J. Shephard, T. Stephens, J. Sutton, & B. McPherson (Eds.), *Exercise, fitness and health* (pp. 491-495). Champaign, IL: Human Kinetics.

Bergh, U., & Forsberg, A. (1992). Cross-country ski racing. In R.J. Shephard & P.O. Åstrand (Eds.), *Endurance in sport* (pp. 570-581). Oxford: Blackwell Scientific.

Berglund, B., & Hemmingson, P. (1987). Effect of reinfusion of autologous blood on exercise performance in cross-country skiers. *International Journal of Sports Medicine*, **8**, 231-233.

Berglund, B., & Hemmingson, P. (1990). Infectious disease in elite cross-country skiers: A one-year incidence study. *Clinical Sports Medicine*, **2**, 19-23.

Bergman, S.A., Hoffler, G.W., Johnson, R.L., & Wolthuis, R.A. (1976). Pre- and post-flight systolic time intervals during LBNP: The second manned Skylab mission. *Aviation, Space and Environmental Medicine*, **47**, 359-362.

Berkowitz, G.S., Kelsey, J.L., Holford, T.R., & Berkowitz, R.L. (1983). Physical activity and the risk of spontaneous pre-term delivery. *Journal of Reproductive Medicine*, **28**, 581-588.

Berman, J.A., Wynne, J., Mallis, G., & Cohn, P.F. (1983). Improving diagnostic accuracy of the exercise test by combining R wave changes with duration of ST depression in a simplified index. *American Heart Journal*, **105**, 60-66.

Bevegard, B.S., & Shepherd, J. (1967). Regulation of circulation during exercise. *Physiological Reviews*, **47**, 178-213.

Bezucha, G.R., Lenser, M.C., Hanson, P.G., & Nagle, F.J. (1982). Comparison of hemodynamic responses to static and dynamic exercise. *Journal of Applied Physiology*, **53**, 1589-1593.

Bhambani, Y.N., Eriksson, P., & Gomes, P.S. (1991). Transfer effects of endurance training with the arms and legs. *Medicine and Science in Sports and Exercise*, **23**, 1035-1041.

Balanin, J.E., Blanchard, M.S., & Russek-Cohen, E. (1989). Lower vertebral bone density in male long distance runners. *Medicine and Science in Sports and Exercise*, **21**, 66-70.

Björntorp, P. (1981). The effects of exercise on plasma insulin. *International Journal of Sports Medicine*, **2**, 125-129.

Blackburn, H., Taylor, H.L., Hamrell, B., Buskirk, E., Nicholas, W.C., & Thorsen, R.D. (1973). Premature ventricular complexes induced by stress testing. *American Journal of Cardiology*, **31**, 441-449.

Blackburn, H., Taylor, H.L., Okamoto, N., Rautaharju, P., Mitchell, P.L., & Kerkhof, A. (1967). Standardization of the exercise electrocardiogram. A systematic comparison of chest lead configurations employed for monitoring during exercise. In M.J. Karvonen & A.J. Barry (Eds.), *Physical activity and the heart*. Springfield, IL: Charles C Thomas.

Blair, D., Habicht, J-P., & Alekel, L. (1989). Assessments of body composition, dietary patterns, and nutritional status in the National Health Examination Surveys and National Health and Nutrition Examination Surveys (DHSS Publication No. 89:1253). In T. Drury (Ed.), *Assessing physical fitness and physical activity in population-based surveys* (pp. 79-104). Hyattsville, MD: U.S. Public Health Service.

Blair, S.N., Jacobs, D.R., & Powell, K.E. (1985). Relationships between exercise and other health behaviors. *U.S. Public Health Reports*, **100**, 172-179.

Blair, S.N., Kohl, H.W., & Goodyear, N.N. (1987). Rates and risks for running and exercise injuries: Studies in three populations. *Research Quarterly*, **58**, 221-228.

Blair, S.N., Kohl, H.W., Paffenbarger, R.S., Clark, D.G., Cooper, K.H., & Gibbons, L.W. (1989). Physical fitness and all-cause mortality: A prospective study of healthy men and women. *Journal of the American Medical Association*, **262**(17), 2395-2401.

Blair, S.N., Ludwig, D.A., & Goodyear, N.N. (1988). A canonical analysis of central and peripheral subcutaneous fat distribution and coronary heart disease risk factors in men and women aged 18-65 years. *Human Biology*, **60**, 111-122.

Blair, S.N., Piserchia, P.V., Wilbur, C.S., & Crowder, J.H. (1986). A public health intervention model for work site health promotion: Impact on exercise and physical fitness in a health promotion plan after 24 months. *Journal of the American Medical Association*, **255**, 921-926.

Blimkie, C.J., Cunningham, D.A., & Leung, F.Y. (1977). Urinary catecholamine excretion and lactate concentrations in competitive hockey players aged 11 to 23 years. In H. Lavallée & R.J. Shephard (Eds.), *Frontiers of activity and child health* (pp. 313-321). Quebec City: Editions du Pélican.

Blomqvist, C.G. (1974). Exercise physiology related to diagnosis of coronary artery disease. In S. Fox (Ed.) *Coronary artery disease: Prevention, detection, rehabilitation with emphasis on exercise testing* (pp. 2-1 to 2-26). Denver: International Medical.

Blomqvist, C.G., & Saltin, B. (1983). Cardiovascular adaptations to physical training. *Annual Review of Physiology*, **45**, 169-189.

Blomqvist, C.G., & Stone, H.L. (1982). Cardiovascular adjustments to gravitational stress. In J.T. Shepherd, F.M. Abboud, & S.R. Geiger (Eds.), *Handbook of physiology: The cardiovascular system*. Bethesda, MD: American Physiological Society.

Blood, S.M., & Ades, P.A. (1988). Effect of beta-adrenergic blockade on exercise conditioning in coronary patients: A review. *Journal of Cardiopulmonary Rehabilitation*, **8**, 141-144.

Bloom, S.R., Johnson, R.H., Park, D.M., Rennie, M.J., & Sulaiman, W.R. (1976). Differences in the metabolic and hormonal response to exercise between racing cyclists and untrained individuals. *Journal of Physiology*, **258**, 1-18.

Bly, J.L., Jones, R.C., & Richardson, J.E. (1986). Impact of worksite health promotion on health care costs and utilization: Evaluation of Johnson & Johnson's Live for Life program. *Journal of the American Medical Association*, **256**, 3235-3240.

Bogardus, C., Ravussin, E., Robbins, D.C., Wolfe, R.R., Horton, E.S., & Sims, E.A.H. (1984). Effects of physical training and diet therapy on carbohydrate metabolism in patients with glucose intolerance and non-insulin dependent diabetes mellitus. *Diabetes*, **33**, 311-318.

Bohr, C. (1909). Uber die spezifische Tätigkeit der Lungen bei der respiratorischen Gasaufnahme [On the specific function of the lungs during respiratory gas uptake]. *Skandinavisches Archiv für Physiologie*, **22**, 221-280.

Boileau, R.A., Mayhew, J.L., Riner, W.F., & Lussier, L. (1982). Physiological characteristics of elite middle and long distance runners. *Canadian Journal of Applied Sport Sciences*, **7**, 167-172.

Boileau, R.A., Misner, J.E., Dykstra, G.L., & Spitzer, T.A. (1983). Blood lactic acid removal during treadmill and bicycle exercise at various intensities. *Journal of Sports Medicine and Physical Fitness*, **23**, 159-167.

Boldin, E.M., & Lundegren, H.L. (1985). Comparative aerobic training effects of arm versus wheelchair ergometry. *Medicine and Science in Sports and Exercise*, **17**, 288-289.

Böning, D., Schweigart, V., Tibes, V., Hammer, B., & Meier, V. (1974). Oxygen transport of the exercise muscle: Importance of the "in vivo" oxygen dissociation curve. IUPS Satellite Symposium on Exercise Physiology, Patiala, India.

Bonjer, F.H. (1968). Relationship between physical working capacity and allowable caloric expenditure. In W. Rohmert (Ed.), *International colloquium on muscular exercise and training* (pp. 86-98). Darmstadt: Gentner Verlag.

Booth, F.W., & Watson, P.A. (1985). Control of adaptations in protein levels in response to exercise. *Federation Proceedings*, **44**, 2293-2300.

Borg, G. (1971). The perception of physical performance. In R.J. Shephard (Ed.), *Frontiers of fitness* (pp. 280-294). Springfield, IL: Charles C Thomas.

Boshoff, W.H. (1965). Ergonomic aspects of traditional and modern cultivation tasks in Uganda. Paper presented at 4th International Congress on Rural Medicine, Usada, Japan.

Bouchard, C. (1990). Discussion: Heredity, fitness, and health. In C. Bouchard, R.J. Shephard, T. Stephens, J. Sutton, & B. McPherson (Eds.), *Exercise, fitness, and health* (pp. 147-154). Champaign, IL: Human Kinetics.

Bouchard, C. (1992). Genetic determinants of endurance performance. In R.J. Shephard & P.O. Åstrand (Eds.), *Endurance in sports* (pp. 149-159). Oxford: Blackwell Scientific.

Bouchard, C., & Després, J-P. (1989). Variation in fat distribution with age and health implications. In W. Spirduso & H. Eckert (Eds.), *Physical activity and aging: The Academy papers* (pp. 78-106). Champaign, IL: Human Kinetics.

Bouchard, C., Hollmann, W., Venrath, H., Herkenrath, G., & Schlüssel, H. (1966). Minimalbelastungen zur Prävention kardiovaskular Erkrankungen [Minimal work level for prevention of cardiovascular illness]. *Sportarzt und Sportmedizin*, **7**, 348-357.

Bouchard, C., Lesage, R., Lortie, G., Simoneau, J.A., Hamel, P., Boulay, M.R., Pérusse, L., Thériault, G., & LeBlanc, C. (1986). Aerobic performance in brothers, dizygotic and monozygotic twins. *Medicine and Science in Sports and Exercise*, **18**, 639-646.

Bouchard, C., Lortie, G., Simoneau, J.A., LeBlanc, C., Thériault, G., & Tremblay, A. (1984). Submaximal power output in adopted and biological siblings. *Annals of Human Biology*, **11**, 303-309.

Bouchard, C., & Malina, R. (1983). Genetics for the sports scientist: Selected methodological considerations. *Exercise and Sport Sciences Reviews*, **11**, 275-305.

Bouchard, C., Shephard, R.J., Stephens, T., Sutton, J., & McPherson, B. (1990). *Exercise, fitness, and health*. Champaign, IL: Human Kinetics.

Bouhour, J.B., & Borgat, C. (1985). Sudden death and myocarditis during activities and sports performance. *Journal of Sports Cardiology*, **2**, 81-85.

Bourey, R.E., & Santorio, S.A. (1988). Interaction of exercise, coagulation, platelets, and fibrinolysis: A brief review. *Medicine and Science in Sports and Exercise*, **20**, 439-446.

Bowne, D.W., Russell, M.L., Morgan, J.L., Optenberg, S.A., & Clarke, A.E. (1984). Reduced disability and health care costs in an industrial fitness program. *Journal of Occupational Medicine*, **26**, 809-816.

Bozner, A., & Meessen, H. (1969). Die Feinstruktur des Herzmuskels der Ratte nach einmaligem und nach wiederholtem Schwimmtraining [The fine structure of rat heart muscle with single and repeated bouts of swim training]. *Virchows Archiv B, Cell Pathology*, **3**, 248-269.

Braith, R.W., Graves, J.E., Pollock, M.L., Leggett, S.L., Carpenter, D.M., & Colvin, A.B. (1989). Comparison of two versus three days per week of variable resistance training during 10 and 18 week programs. *International Journal of Sports Medicine*, **10**, 450-454.

Bray, G.A. (1979). An overview. In G.A. Bray (Ed.), *Obesity in America: A conference* (pp. 1-19). Bethesda, MD: U.S. Dept. of Health, Education, & Welfare, Public Health Service, NIH Publ. 79-359.

Bray, G.A. (1990). Exercise and obesity. In C. Bouchard, R.J. Shephard, T. Stephens, J. Sutton, & B. McPherson (Eds.), *Exercise, fitness, and health* (pp. 497-510). Champaign, IL: Human Kinetics.

Brenner, I., Monga, M., Webb, K., McGrath, M., & Wolfe, L. (1991). Controlled prospective study of aerobic conditioning effects on pregnancy outcome. *Medicine and Science in Sports and Exercise*, **23**, S169.

Brenner, I., & Wolfe, L. (in press). Exercise in pregnancy. *Sports Medicine*.

Brewer, V., Meyer, B.M., Keele, M.S., Upton, J., & Hagan, R.D. (1983). Role of exercise in prevention of involutional bone loss. *Medicine and Science in Sports and Exercise*, **15**, 445-449.

Brien, A.J., & Simon, T.L. (1987). The effects of red blood cell infusion on 10 km race times. *Journal of the American Medical Association*, **257**, 2761-2765.

Brodthagen, U.A., Hansen, K.A., Knudsen, J.B., Jordal, R., Kristensen, O., & Paulev, P.E. (1985). Red cell 2-3 DPG, ATP, and mean cell volume in highly trained athletes: Effect of long-term submaximal exercise. *European Journal of Applied Physiology*, **53**, 334-338.

Brown, J.R., & Crowden, J.P. (1963). Energy expenditure ranges and muscular work grades. *British Journal of Industrial Medicine*, **20**, 277-283.

Brown, J.R. & Shephard, R.J. (1967). Some measurements of fitness in older female employees of a Toronto department store. *Canadian Medical Association Journal*, **97**, 1208-1213.

Brown, S. (1965, June). *The energy cost of 5BX exercises*. Paper presented at the convention of the Canadian Association for Health, Physical Education and Recreation. Fredericton, NB.

Brown, S.E., King, R.R., Termerlin, S.M., Stansbury, D.W., Mahutte, C.K., & Light, R.W. (1984). Exercise performance with added dead space in chronic airflow obstruction. *Journal of Applied Physiology*, **56**, 1020-1026.

Brownell, K.D., & Kaye, F.S. (1982). A school-based behavior modification, nutrition education, and physical activity program for obese children. *American Journal of Clinical Nutrition*, **35**, 277-283.

Brownell, K.D., Stundard, A.J., & Albaum, J.M. (1980). Evaluation and modification of exercise patterns in the natural environment. *American Journal of Psychiatry*, **137**, 1540-1545.

Brundin, T., & Cernigliaro, C. (1975). The effect of physical training on the sympathoadrenal response to exercise. *Scandinavian Journal of Clinical and Laboratory Investigation*, **35**, 525-530.

Brunner, B.C. (1969). Personality and motivating factors influencing adult participation in vigorous physical activity. *Research Quarterly*, **40**, 464-469.

Bryan, A.C., Bentivoglio, L.G., Beerel, F., MacLeish, H., Zidulka, A., & Bates, D.V. (1964). Factors affecting regional distribution of ventilation and perfusion in the lung. *Journal of Applied Physiology*, **19**, 395-402.

Buderer, M.C., Rummel, J.A., Michel, E.L., Mauldin, D.G., & Sawin, C.F. (1976). Exercise cardiac output following Skylab missions: The second manned Skylab mission. *Aviation, Space and Environmental Medicine*, **47**, 365-372.

Bull, R.K., Davies, C.T.M., Lind, A.R., & White, M.J. (1989). The human pressor response during and following voluntary and evoked isometric contractions with occluded local blood supply. *Journal of Physiology*, **411**, 63-70.

Bullen, B.A., Reed, R.B., & Mayer, J. (1964). Physical activity of obese and non-obese adolescent girls: Appraised by motion picture samples. *American Journal of Clinical Nutrition*, **14**, 211-223.

Bunc, V., Heller, J., & Leso, J. (1988). Kinetics of heart rate responses to exercise. *Journal of Sports Science*, **6**, 39-48.

Bunc, V., Heller, J., Moravec, P., & Sprynarova, S. (1989). Ventilatory threshold and mechanical efficiency in endurance runners. *European Journal of Applied Physiology*, **58**, 693-698.

Buono, M.J., & Sjoholm, N.T. (1988). Effect of physical training on peripheral sweat production. *Journal of Applied Physiology*, **65**, 811-814.

Buono, M.J., Wilmore, D.H., & Roby, F.B. (1983). Indirect assessment of thoracic fluid balance following maximal exercise in man. *Journal of Sports Science*, **1**, 217-226.

Burke, E.R., Faria, I.E., & White, J.A. (1990). Cycling. In T. Reilly, N. Secher, P. Snell, & C. Williams, *Physiology of sports* (pp. 173-216). London: E & F Spon.

Burt, J.J., & Jackson, R. (1965). The effects of physical exercise on the coronary collateral circulation of dogs. *Journal of Sports Medicine and Physical Fitness*, **5**, 203-206.

Burton, A.C. (1965). *Physics and biophysics of the circulation*. Chicago: Year Book Medical.

Butterfield, G.E., & Tremblay, A. (in press). Physical activity and nutrition in the context of fitness and health. In C. Bouchard, R.J. Shephard, & T. Stephens (Eds.), *Physical activity, fitness, and health*. Champaign, IL: Human Kinetics.

Buyze, M.T., Foster, C., Pollock, M.L., Sennett, S.M., Hare, J., & Sol, N. (1986). Comparative training responses to rope skipping and jogging. *The Physician and Sportsmedicine*, **14**(11), 65-69.

Byrne-Quinn, E., Weil, J., Sodal, I.E., Filley, G.F., & Grover, R.F. (1971). Ventilatory control in the athlete. *Journal of Applied Physiology*, **30**, 91-98.

Byström, S.E.G., & Kilböm, A. (1990). Physiological response in the forearm during and after isometric intermittent handgrip. *European Journal of Applied Physiology*, **60**, 457-466.

Cade, R., Conte, M., Zauner, C., Mars, D., Peterson, J., Lunne, D., Hommen, N., & Packer, D. (1984). Effects of phosphate loading on 2,3-diphosphoglycerate and maximal oxygen uptake. *Medicine and Science in Sports and Exercise*, **16**, 263-268.

Cady, L.D., Thomas, P.C., & Karwasky, R.J. (1985). Program for increasing health and physical fitness of firefighters. *Journal of Occupational Medicine*, **27**, 110-114.

Caiozzo, V.J., & Kyle, C.R. (1980). The effect of external loading upon power output in stair-climbing. *European Journal of Applied Physiology*, **44**, 217-222.

Campbell, W.R. & Pohndorf, R.H. (1961). Physical fitness of British and United States children. In L.A. Larson (Ed.), *Health and fitness in the modern world*. Washington, D.C.: Athletic Institute.

Canada Health Survey. (1982). Ottawa: Health and Welfare Canada.

Canada's Health Promotion Survey. (1988). Ottawa: Health and Welfare Canada.

Canadian Association for Health, Physical Education and Recreation. (1980). *Fitness performance II. Test manual*. Ottawa: Author.

Canada Fitness Survey. (1983). *Fitness and lifestyle in Canada*. Ottawa: Fitness and Lifestyle Research Institute.

Cann, C.E., Martin, M.C., Genant, H.K., & Jeffe, R.B. (1984). Decreased spinal mineral content in amenorrheic women. *Journal of the American Medical Association*, **251**, 626-629.

Cannon, J.G., & Kluger, M.J. (1984). Exercise enhances survival rate in mice infected with *Salmonella typhi murium* (41830). *Proceedings of the Society for Experimental Biology and Medicine*, **175**, 518-521.

Cardus, D. (1967). O_2 alveolar-arterial tension difference after 10 days recumbency in man. *Journal of Applied Physiology*, **23**, 934-937.

Carpenter, M.W., Sady, S.P., Hoegsberg, B., Sady, M.A., Haydon, B., Cullinane, E.M., Coustan, D.R., & Thompson, P.D. (1988). Fetal response to maternal exertion. *Journal of the American Medical Association*, **259**, 3006-3009.

Carswell, S.H. (1975). Changes in aerobic power in patients undergoing elective surgery. *Journal of Physiology* (London), **251**, 42P-43P.

Carswell, S.H., Holman, B.D., Thompson, J., & Walker, W.F. (1978). Acceptable levels of aerobic power for patients undergoing elective surgery. *Journal of Physiology* (London), **285**, 13P.

Casaburi, R., Patessio, A., Ioli, F., Zanaboni, S., Donner, C.F., & Wasserman, K. (1991). Reductions in exercise lactic acidosis and ventilation as a result of exercise training in patients with obstructive lung disease. *American Review of Respiratory Diseases*, **143**, 9-18.

Caspersen, C.J., Powell, K.E., & Christenson, G.M. (1985). Physical activity, exercise, and physical fitness: Definitions and distinctions for health-related research. *Public Health Reports*, **100**, 126-131.

Celsing, F., Svedenhag, J., Philstedt, P., & Ekblöm, B. (1986). Effects of anemia and stepwise-induced polycythaemia on maximal aerobic power in individuals with high and low haemoglobin concentrations. *Acta Physiologica Scandinavica*, **129**, 47-54.

Chagnon, Y.C., Allard, C., & Bouchard, C. (1984). Red blood cell genetic variation in Olympic endurance athletes. *Journal of Sport Science*, **2**, 121-129.

Chance, B. (1957). Cellular oxygen requirements. *Federation Proceedings*, **16**, 671-680.

Chance, B. (1977). Molecular basis of O_2 affinity for cytochrome oxidase. In F. Jöbsis (Ed.), *Oxygen and physiological function* (pp. 14-25). Dallas: Professional Information Library.

Chance, B., & Pring, M. (1968). Logic in the design of the respiratory chain. In B. Hess & H. Standinger (Eds.), *Biochimie des Sauerstoffs* (pp. 120-130). Berlin: Springer-Verlag.

Chantraine, A. (1985). Knee joint in soccer players: Osteoarthritis and axis deviation. *Medicine and Science in Sports and Exercise*, **17**, 434-439.

Chapman, E.A., DeVries, H.A., & Swezey, R. (1972). Joint stiffness: Effect of exercise on young and old men. *Journal of Gerontology*, **27**, 218-221.

Chen, J.D. (1991). Growth, exercise, fitness, and nutrition in China. In R.J. Shephard & J. Pařízková (Eds.), *Human growth, physical fitness and nutrition* (pp. 19-32). Basel, Switzerland: Karger.

Cheraskin, E., & Ringsdorf, W.M. (1971). Predictive medicine X: Physical activity. *Journal of the American Geriatric Society*, **19**, 969-973.

Chirico, A.M., & Stunkard, A.J. (1960). Physical activity and human obesity. *New England Journal of Medicine*, **263**, 935-940.

Chisholm, D.M., Collis, M.L., Kulak, L.L., Davenport, W., & Gruber, N. (1975). Physical activity readiness. *British Columbia Medical Journal*, **17**, 375-378.

Chow, R.K., Harrison, J.E., Brown, C.F., & Hajek, V. (1986). Physical fitness effect on bone mass in postmenopausal women. *Archives of Physical Medicine and Rehabilitation*, **67**, 231-234.

Chow, R.K., Harrison, J.E., & Notarius, C. (1987). Effect of two randomized exercise programmes on bone mass of healthy post-menopausal women. *British Medical Journal*, **295**, 1441-1444.

Christensen, E.H., & Hansen, O. (1939). Zur Methodik der Respiratorischer Quotient: Bestimmungen in Rühe und Arbeit. *Skandinavisches Archiv für Physiologie*, **81**, 137-151.

Christian, J.C. (1979). Testing twin means and estimating genetic variance: Basic methodology for the analysis of quantitative data. *Acta Geneticae Medicae et Gemellologicae* (Roma), **28**, 35-40.

Chumlea, W.C., & Baumgartner, R.N. (1990). Bioelectric impedance methods for the estimation of body composition. *Canadian Journal of Sport Sciences*, **15**, 172-179.

Clanton, T.L., Dixon, G.F., Drake, J., & Gadek, J.E. (1987). Effects of swim training on lung volumes and inspiratory muscle conditioning. *Journal of Applied Physiology*, **62**, 39-46.

Clapp, J.F. (1989a). The effects of exercise on utero-placental blood flow. In C. Rosenfeld (Ed.), *Reproductive and perinatal medicine: Vol. X. The uterine circulation* (pp. 299-311). Ithaca, NY: Perinatology Press.

Clapp, J.F. (1989b). The effects of maternal exercise in early pregnancy outcome. *American Journal of Obstetrics and Gynecology*, **161**, 1453-1457.

Clapp, J.F., & Capeless, E.L. (1990). Neonatal morphometrics after endurance exercise during pregnancy. *American Journal of Obstetrics and Gynecology*, **163**, 1805-1811.

Clapp, J.F., & Dickstein, S. (1984). Endurance exercise and pregnancy outcome. *Medicine and Science in Sports and Exercise*, **16**, 556-562.

Clapp, J.F., Wesley, M., & Sleamaker, R.H. (1987). Thermoregulatory and metabolic responses to jogging prior to and during pregnancy. *Medicine and Science in Sports and Exercise*, **19**, 124-130.

Clarke, C.R., Schrott, H.G., Leaverton, P.E., Connor, W.E., & Lauer, R.M. (1978). Tracking of blood lipids and blood pressures in school-age children: The Muscatine study. *Circulation*, **58**, 626-634.

Clausen, J.P. (1973). Muscle blood flow during exercise and its significance for maximal performance. In J. Keul (Ed.), *Limiting factors of physical performance* (pp. 253-266). Stuttgart: Thieme.

Clausen, J.P. (1977). Effects of physical training on cardiovascular adjustments to exercise in man. *Physiological Reviews*, **57**, 779-815.

Clausen, J.P., Klausen, K., Rasmussen, B., & Trap-Jensen, J. (1973). Central and peripheral circulatory changes after training of the arms and legs. *American Journal of Physiology*, **225**, 675-682.

Clement, D.B., & Asmundson, R.C. (1982). Nutritional intake and hematological parameters in endurance runners. *The Physician and Sportsmedicine*, **10**(3), 37-43.

Clement, D.B., Asmundson, R.C., & Medhurst, C.W. (1977). 3: Hemoglobin values: Comparative survey of the 1976 Canadian Olympic team. *Canadian Medical Association Journal*, **117**, 614-616.

Coast, J.R., Clifford, P.S., Henrich, T.W., Stray-Gunderson, J., & Johnson, R.L. (1990). Maximal inspiratory pressure following maximal exercise in trained and untrained subjects. *Medicine and Science in Sports and Exercise*, **22**, 811-815.

Coates, G., O'Brodovich, H., Jeffries, A.L., & Gray, G.W. (1984). Effects of exercise on lung lymph flow in sheep and goats during normoxia and hypoxia. *Journal of Clinical Investigation*, **74**, 133-141.

Cobley, A.J., Cooke, N.T., Freedman, S., & Moxham, J. (1981). Increase in blood lactate following maximum voluntary ventilation. *Journal of Physiology*, **315**, 35P.

Coburn, R.F., & Mayers, L.B. (1971). Myoglobin O_2 tension determined from measurements of carboxymyoglobin in skeletal muscle. *American Journal of Physiology*, **220**, 66-74.

Cockcroft, A., Beaumont, A., Adams, L., & Guz, A. (1985). Arterial oxygen desaturation during treadmill and bicycle exercise in patients with chronic obstructive airway disease. *Clinical Science*, **68**, 327-332.

Cohen, J.L., & Segal, K.R. (1985). Left ventricular hypertrophy in athletes: An exercise-electrocardiographic study. *Medicine and Science in Sports and Exercise*, **17**, 695-700.

Collings, C.A., Curet, L.B., & Mullin, J.P. (1983). Maternal and fetal responses to a maternal exercise program. *American Journal of Obstetrics and Gynecology*, **145**, 702-707.

Collins, K.J., & Roberts, D.F. (1988). *Capacity for work in the tropics*. Cambridge: Cambridge University Press.

Comstock, G.W. (1957). An epidemiological study of blood pressure levels in a bi-racial community in the southern United States. *American Journal of Hygiene*, **65**, 271-315.

Conconi, F., Borsetto, C., Casoni, I., & Farrari, M. (1988). Noninvasive determination of anaerobic threshold in cyclists. In E.R. Burke & M.M. Newson (Eds.), *Medical and scientific aspects of cycling* (pp. 79-91). Champaign, IL: Human Kinetics.

Conger, P.R., Quinney, H.A., Gauthier, R., & Massicotte, D. (1982). A comparison of the CAHPER performance test 1966-1980. *CAHPER Journal*, **49**(2), 6-11, 12-16.

Conley, D.L., & Krahenbuhl, G.S. (1980). Running economy and distance running performance of highly trained athletes. *Medicine and Science in Sports and Exercise*, **12**, 357-360.

Connett, R.J., Gayeski, T.E., & Honig, C.R. (1984). Lactate accumulation in fully aerobic, working-dog gracilis muscle. *American Journal of Physiology*, **246**, H120-H128.

Constable, S.H., Favier, R.J., & Holloszy, J.O. (1986). Exercise and glycogen depletion: Effects on ability to activate muscle phosphorylase. *Journal of Applied Physiology*, **60**, 1518-1523.

Convertino, V., Hung, J., Goldwater, D., & DeBusk, R.F. (1982). Cardiovascular responses to exercise in middle-aged men after ten days of bedrest. *Circulation*, **65**, 134-140.

Convertino, V., Sandler, H.A., Webb, P.A., & Annis, J.F. (1982). Induced venous pooling and cardiorespiratory responses to exercise after bed rest. *Journal of Applied Physiology*, **52**, 1343-1348.

Convertino, V.A. (1991). Blood volume: Its adaptation to endurance training. *Medicine and Science in Sports and Exercise*, **23**, 1338-1348.

Cooper, K.H. (1968). *Aerobics*. New York: Evans.

Cordain, L., Glissan, B.J., Latin, R.W., Tucker, A., & Stager, J. (1987). Maximal respiratory pressures and pulmonary function in male runners. *British Journal of Sports Medicine*, **21**, 18-22.

Cordain, L., Latin, R.W., & Behnke, J.J. (1986). The effects of an aerobic running program on bowel transit time. *Journal of Sports Medicine*, **26**, 101-104.

Cordain, L., & Stager, J. (1988). Pulmonary structure and function in swimmers. *Sports Medicine*, **6**, 271-278.

Cordain, L., Tucker, A., Moon, D., & Stager, J. (1990). Lung volumes and maximal respiratory pressures in collegiate swimmers and runners. *Research Quarterly*, **61**, 70-74.

Costill, D.L., Fink, W.J., Hargreaves, M., King, D.S., Thomas, R., & Fielding, R. (1985). Metabolic characteristics of skeletal muscle during detraining from competitive swimming. *Medicine and Science in Sports and Exercise*, **17**, 339-343.

Costill, D.L., Sharp, R.L., Fink, W.J., & Katz, A. (1982). Determination of human muscle pH in needle biopsy specimens. *Journal of Applied Physiology*, **53**, 1310-1313.

Cotes, J.E. (1965). *Lung function: Assessment and application in medicine*. Oxford: Blackwell Scientific.

Cotes, J.E., & Woolmer, R.F. (1962). A comparison between twenty-seven laboratories of the results of analysis of an expired gas sample. *Journal of Physiology*, **163**, 36P-37P.

Couture, L., Chagnon, M., Allard, C., & Bouchard, C. (1986). More on the red blood cell genetic variation in Olympic athletes. *Canadian Journal of Applied Sport Sciences*, **11**, 16-18.

Cox, M., Shephard, R.J., & Corey, P. (1981). Influence of an employee fitness programme upon fitness, productivity, and absenteeism. *Ergonomics*, **24**, 795-806.

Cox, M.L., Bennett, J.B., & Dudley, G.A. (1986). Exercise training-induced alterations of cardiac morphology. *Journal of Applied Physiology*, **61**, 926-931.

Coyle, E.F. (1988). Detraining and retention of training-induced adaptations. In American College of Sports Medicine (Eds.), *Resource manual for guidelines for exercise testing and exercise prescription* (pp. 83-89). Philadelphia: Lea & Febiger.

Coyle, E.F., Hemmert, M.K., & Coggan, A.R. (1986). Effects of detraining on cardiovascular responses to exercise: Role of blood volume. *Journal of Applied Physiology*, **60**, 95-99.

Coyle, E.F., Martin, W.H., Sinacore, D.R., Joyner, M.J., Hagberg, J.M., & Holloszy, J.O. (1984). Time course of loss of adaptation after stopping prolonged intense endurance training. *Journal of Applied Physiology*, **57**(6), 1857-1864.

Crenshaw, A.G., Friden, J., Thornell, L-E., & Hargens, A.R. (1991). Extreme endurance training: Evidence of capillary and mitochondria compartmentization in human skeletal muscle. *European Journal of Applied Physiology*, **63**, 173-178.

Criqui, M. (1985). The problem of response bias. In R.M. Kaplan & M.H. Criqui (Eds.), *Behavioral epidemiology and disease prevention*. New York: Plenum Press.

Crone, P.B., & Tee, G.H. (1974). Staphylococci in swimming pool water. *Journal of Hygiene* (Cambridge), **73**, 213-220.

Cullen, K., Wearne, K.L., Stenhouse, N.S., & Cumpston, G.N. (1983). Q waves and ventricular extrasystoles in resting electrocardiograms: A 16-year follow-up in Busselton study. *British Heart Journal*, **50**, 465-468.

Cullinane, E.L., Sady, S.P., Vadeboncoeur, L., Burke, M., & Thompson, P.D. (1986). Cardiac size and VO2max do not decrease after short-term exercise cessation. *Medicine and Science in Sports and Exercise*, **18**, 420-424.

Cumming, D.C. (1989). Menstrual disturbances caused by exercise. In K.M. Pirke, W. Wuttke, & U. Schweiger (Eds.), *The menstrual cycle and its disorders* (p. 150). New York: Springer-Verlag.

Cumming, G.R. (1971). Correlation of physical performance with laboratory measures of fitness. In R.J. Shephard (Ed.), *Frontiers of fitness* (pp. 265-279). Springfield, IL: Charles C Thomas.

Cumming, G.R. (1978). Body size and the assessment of physical performance. In R.J. Shephard & H. Lavallée (Eds.), *Physical fitness assessment: Principles, practice, and application* (pp. 18-31). Springfield, IL: Charles C. Thomas.

Cumming, G.R. (1989). Exercise therapy in pediatric cardiology. In J. Torg, P. Welsh, & R.J. Shephard (Eds.), *Current therapy in sports medicine 2* (pp. 39-45). Burlington, ON: Decker.

Cunningham, D.A., Rechnitzer, P.A., & Donner, A. (1986). Exercise training and the speed of self-selected walking pace in retirement. *Canadian Journal on Aging*, **5**, 19-26.

Dalen, N., & Olsson, K.E. (1974). Bone mineral content and physical activity. *Acta Orthopaedica Scandinavica*, **45**, 170-174.

Dal Monte, A., Faina, M., & Menchinelli, C. (1992). Sport-specific ergometric equipment. In R.J. Shephard & P.O. Åstrand (Eds.), *Endurance in sport* (pp. 201-207). Oxford: Blackwell Scientific.

Danforth, W.H. (1965). Activation of glycolytic pathway in muscle. In B. Chance, R.W. Estabrook, & J.R. Williamson (Eds.), *Control of energy metabolism* (pp. 287-298). New York: Academic Press.

Daniels, J.T. (1992). Triathlon training and competition. In R.J. Shephard & P.O. Åstrand (Eds.), *Endurance in sport* (pp. 602-611). Oxford: Blackwell Scientific.

Danielson, R., & Danielson, K. (1982). *Exercise program effects on firefighters*. Toronto: Ontario Ministry of Tourism & Recreation.

Darling, R.C. (1946). The significance of physical fitness. *Archives of Physical Medicine*, **28**, 140-145.

Daub, W.B., Green, H.J., Houston, M.E., Thomson, J.A., Fraser, I.G., & Ranney, D.A. (1983). Specificity of physiological adaptations resulting from ice-hockey training. *Medicine and Science in Sports and Exercise*, **15**, 290-294.

Davies, C.T.M., & Sargeant, A.J. (1974). Physiological responses to standardized arm work. *Ergonomics*, **17**, 41-49.

Davies, C.T.M., & Sargeant, A.J. (1975). Effects of training on the responses to one- and two-leg work. *Journal of Applied Physiology*, **38**, 375-385.

Davies, C.T.M., & Starkie, D.W. (1985). The pressor response to voluntary and electrically-evoked isometric contractions in man. *European Journal of Applied Physiology*, **53**, 359-363.

Davies, C.T.M., & Van Haaren, J.P.M. (1973a). Effect of treatment on physiological responses to exercise in East African industrial workers with iron-deficiency anaemia. *British Journal of Industrial Medicine*, **30**, 335-340.

Davies, C.T.M., & Van Haaren, J.P.M. (1973b). Maximum aerobic power and body composition in healthy East African older male and female subjects. *American Journal of Physical Anthropology*, **39**, 395-401.

Davies, C.T.M., von Döbeln, W., Fohlin, L., Freyschuss, U., & Thorén, C. (1978). Total body potassium, fat free weight, and maximal aerobic power in children with anorexia nervosa. *Acta Paediatrica Scandinavica*, **67**, 229-234.

Davies, E.C., Logan, G.A., & McKinney, W.C. (1961). *Biophysical values of muscular activity*. Dubuque, IA: Brown.

Davis, G.M., Plyley, M.J., & Shephard, R.J. (1991). Gains of cardio-respiratory fitness with arm crank training in spinally disabled men. *Canadian Journal of Sport Sciences*, **16**, 64-72.

Davis, G.M., & Shephard, R.J. (1990). Strength training for wheelchair users. *British Journal of Sports Medicine*, **24**, 25-30.

Davis, R.B., Boyd, D.G., McKinney, M.E., & Jones, C.C. (1990). Effects of exercise and exercise conditioning on blood platelet function. *Medicine and Science in Sports and Exercise*, **22**, 49-53.

Dawber, T.R. (1980). *The Framingham study: The epidemiology of atherosclerotic disease.* Cambridge, MA: Harvard University Press.

DeBusk, R.F., Valdez, R., Houston, N., & Haskell, W. (1978). Cardiovascular responses to dynamic and static effort soon after myocardial infarction: Application to occupational work assessment. *Circulation*, **58**, 368-375.

DeBusk, R.F., Stenestrand, U., Sheehan, M., & Haskell, W.L. (1990). Training effects of long versus short bouts of exercise in healthy subjects. *American Journal of Cardiology*, **65**, 1010-1013.

Dedmon, R.E. (1988). Barriers and opportunities in providing wellness programs for hourly and salaried employees. In J.H. Myers (Ed.), *Decreasing barriers: A blueprint for workplace health in the nineties* (pp. 23-42). Dallas: American Heart Association.

Dekkar, N. (1991). Growth, nutrition, and physical performance in Algeria. In R.J. Shephard & J. Pařízková (Eds.), *Human growth, physical fitness, and nutrition* (pp. 41-60). Basel: S. Karger.

Demedts, M., & Anthonisen, N.R. (1973). Effects of increased external airway resistance during steady state exercise. *Journal of Applied Physiology*, **35**, 361-366.

Demirjian, A., Jenicek, J., & Dubuc, M.B. (1972). Les normes staturo-pondérales de l'enfant urbain Canadien-français d'âge scolaire [Height-weight norms for urban French Canadian Schoolchildren]. *Canadian Journal of Public Health*, **67**, 209-216.

Dempsey, J.A. (1986). Is the lung built for exercise? *Medicine and Science in Sports and Exercise*, **18**, 143-155.

Dempsey, J.A., & Babcock, M. (in press). Pulmonary adaptation to physical activity. In C. Bouchard, R.J. Shephard, & T. Stephens (Eds.), *Physical activity, fitness, and health.* Champaign, IL: Human Kinetics.

Dempsey, J.A., & Manohar, M.A. (1992). Pulmonary system. In R.J. Shephard & P.O. Åstrand (Eds.), *Endurance in sport* (pp. 61-71). Oxford: Blackwell Scientific.

Denison, D.M., Waller, J.F., Turton, C.W.G., & Sopwith, T. (1982). Does the lung work? 5. Breathing in and frequency out. *British Journal of Diseases of the Chest*, **76**, 237-252.

Deroanne, R., Juchmes, J., Hausman, A., Pirnay, F., & Petit, J.M. (1968). Résistance inspiratoire et tolérance à l'exercice musculaire chez l'homme normal [Inspiratory resistance and exercise tolerance in normal men]. *Archives Internationales de Physiologie et Biochimie*, **76**, 163-164.

Després, J-P. (in press). Physical activity and adipose tissue. In C. Bouchard, R.J. Shephard, & T. Stephens (Eds.), *Physical activity, fitness, and health.* Champaign, IL: Human Kinetics.

Després, J-P, Bouchard, C., & Malina, R.M. (1990). Physical activity and coronary heart disease risk factors during childhood and adolescence. *Exercise and Sport Sciences Reviews*, **18**, 243-261.

Després, J-P., Bouchard, C., Tremblay, A., Savard, R., & Marcotte, M. (1985). Effects of aerobic training on fat distribution in male subjects. *Medicine and Science in Sports and Exercise*, **17**, 113-118.

Després, J-P., Moorjani, S., Tremblay, A., Pehlman, E.T., Lupien, P.J., Nadeau, A., & Bouchard, C. (1988). Heredity and changes in plasma lipids and lipoproteins and short-term exercise training in men. *Arteriosclerosis*, **8**, 402-409.

DeStephano, F., Coulehan, J., & Kennethewiant, M. (1979). Blood pressure survey on the Navajo Indian reservation. *American Journal of Epidemiology*, **109**, 335-345.

de Troyer, A., & Yernault, J. (1980). Inspiratory muscle force in normal subjects and patients with interstitial lung disease. *Thorax*, **35**, 92-100.

Detry, J.M., Brengelmann, G.L., Rowell, L.B., & Wyss, C. (1972). Skin and muscle components of forearm flow in directly heated resting man. *Journal of Applied Physiology*, **32**, 506-511.

DeVries, H.A. (1970). Physiological effects of exercise training regimen upon men aged 52 to 88. *Journal of Gerontology*, **24**, 325-336.

DeVries, H.A. (1980). *Physiology of exercise for physical education and athletics* (3rd ed.). Dubuque, IA: Brown.

Dick, F. (1992, February). Altitude training. Paper presented at the conference on "Sport et Montagne," Chamonix, France.

Dicker, S., Lofthus, G., Thornton, N., & Brooks, G. (1980). Respiratory and heart rate responses to tethered, controlled frequency breathing swimming. *Medicine and Science in Sports*, **12**, 20-23.

Dickuth, H.H., Horstman, T., Staiger, J., Reindell, H., & Keul, J. (1989). The long-term involution of physiological cardiomegaly and cardiac hypertrophy. *Medicine and Science in Sports and Exercise*, **21**, 244-249.

Dietrick, J.E., Whedon, G.D., & Shore, E. (1948). Effects of immobilization upon various metabolic and physiologic functions of normal men. *American Journal of Medicine*, **4**, 3-35.

diNatale, J., Lee, M., Ward, G., & Shephard, R.J. (1985). Loss of physical condition in sightless adolescents during a summer vacation. *Adapted Physical Education Quarterly*, **2**, 144-150.

diPrampero, P.E. (1971). Anaerobic capacity and power. In R.J. Shephard (Ed.), *Frontiers of fitness* (pp. 155-173). Springfield, IL: Charles C Thomas.

diPrampero, P.E. (1992). The energetics of running. In R.J. Shephard & P.O. Åstrand (Eds.), *Endurance in sport* (pp. 542-549). Oxford: Blackwell Scientific.

diPrampero, P.E., Cortilo, G., Mognoni, P., & Saibene, F. (1976). Energy cost of speed skating and efficiency of work against resistance. *Journal of Applied Physiology*, **40**, 584-591.

Disch, J., Frankiewicz, R., & Jackson, A. (1975). Construct validation of distance run tests. *Research Quarterly*, **46**, 169-176.

Doll, E., Keul, J., & Maiwald, C. (1968). Oxygen tension and acid-base equilibria in venous blood of working muscle. *American Journal of Physiology*, **215**, 23-29.

Doubt, T.J., & Shieh, S.S. (1991). Additive effects of caffeine and cold water during submaximal exercise. *Medicine and Science in Sports and Exercise*, **23**, 435-442.

Douglas, P.S., Hiller, D.B., & O'Toole, M.L. (1987). Left ventricular structure and function in endurance athletes: Results of 1984 Labman study. *Annals of Sports Medicine*, **3**, 109-110.

Douglas, P.S., O'Toole, M.L., & Woolard, J. (1990). Regional wall motion abnormalities after prolonged exercise in the normal left ventricle. *Circulation*, **82**, 2108-2114.

Doyle, F., Brown, J., & Lachance, C. (1970). Relation between bone mass and muscle weight. *Lancet*, **1**, 391-393.

Drake, V., Jones, G., Brown, J.R., & Shephard, R.J. (1968). Fitness performance tests and their relationship to maximum oxygen uptake. *Canadian Medical Association Journal*, **99**, 844-848.

Drake, V., White, D., & Shephard, R.J. (1969). The fitness performance of Canadian working men: With some comments on the adaptation of performance tests to a small gymnasium. *Journal of Sports Medicine and Physical Fitness*, **9**, 152-161.

Dressendorfer, R.E., & Wade, C.E. (1991). Effects of a 15-d race on plasma steroid levels and leg muscle fitness in runners. *Medicine and Science in Sports and Exercise*, **23**, 954-958.

Dreyer, G. (1920). *The assessment of physical fitness*. London: Cassell.

Drinkwater, B.L. (1984). Women and exercise: Physiological aspects. *Exercise and Sport Sciences Reviews*, **12**, 21-52.

Drinkwater, B.L., Nilson, K., Ott, S., & Chesnut, C.H. (1986). Bone mineral density after resumption of menses in amenorrheic athletes. *Journal of the American Medical Association*, **256**, 380-382.

Drinkwater, B.L., Nilson, K., Chesnut, C.H., Bremmer, W.J., Shainholtz, S., & Southworth, M.B. (1984). Bone mineral content of amenorrheic and eumenorrheic athletes. *New England Journal of Medicine*, **311**, 277-281.

Drygas, W.K. (1988). Changes in blood platelet function, coagulation, and fibrinolytic activity in response to moderate, exhaustive, and prolonged exercise. *International Journal of Sports Medicine*, **9**, 67-72.

Dudley, G.A., & Fleck, S.J. (1987). Strength training and endurance training. *Sports Medicine*, **4**, 79-85.

Durnin, J.V.G.A. (1966). Age, physical activity, and energy expenditure. *Proceedings of the Nutrition Society*, **25**, 107-113.

Durnin, J.V.G.A., & Passmore, R. (1967). *Energy, work, and leisure*. London: Heinemann.

Ebbeling, C.B., & Clarkson, R.M. (1989). Exercise-induced muscle damage and adaptation. *Sports Medicine*, **7**, 207-234.

Ebbeling, C.B., & Clarkson, R.M. (1990). Muscle adaptation prior to recovery following eccentric exercise. *European Journal of Applied Physiology*, **60**, 26-31.

Eckstein, R.W. (1957). Effect of exercise and coronary artery narrowing on coronary collateral circulation. *Circulation Research*, **5**, 230-235.

Eddy, D.O., Sparks, K.L., & Adelizi, D.A. (1977). The effects of continuous and interval training in women and men. *European Journal of Applied Physiology*, **37**, 83-92.

Edholm, O.G. (1970). The changing patterns of human activity. *Ergonomics*, **13**, 625-643.

Edholm, O.G., Adam, J.M., Healy, M.J.R., Wolff, H.S., Goldsmith, R., & Best, T.W. (1970). Food intake and energy expenditure of army recruits. *British Journal of Nutrition*, **24**, 1091-1107.

Edin, J.B., Gerberich, S.G., Leon, A.S., McNally, C., Serfass, R., Shaw, G., Moy, J., & Casal, D. (1990). Analysis of the training effects of minitrampoline rebounding on physical fitness, body composition, and blood lipids. *Journal of Cardiopulmonary Rehabilitation*, **10**, 401-408.

Edwards, D.A.W., Hammond, W.H., Healy, M.J.R., Tanner, J.M., & Whitehouse, R.H. (1955). Design and accuracy of calipers for measuring subcutaneous tissue thickness. *British Journal of Nutrition*, **2**, 133-143.

Ehn, L., Carlmark, B., & Höglund, S. (1980). Iron status in athletes involved in intense activity. *Medicine and Science in Sports*, **12**, 61-64.

Ehsani, A.A., Hagberg, J.M., & Hickson, R.C. (1978). Rapid changes in left ventricular dimensions and mass in response to physical conditioning and deconditioning. *American Journal of Cardiology*, **42**, 52-56.

Eichna, L.W., Park, C.R., Nelson, N., Horvath, S.M., & Palmes, E.D. (1950). Thermal regulation during acclimatization in a hot, dry (desert-type) environment. *American Journal of Physiology*, **163**, 585-597.

Eichner, R. (1989). Gastro-intestinal bleeding in athletes. *The Physician and Sportsmedicine*, **17**(5), 128-140.

Eichner, R. (in press). Physical activity and free radicals. In C. Bouchard, R.J. Shephard, & T. Stephens (Eds.), *Physical activity, fitness, and health*. Champaign, IL: Human Kinetics.

Eisenman, P.A., Johnson, S.C., Bainbridge, C.N., & Zupan, M.F. (1988). Applied physiology of cross-country skiing. *Sports Medicine*, **8**, 67-79.

Ekblom, B., & Gjessing, E. (1968). Maximal oxygen uptake of the Easter Island population. *Journal of Applied Physiology*, **25**, 124-129.

Ekblom, B., Hermansen, L., & Saltin, B. (1967). *HastighertsÅkning pÅ Skridsko. Idrottsfysiologi report #5* [Velocity of speed skaters. Sports Physiology Report #5]. Framtiden, Stockholm.

Ekblom, B., & Huof, R. (1972). Response to submaximal and maximal exercise at different levels of carboxyhaemoglobin. *Acta Physiologica Scandinavica*, **86**, 474-482.

Ekblom, B.T. (1985). Exercise and rheumatoid arthritis. In P. Welsh & R.J. Shephard (Eds.), *Current therapy in sports medicine, 1985-1986* (pp. 108-109). Burlington, ON: Decker.

Ekelund, L.G., Haskell, W.L., Johnson, J.L., Whaley, F.S., Criqui, M.H., & Sheps, D.S. (1988). Physical fitness as a predictor of cardiovascular mortality in asymptomatic North American men: The Lipid Research Clinics mortality follow-up study. *New England Journal of Medicine*, **319**, 1379-1384.

Ekelund, L.G., & Holmgren, A. (1967). Central hemodynamics during exercise. *Circulation Research*, **21**(Suppl. 1), 133-143.

Elias, B.A., Berg, K.E., Latin, R.W., Mellion, M.B., & Hofschire, P.J. (1991). Cardiac structure and function in weight trainers, runners, and runner/weight trainers. *Research Quarterly*, **62**, 326-332.

Ellis, G. (1971). *Units, symbols, and abbreviations: A guide for biological and medical editors and authors*. London: Royal Society of Medicine.

Engel, L.A., Wood, L.D.H., Utz, G., & Macklem, P.T. (1973). Gas mixing during inspiration. *Journal of Applied Physiology*, **35**, 18-24.

Engström, L.M., & Fischbein, S. (1977). Physical capacity in twins. *Acta Medicae Geneticae et Gemellologicae* (Roma), **26**, 159-165.

Enos, W.F., Holmes, R.H., & Bayer, J.C. (1953). Coronary artery sclerosis in American soldiers killed during the Korean war. *Journal of the American Medical Association*, **152**, 1090-1093.

Epp, J. (1986). *Achieving health for all: A framework for health promotion*. Ottawa: Health and Welfare Canada.

Eriksson, L.I., Jorfeldt, L., & Ekstrand, J. (1986). Overuse and distortion soccer injuries related to the player's estimated maximal aerobic capacity. *International Journal of Sports Medicine*, **7**, 214-216.

Erkkola, R. (1976). The physical work capacity of the expectant mother and its effect on pregnancy, labor, and the newborn. *International Journal of Gynaecology and Obstetrics*, **14**, 153-159.

Ernsting, J., & Shephard, R.J. (1951). Respiratory adaptations in congenital heart disease. *Journal of Physiology*, **112**, 332-343.

Essfeld, D., Hoffmann, U., & Stegemann, J. (1991). A model for studying the distortion of muscle oxygen uptake patterns by circulation parameters. *European Journal of Applied Physiology*, **62**, 83-90.

Evans, J. (1987). *Toward a shared direction for health in Ontario*. Toronto: Ontario Ministry of Health.

Fagard, R., Van den Broeke, C., Bielen, E., & Amery, A. (1987). Maximum oxygen uptake and cardiac size and function in twins. *American Journal of Cardiology*, **60**, 1362-1367.

Fagard, R., Van den Broeke, C., & Amery, A. (1989). Left ventricular dynamics during exercise in elite marathon runners. *Journal of the American College of Cardiology*, **14**, 112-118.

Faigenbaum, A.D., Skrinar, G.S., Cesare, W.F., Kraemer, W.J., & Thomas, H.E. (1990). Physiologic and symptomatic responses of cardiac patients to resistance exercise. *Archives of Physical Medicine and Rehabilitation*, **71**, 395-398.

Faria, I.E. (1984). Applied physiology of cycling. *Sports Medicine*, **1**, 187-204.

Faria, I.E., Faria, E.W., Roberts, S., & Yoshimura, D. (1989). Comparison of physical and physiological characteristics in elite young and mature cyclists. *Research Quarterly*, **60**, 388-395.

Faulkner, J.A., Green, H.J., & White, T.P. (in press). Skeletal muscle adaptation to acute and chronic physical activity. In C. Bouchard, R.J. Shephard, & T. Stephens (Eds.), *Physical activity, fitness, and health*. Champaign, IL: Human Kinetics.

Feicht, C.B., Johnson, T.S., Martin, B.J., Sparkes, K.E., & Wagner, W.W. (1978). Secondary amenorrhoea in athletes. *Lancet*, (2), 1145-1146 [letter].

Ferland, Y. (1980, November). Schooling and leisure activities. *Canadian Statistical Review*, pp. vi-ix.

Fernhall, B., & Kohrt, W. (1990). The effect of training specificity on maximal and submaximal physiological responses to treadmill and cycle ergometry. *Journal of Sports Medicine and Physical Fitness*, **30**, 268-275.

Findlay, I.N., Taylor, R.S., Dargie, H.J., Grant, S., Pettigrew, A.R., Wilson, J.T., Aitchison, T., Cleland, J.G., Elliott, A.T., Fisher, B.M., et al. (1987). Cardiovascular effects of training for a marathon run in unfit middle-aged men. *British Medical Journal*, **295**, 521-524.

Fisher, B.D., Baracos, V.E., Shnitka, T.K., Mendryk, S.W., & Reid, D.C. (1990). Ultrastructural events following acute muscle trauma. *Medicine and Science in Sports and Exercise*, **22**, 185-193.

Fisher, N.L. & Smith, D.W. (1981). Occipital encephalocele and early gestational hyperthermia. *Pediatrics*, **68**, 480-483.

Fitness Canada. (1983). *Fitness and lifestyle in Canada*. Ottawa: Fitness Canada.

Fitness Canada. (1986). *Canadian standardized test of fitness (CSTF) operations manual* (3rd ed.). Ottawa: Fitness Canada.

Fitness Ontario. (1983). *Physical activity patterns in Ontario: Part II*. Toronto: Fitness Ontario.

Fleck, S.J. (1988). Cardiovascular adaptations to resistance training. *Medicine and Science in Sports and Exercise*, **20**(Suppl.), S146-S151.

Fleck, S.J., & Kraemer, W.J. (1987). *Designing resistance training programs*. Champaign, IL: Human Kinetics Books.

Flenley, D.C., Fairweather, L.J., Cooke, N.J., & Kirby, B.J. (1973). The effects of variations in P_{50} on oxygen transport in chronic hypoxic lung disease. *Clinical Science and Molecular Biology*, **46**, 18P.

Flook, V., & Kelman, G.R. (1973). Submaximal exercise with increased respiratory resistance to breathing. *Journal of Applied Physiology*, **35**, 379-384.

Florey, V.C. Du, Melia, R.J.W., & Darby, S.C. (1978). Changing mortality from ischaemic heart disease in Great Britain 1966-76. *British Medical Journal*, (i), 635-637.

Fohlin, L. (1978). Exercise performance and body dimensions in anorexia nervosa before and after rehabilitation. *Acta Medica Scandinavica*, **204**, 61-65.

Folinsbee, L.J. (1990). Discussion: Exercise and the environment. In C. Bouchard, R.J. Shephard, T. Stephens, J. Sutton, & B. McPherson (Eds.), *Exercise, fitness, and health* (pp. 179-184). Champaign, IL: Human Kinetics.

Folinsbee, L.J., Wallace, E.S., Bedi, J.F., & Horvath, S.M. (1983). Exercise respiratory pattern in elite cyclists and sedentary subjects. *Medicine and Science in Sports and Exercise*, **15**, 503-509.

Forbes, G.B. (1990). The abdomen-hip ratio: Normative data and observations on selected patients. *International Journal of Obesity*, **14**, 149-157.

Forgraeus, L. (1973). Oxygen uptake in work at lowered and raised ambient air pressures. *Acta Physiologica Scandinavica*, **87**, 411-421.

Fox, S.M., & Haskell, W. (1968). Exercise and stress testing workshop report: National Conference on Exercise in the Prevention, in the Evaluation and in the Treatment of Heart Disease. *Journal of the South Carolina Medical Association*, **65**(Suppl. 1), 75-78.

Francis, K., & Hoobler, T. (1986). Changes in oxygen consumption associated with treadmill walking and running with light, hand-carried weights. *Ergonomics*, **29**, 999-1004.

Franklin, B.A., Bonzheim, K., Gordon, S., & Timmis, G.C. (1991). Resistance training in cardiac rehabilitation. *Journal of Cardiac Rehabilitation*, **11**, 99-107.

Fredberg, J.J. (1980). Spatial considerations in oscillation mechanics of the lungs. *Federation Proceedings*, **39**, 2747-2754.

Fredrickson, C., Puhl, J., & Runyan, W. (1980). Iron status of high school women cross-country runners. *Medicine and Science in Sports*, **12**, 81 (abstract).

Freedman, S. (1970). Sustained maximal voluntary ventilation. *Respiratory Physiology*, **8**, 230-244.

Fregosi, R.F., & Dempsey, J.A. (1986). Effects of exercise in normoxia and acute hypoxia on respiratory muscle metabolites. *Journal of Applied Physiology*, **60**, 1274-1283.

Frenkl, R., Györe, A., Meszaros, J., & Szeberenyi, S. (1980). A study of the enzyme-inducing effect of physical exercise on man: "The trained liver." *Journal of Sports Medicine and Physical Fitness*, **20**, 371-376.

Freund, B.J., Allen, D., & Wilmore, J.H. (1986). Interaction of test protocol and inclined run training on maximal oxygen uptake. *Medicine and Science in Sports and Exercise*, **18**, 588-592.

Frick, M.H., Elo, O., Haapa, K., Heinonen, O.P., Heinsalmi, P., Helo, P., Huttunen, J.K., Kaitaniemi, P., Koskinen, P., Manninen, V., Mäenpää, H., Mälkönen, M., Mänttari, M., Norola, S., Pasternak, A., Pikkarainen, J., Romo, M., Sjösblom, T., & Nikkila, E.A. (1987). Helsinki Heart Study: Primary prevention trial with gemfibrozil in middle-aged men with dyslipidemia. *New England Journal of Medicine*, **317**, 1237-1245.

Fried, T., & Shephard, R.J. (1969). Deterioration and restoration of physical fitness after training. *Canadian Medical Association Journal*, **100**, 831-837.

Fried, T., & Shephard, R.J. (1970). Assessment of a lower extremity training programme. *Canadian Medical Association Journal*, **103**, 260-266.

Friedman, E.H., & Rosenman, R.H. (1974). *Type A behavior and your heart*. Greenwich, CT: Fawcett Books.

Friedman, M., Rosenman, R.H., & Brown, A.E. (1963). The continuous heart rate in men exhibiting an overt behavior pattern associated with an increased incidence of clinical coronary artery disease. *Circulation*, **28**, 861-866.

Friman, G. (1976). Effects of acute infectious disease on circulatory function. *Acta Medica Scandinavica*, (Suppl. 592), 1-62.

Fringer, M.N., & Stull, A.G. (1974). Changes in cardiorespiratory parameters during periods of training and detraining in young female adults. *Medicine and Science in Sports*, **6**, 20-25.

Frisch, R.E., Gotz-Welbergen, A.V., McArthur, J.W., Albright, T.E., Witischi, J., & Bullen, B.A. (1981). Delayed menarche and amenorrhea of college athletes in relation to age of onset of training. *Journal of the American Medical Association*, **246**, 1559-1563.

Frisch, R.E., Hall, G.M., Aoki, T.T., Birnholz, J., Jacob, R., Landsberg, L., Munro, H., Parker-Jones, K., Tulchinskly, D., & Young, J. (1984). Metabolic, endocrine, and reproductive changes of a woman channel-swimmer. *Metabolism*, **33**, 1106-1111.

Frisch, R.E., Wyshak, G., Albright, N.L., Albright, T.E., & Schiff, I. (1989). Lower prevalence of non-reproductive system cancers among female former college athletes. *Medicine and Science in Sports and Exercise*, **21**, 250-253.

Frisch, R.E., Wyshak, G., Albright, N.L., Albright, T.E., Schiff, I., Jones, K.P., Witschi, J., Shiang, E., Koff, E., & Margulis, M. (1985). Lower prevalence of breast cancer and cancers of the reproductive system among former college athletes compared to non-athletes. *British Journal of Cancer*, **52**, 885-891.

Frisk-Holmberg, M., Essén, B., Fredrickson, M., Ström, G., & Witell, L. (1983). Muscle fibre composition in relation to blood pressure response to isometric exercise in normotensive and hypertensive subjects. *Acta Medica Scandinavica*, **213**, 21-26.

Fry, R.W., & Morton, A.R. (1991). Physiological and kinanthropometric attributes of elite flatwater kayakists. *Medicine and Science in Sports and Exercise*, **23**, 1297-1301.

Fry, R.W., Morton, A.R., & Keast, D. (1991). Overtraining in athletes. *Sports Medicine*, **12**, 32-65.

Fuller, J.H., Bernauer, E.M., & Adams, W.C. (1970). Renal function, water, and electrolyte exchange during bed rest with daily exercise. *Aerospace Medicine*, **41**, 60-72.

Gaesser, G.A., & Brooks, G.A. (1984). Metabolic bases of excess post-exercise oxygen consumption: A review. *Medicine and Science in Sports and Exercise*, **16**, 29-43.

Gallagher, G.G., Huda, W., Rigby, M., Greenberg, D., & Younes, M. (1988). Lack of radiographic evidence of interstitial pulmonary edema after maximal exercise in normal subjects. *American Review of Respiratory Diseases*, **137**, 474-476.

Gallanti, G., Toncelli, L., Comeglio, M., Bisi, G., & Gallini, C. (1989). Non-invasive evaluation of cardiac performance at rest and during handgrip in bicyclists and weightlifters after deconditioning. *Sports Training, Medicine, and Rehabilitation*, **1**, 237-248.

Gandevia, S.C., & Hobbs, S.F. (1990). Cardiovascular responses to static exercise in man: Central and reflex contributions. *Journal of Physiology*, **430**, 105-117.

Garabrant, D.H., Peters, J.M., Mack, T.M., & Bernstein, L. (1984). Job activity and colon cancer risk. *American Journal of Epidemiology*, **119**, 1005-1014.

Garfinkel, P., & Garner, D.M. (1982). *Anorexia nervosa: A multidimensional perspective*. New York: Brunner, Mazel.

Garrick, J.G., Gillian, D.M., & Whiteside, P. (1986). The epidemiology of aerobic dance injuries. *American Journal of Sports Medicine*, **14**, 67-72.

Gauthier, M.M. (1986). Guidelines for exercise during pregnancy: Too little or too much? *The Physician and Sportsmedicine*, **14**(4), 162-169.

Gauthier, R., Massicotte, D., Hermiston, R., & MacNab, R. (1983). The physical work capacity of Canadian children, aged 7 to 17, in 1983: A comparison with 1968. *CAHPER Journal*, **50**(2), 1-9.

Geijsel, J.S.M. (1980). The endurance time on a bicycle ergometer as a test for marathon speed skaters. *Journal of Sports Medicine and Physical Fitness*, **20**, 333-340.

Geijsel, J.S.M., Bomhoff, G., van Vezen, J., de Groot, J., & van Ingen Schenau, G.J. (1984). Bicycle ergometry and speed skating performance. *International Journal of Sports Medicine*, **5**, 241-245.

George, K.P., Wolfe, L.A., & Burggaf, G.W. (1991). The "Athletic Heart Syndrome": A critical review. *Sports Medicine*, **11**, 300-331.

Gerberich, S.G., Leon, A.S., McNally, C., Serfass, R., & Edin, J.B. (1990). Analysis of the acute physiologic effects of minitrampoline rebounding exercise. *Journal of Cardiopulmonary Rehabilitation*, **10**, 395-400.

Gerhardsson, M., Norell, S.E., Kiviranta, H., Pedersen, N.L., & Ahlbom, A. (1986). Sedentary jobs and colon cancer. *American Journal of Epidemiology*, **123**, 775-780.

Gettman, L., & Pollock, M.L. (1981). Circuit weight training: A critical review of its physiological benefits. *The Physician and Sportsmedicine*, **9**(1), 44-60.

Gettman, L., Pollock, M.L., Durstine, J.L., Ward, A., Ayres, J., & Linnerud, A.C. (1976). Physiological responses of men to 1-, 3-, and 5-days-per-week training programs. *Research Quarterly*, **47**, 638-646.

Giagnoni, E., Secchi, M.B., Wu, S.C., Marabito, A., Ottrona, L., Mancarella, S., Volpin, N., Fossa, L., Bettazzi, L., Arangio, G., Sachero, A., & Folli, G. (1983). Prognostic value of exercise EKG testing in asymptomatic normotensive subjects: A prospective matched study. *New England Journal of Medicine*, **309**, 1085-1089.

Gibbs, J.O., Mulvaney, D., Henes, C., & Reed, R.W. (1985). Work-site health promotion: Five-year trend in employee health costs. *Journal of Occupational Medicine*, **27**, 826-830.

Gibson, J.N.A., Halliday, D., Morrison, W.L., Stoward, P.J., Hornsby, G.A., Watt, P.W., Murdoch, G., & Rennie, A.J. (1987). Decrease in human quadriceps muscle protein turnover consequent upon leg immobilization. *Clinical Science*, **72**, 503-509.

Gilbert, R., & Auchincloss, J.H. (1969). Mechanics of breathing in normal subjects during brief, severe exercise. *Journal of Laboratory and Clinical Medicine*, **73**, 439-450.

Gilli, P., DePaoli-Vitali, E., Tataranni, G., & Farinelli, A. (1984). Exercise-induced urinary abnormalities in long-distance runners. *International Journal of Sports Medicine*, **5**, 237-240.

Gilliam, T.B., Katch, V.L., Thorland, W., & Weltman, A. (1977). Prevalence of coronary heart disease risk factors in active children, 7 to 12 years of age. *Medicine and Science in Sports*, **9**, 21-25.

Gilson, J.C., & Hugh-Jones, P. (1955). Lung function in coalworkers' pneumoconiosis. *MRC Special Report Series*, **290**, 1-266.

Gisolfi, C.V. (1973). Work-heat tolerance derived from interval training. *Journal of Applied Physiology*, **35**, 349-354.

Glaser, E.M. (1966). *The physiological basis of habituation*. Oxford: Oxford University Press.

Gledhill, N. (1992). Haemoglobin and blood volume. In R.J. Shephard & P.O. Åstrand (Eds.), *Endurance in sport* (pp. 210-215). Oxford: Blackwell Scientific.

Gledhill, N., Spriet, N.L., Froese, A.B., Wilkes, D.L., & Meyers, E.C. (1980). Acid-base status with induced erythrocythemia and its influence on arterial oxygenation during heavy exercise. *Medicine and Science in Sports and Exercise*, **12**, 122 (abstract).

Godin, G., & Shephard, R.J. (1973a). Activity patterns of the Canadian Eskimo. In O.G. Edholm & E.K.E. Gunderson (Eds.), *Human polar biology* (pp. 193-215). London: Heinemann.

Godin, G., & Shephard, R.J. (1985). A simple method to assess exercise behavior in the community. *Canadian Journal of Applied Sport Sciences*, **10**, 141-146.

Godin, G., & Shephard, R.J. (1990). Use of attitude-behaviour models in exercise promotion. *Sports Medicine*, **10**, 103-121.

Godin, G., Cox, M., & Shephard, R.J. (1983). The impact of physical fitness evaluation on the behavioral intentions towards regular exercise. *Canadian Journal of Applied Sport Sciences*, **8**, 240-245.

Godin, G., Desharnais, R., Jobin, J., & Cook, J. (1987). The impact of physical fitness and health age appraisal upon exercise intentions and behavior. *Journal of Behavioral Medicine*, **10**, 241-250.

Goldberg, A.P. (1989). Aerobic and resistive exercise modify risk factors for coronary heart disease. *Medicine and Science in Sports and Exercise*, **21**, 669-674.

Goldberg, D.I., & Shephard, R.J. (1980). Stroke volume during recovery from upright bicycle exercise. *Journal of Applied Physiology*, **48**, 833-837.

Goldbourt, U., & Medalie, J.H. (1979). High density lipoprotein cholesterol and incidence of coronary heart disease: The Israeli Ischaemic Heart Disease Study. *American Journal of Epidemiology*, **109**, 296-308.

Goldsmith, R., & Hale, T. (1971). Relationship between habitual physical activity and physical fitness. *American Journal of Clinical Nutrition*, **24**, 1489-1493.

Gollnick, P. (1971). Cellular adaptations to exercise. In R.J. Shephard (Ed.), *Frontiers of fitness* (pp. 112-126). Springfield, IL: Charles C Thomas.

Gollnick, P., & Hermansen, L. (1973). Biochemical adaptations to exercise: Anaerobic metabolism. *Exercise and Sport Sciences Reviews*, **1**, 1-43.

Goode, R.C., Virgin, A., Romet, T.T., Crawford, D., Duffin, J., Pallandi, T., & Woch, Z. (1976). Effects of a short period of physical activity in adolescent boys and girls. *Canadian Journal of Applied Sport Sciences*, **1**, 241-250.

Goodman, J. (1989). Exercise rehabilitation for coronary artery bypass graft patients. In J. Torg, P. Welsh, & R.J. Shephard (Eds.), *Current therapy in sports medicine 2* (pp. 119-122). Burlington, ON: Decker.

Göranzon, H., & Forsum, E. (1985). Effect of reduced energy intake versus increased physical activity on the outcome of nitrogen balance experiments in man. *American Journal of Clinical Nutrition*, **41**, 919-928.

Gordon, N.F., van Rensburg, J.P., Russell, H.M.S., Karolczak, I., Celliers, C.P., & Myburgh, D.P. (1987). Comparison of continuous and intermittent multistage maximal exercise testing during beta-adrenoceptor blockade in physically active men. *International Journal of Sports Medicine*, **8**, 6-10.

Gordon, N.F., van Rensburg, J.P., Russell, H.M.S., Kielblock, A.J., & Myburgh, D.P. (1987). Effect of beta-adrenoceptor blockade and calcium antagonism, alone and in combination, on thermoregulation during prolonged exercise. *International Journal of Sports Medicine*, **8**, 1-5.

Gore, C.J., & Withers, R.T. (1990). The effects of exercise intensity and duration on the oxygen deficit and excess post-exercise oxygen consumption. *European Journal of Applied Physiology*, **60**, 169-174.

Gorski, J., Namiot, Z., & Giedrojc, J. (1978). Effect of exercise on metabolism of glycogen and triglycerides in the respiratory muscles. *Pflügers Archiv*, **377**, 251-254.

Gorski, J., Oscai, L.B., & Palmer, W.K. (1990). Hepatic lipid metabolism in exercise and training. *Medicine and Science in Sports and Exercise*, **22**, 213-221.

Gottheiner, V. (1960). Herzinfarct und Sport. In *Proceedings of Sports Medical Symposium of Seventeenth Olympic Games*, Rome, 1960.

Gottheiner, V. (1968). Long-range strenuous sports training for cardiac reconditioning and rehabilitation. *American Journal of Cardiology*, **34**, 48-55.

Granger, H.J., Goodman, A.H., & Cook, B.H. (1975). Metabolic models of microcirculatory regulation. *Federation Proceedings*, **34**, 2025-2030.

Graves, J.E., Pollock, M.L., Jones, A.E., Colvin, A.B., & Leggett, S.H. (1989). Specificity of limited range of motion, variable resistance training. *Medicine and Science in Sports and Exercise*, **21**, 84-89.

Graves, J.E., Pollock, M.L., Leggett, S.H., Braith, R.W., Carpenter, D.M., & Bishop, L.M. (1988). Effect of reduced training frequency on muscular strength. *International Journal of Sports Medicine*, **9**, 316-319.

Graves, J.E., Pollock, M.L., Montain, S.J., Jackson, A.C., & O'Keefe, J.M. (1987). The effect of hand-held weights on the physiological responses to walking exercise. *Medicine and Science in Sports and Exercise*, **19**, 260-265.

Green, H.J., Jones, L.L., Hughson, R.L., Painter, D.C., & Farrance, B.W. (1987). Training-induced hypervolemia: Lack of an effect on oxygen utilization during exercise. *Medicine and Science in Sports and Exercise*, **19**, 202-206.

Green, H.J., Jones, L.L., & Painter, D.C. (1990). Effects of short-term training on cardiac function during prolonged exercise. *Medicine and Science in Sports and Exercise*, **22**, 488-493.

Green, H.J., Thomson, J.A., Ball, M.E., Hughson, R.L., Houston, M.S., & Sharratt, M.T. (1984). Alterations in blood volume following short-term supramaximal exercise. *Journal of Applied Physiology*, **56**, 145-149.

Green, J.H., Cable, N.T., & Elms, N. (1990). Heart rate and oxygen consumption during walking on land and in deep water. *Journal of Sports Medicine and Physical Fitness*, **30**, 49-52.

Greenleaf, J.E., Bernauer, E.M., Young, H.L., Morse, J.T., Staley, R.W., Juhos, L.T., & Van Beaumont, W. (1977). Fluid and electrolyte shifts during bed rest with isometric and isotonic exercise. *Journal of Applied Physiology*, **42**, 59-66.

Greenleaf, J.E., & Kozlowski, S. (1982). Physiological consequences of reduced physical activity and bed rest. *Exercise and Sport Sciences Reviews*, **10**, 84-119.

Greksa, L.P., & Baker, P.T. (1982). Aerobic capacity of modernizing Samoan man. *Human Biology*, **54**, 777-799.

Grogan, J.W., & Kelly, J.M. (1985). Metabolic responses of upper body training on arm, leg, and combined arm-leg exercise. *Medicine and Science in Sports and Exercise*, **17**, 268-269.

Guerrera, G., Melina, D., Colivicchi, F., Santoliquido, A., Guerrera, G., & Folli, G. (1991). Abnormal blood pressure response to exercise in borderline hypertension: A two-year follow-up study. *American Journal of Hypertension*, **4**, 271-273.

Gullstrand, L. (1992). Swimming as an endurance sport. In R.J. Shephard & P.O. Åstrand (Eds.), *Endurance in sport* (pp. 531-541). Oxford: Blackwell Scientific.

Gwirtz, P.A., Brandt, M.A., Mass, H.J., & Jones, C.E. (1990). Endurance training alters arterial baroreflex function in dogs. *Medicine and Science in Sports and Exercise*, **22**, 200-206.

Haab, P. (1982). A model for the study of diffusion and perfusion limitation. *Federation Proceedings*, **41**, 2119-2121.

Haas, F., Simnowitz, M., Axen, K., Gaudino, D., & Haas, A. (1982). Effect of upper body posture on forced inspiration and expiration. *Journal of Applied Physiology*, **52**, 879-886.

Hagan, R.D., Laird, W.P., & Gettman, L.R. (1985). The problems of per surface area and per weight standardization indices in the determination of cardiac hypertrophy in endurance trained athletes. *Journal of Cardiac Rehabilitation*, **5**, 554-560.

Hagberg, J.M. (1990). Exercise, fitness, and hypertension. In C. Bouchard, R.J. Shephard, T. Stephens, J. Sutton, & B. McPherson (Eds.), *Exercise, fitness, and health* (pp. 455-456). Champaign, IL: Human Kinetics.

Hagberg, J.M., Goldring, D., Ehsani, A.A., Heath, G.W., Hernandez, A., Schechtman, K., & Holloszy, J.O. (1983). Effect of exercise training on the blood pressure and hemodynamic features of hypertensive adolescents. *American Journal of Cardiology*, **52**, 763-768.

Hagerman, F.C. (1984). Applied physiology of rowing. *Sports Medicine*, **1**, 303-326.

Haines, R.F. (1974). Effect of bed rest and exercise on body balance. *Journal of Applied Physiology*, **36**, 323-327.

Hall, D.C., & Kaufmann, D.A. (1987). Effects of aerobic and strength conditioning on pregnancy outcomes. *American Journal of Obstetrics and Gynecology*, **157**, 1199-1203.

Hall, P.E., Smith, S.R., & Kendall, M.J. (1987). The effect of beta-adrenoceptor antagonists during modest exercise on plasma ammonia and heart rate. *Clinical Science*, **72**, 679-682.

Hammond, H.K., White, P.C., Brunton, L.L., & Longhurst, J.C. (1987). Association of decreased myocardial beta-receptors and chronotropic response to isoproterenol and exercise in pigs following chronic dynamic exercise. *Circulation Research*, **60**, 720-726.

Hammond, M.D., Gale, G.E., Kapiton, K.S., Ries, A., & Wagner, P.D. (1986). Pulmonary gas exchange in humans during exercise at sea level. *Journal of Applied Physiology*, **60**, 1590-1598.

Hanel, B., & Secher, N.H. (1991). Maximal oxygen uptake and work capacity after inspiratory muscle training: A controlled study. *Journal of Sports Sciences*, **9**, 43-52.

Hanke, H. (1979). *Freizeit in der DDR* [Free time in the German Democratic Republic]. Berlin: Dietz Verlag.

Hanson, P., Claremont, A., Dempsey, J., & Reddan, W. (1982). Determinants and consequences of ventilatory responses to competitive endurance running. *Journal of Applied Physiology*, **52**, 615-623.

Harber, V.J., & Sutton, J.R. (1984). Endorphins and exercise. *Sports Medicine*, **1**, 154-171.

Harmon, M., Maughan, R.J., & Nimmo, M.A. (1987). Human skeletal muscle adaptation to a 6-month endurance training programme. *Journal of Physiology*, **394**, 92P.

Harri, M., Donnenberg, T., Oksanen-Rossi, R., Hohtola, E., & Sundin, U. (1984). Related and unrelated changes in response to exercise and cold in rats: A reevaluation. *Journal of Applied Physiology*, **57**, 1489-1497.

Harris, E.A., Buchanan, P.R., & Whitlock, R.M. (1987). Human alveolar gas-mixing efficiency for gases of differing diffusivity in health and airflow limitation. *Clinical Science*, **73**, 351-359.

Harris, K.A., & Holly, R.G. (1987). Physiological responses to circuit weight training in borderline hypertensive subjects. *Medicine and Science in Sports and Exercise*, **19**, 246-252.

Harrison, G.A. (1979). *Population structure and human variation*. London: Cambridge University Press.

Harrison, M.H. (1986). Heat and exercise: Effects on blood volume. *Sports Medicine*, **3**, 214-223.

Hart-Hansen, J.P., Hancke, S., & Møller-Petersen, J. (1991). Atherosclerosis in Greenland: An ultrasonic investigation. In B. Postl, P. Gilbert, J. Goodwill, M.E.K. Moffatt, J.D. O'Neil, P.A. Sarsfield, & T.K. Young (Eds.), *Circumpolar health 90* (pp. 400-403). Winnipeg: Canadian Society for Circumpolar Health.

Hartley, L.H. (1975). Growth hormone and catecholamine response to exercise in relation to physical training. *Medicine and Science in Sports*, **7**, 34-36.

Hartley, L.H., Mason, J.W., Hogan, R.P., Jones, L.G., Kotchen, T.A., Mougey, E.H., Wherry, F.E., Pennington, L.L., & Ricketts, P.T. (1972). Multiple hormonal responses to graded exercise in relation to physical training. *Journal of Applied Physiology*, **33**, 602-606.

Hartley, L.H., Pernow, B., Haggendal, H., LaCour, J.R., de Lattre, J., & Saltin, B. (1970). Central circulation during submaximal work preceded by heavy exercise. *Journal of Applied Physiology*, **29**, 818-823.

Hartling, O.J., Kelbaek, H., Gjørup, T., Schibye, B., Klausen, K., & Trap-Jensen, J. (1989). Forearm oxygen uptake during maximal forearm dynamic exercise. *European Journal of Applied Physiology*, **58**, 466-470.

Hartung, G.H., & Kirby, T.E. (1980). Energy cost of exercise on a miniature trampoline in cardiac patients and normal subjects. *Medicine and Science in Sports*, **12**, 118 (abstract).

Haskell, W.L. (1984). The influence of exercise on the concentrations of triglyceride and cholesterol in human plasma. *Exercise and Sport Sciences Reviews*, **12**, 205-244.

Haskell, W.L. (1991). Dose-response relationship between physical activity and disease risk factors. In P. Oja & R. Telama (Eds.), *Sport for all* (pp. 125-134). Amsterdam: Elsevier.

Haslam, D.R.S., McCartney, N., McElvie, R.S., & McDougall, J.D. (1988). Direct measurements of arterial blood pressure during formal weight lifting in cardiac patients. *Journal of Cardiopulmonary Rehabilitation*, **8**, 213-225.

Haslam, R.W., & Cobb, R.B. (1982). Frequency of intensive, prolonged exercise as a determinant of relative coronary circumference index. *International Journal of Sports Medicine*, **3**, 118-121.

Hatch, T., & Cook, K.M. (1955). Partitional respirometry. *Archives of Industrial Health*, **11**, 142-158.

Hatt, P.Y., Ledoux, C., Bonvalet, J.P., & Guillemat, H. (1965). Lyse et synthèse des protéines myocardiques au cours de l'insuffisance cardiaque expérimentale: Etude au microscope électronique [Lysis and synthesis of myocardial proteins in the course of experimental cardiac insufficiency (study by electron microscopy)]. *Archives des Maladies du Coeur et des Vaisseaux*, **58**, 1703-1721.

Health and Welfare Canada. (1988). *Canada's health promotion survey*. Ottawa: Author.

Hedin, G., & Friman, G. (1982). Orthostatic reactions and blood volumes after moderate physical activity during acute febrile infections. *International Rehabilitation Medicine*, **4**, 107-109.

Heinrich, C.H., Going, S.B., Pamenter, R.B., Perry, C.D., Boyden, T.W., & Lohman, T.G. (1990). Bone mineral content of cyclically menstruating female resistance- and endurance-trained athletes. *Medicine and Science in Sports and Exercise*, **22**, 558-563.

Hempel, L., & Wells, C.L. (1985). Cardiorespiratory cost of the Nautilus express circuit. *The Physician and Sportsmedicine*, **13**(4), 82-97.

Henriksson, J. (1992a). Cellular metabolic factors. In R.J. Shephard & P.O. Åstrand. *Endurance in sport* (pp. 46-61). Oxford: Blackwell Scientific.

Henriksson, J. (1992b). Metabolism in the contracting skeletal muscle. In R.J. Shephard & P.O. Åstrand (Eds.), *Endurance in sport* (pp. 228-245). Oxford: Blackwell Scientific.

Henriksson, J., & Reitman, J.S. (1977). Time course of changes in human skeletal muscle succinate dehydrogenase and cytochrome oxidase activities and maximal oxygen uptake with physical activity and inactivity. *Acta Physiologica Scandinavica*, **99**, 91-97.

Henson, L.C., Poole, D.C., Donahoe, C.P., & Heber, D. (1987). Effects of exercise training on resting energy expenditure during caloric restriction. *American Journal of Clinical Nutrition*, **46**, 893-899.

Herbert, W.G., & Ribisl, P.M. (1972). Effect of dehydration upon physical working capacity of wrestlers under competitive conditions. *Research Quarterly*, **43**, 416-422.

Hermansen, L., & Stensvold, I. (1972). Production and removal of lactate during exercise in man. *Acta Physiologica Scandinavica*, **86**, 191-201.

Hesser, C.M., Linnarsson, D., & Fagreus, L. (1981). Pulmonary mechanics and work of breathing at maximal ventilation and raised air pressure. *Journal of Applied Physiology*, **50**, 747-753.

Hettinger, T.L. (1961). *Physiology of strength*. Springfield, IL: Charles C Thomas.

Hewitt, D., Jones, G.J.L., Godin, G.J., McComb, K., Breckenridge, W.C., Little, J.A., Steiner, G., Mishkel, M.A., Baillie, J.H., Martin, R.H., Gibson, E.S., Prendergast, W.F., & Parliament, W.J. (1977). Normative standards of plasma cholesterol and triglyceride concentrations in Canadians of working age. *Canadian Medical Association Journal*, **117**, 1020-1024.

Hickson, R.C., Foster, C., Pollock, M.L., Galasi, T.M., & Rich, S. (1985). Reduced training intensities and loss of aerobic power, endurance, and cardiac growth. *Journal of Applied Physiology*, **58**, 492-499.

Hickson, R.C., Kanakis, C., Davis, J.R., Moore, A.M., & Rich, S. (1982). Reduced training duration effects on aerobic power, endurance, and cardiac growth. *Journal of Applied Physiology*, **53**, 225-229.

Hickson, R.C., & Rosenkoetter, M.A. (1981). Reduced training frequencies and maintenance of increased aerobic power. *Medicine and Science in Sports and Exercise*, **13**, 13-16.

Hildes, J.A., Schaefer, O., Sayed, J.E., Fitzgerald, E.J., & Koch, E.A. (1976). Chronic pulmonary disease and associated cardiovascular disease in Igloolimiuts. In R.J. Shephard & S. Itoh (Eds.), *Circumpolar health* (pp. 327-331). Toronto: University of Toronto Press.

Hill, A.V. (1925). The physiological basis of athletic records. *Scientific Monthly*, **21**, 409-428.

Hill, A.V., Long, C.N., & Lupton, H. (1924-1925). Muscular exercise, lactic acid, and the supply and utilization of oxygen: Parts I-VIII. *Proceedings of the Royal Society* (Biology), **96**, 438-475; **97**, 84-138, 155-176.

Hill, E.P., Power, G.G., & Longo, L.D. (1973). Mathematical simulation of pulmonary O_2 and CO_2 exchange. *American Journal of Physiology*, **224**, 904-917.

Hill, J.O. (in press). Physical activity, fitness, overweight, and moderate obesity. In C. Bouchard, R.J. Shephard, & T. Stephens (Eds.), *Physical activity, fitness, and health*. Champaign, IL: Human Kinetics.

Hill, J.O., Sparling, P.B., Shields, T.W., & Heller, P.A. (1987). Effects of exercise and food restriction on body composition and metabolic rate in obese women. *American Journal of Clinical Nutrition*, **46**, 622-630.

Hlastala, M.P. (1982). Diffusion in lung gas and across alveolar membranes in mammalian lungs. *Federation Proceedings*, **41**, 2122-2124.

Ho, H.W., Roy, R.R., Taylor, J.F., Heusner, W.W., & Van Huss, W.D. (1983). Differential effects of running and weight lifting on the rat coronary arterial tree. *Medicine and Science in Sports and Exercise*, **15**, 472-477.

Hoes, M., Binkhorst, R.A., Smeekes-Kuyl, A., & Vissurs, A.C. (1968). Measurement of forces exerted on a pedal crank during work on the bicycle ergometer at different loads. *Internationale Zeitschrift für Angewandte Physiologie*, **26**, 33-42.

Hofer, H.W., & Pette, D. (1968). Wirkungen und Wechselwirkungen von Substraten und Effektoren an der Phosphofructokinase des Kaninchen-skeletmuskeln [Action and exchange of substrates and effectors in the phosphofructokinase of dog skeletal muscle]. *Zeitschrifte für Physiologische Chimie*, **349**, 1378-1392.

Holdstock, D.J., Misiewicz, J.J., Smith, T., & Rowlands, E.N. (1970). Propulsion (mass movements) in the human colon and its relationship to meals and somatic activity. *Gut*, **11**, 91-99.

Hollenberg, M., Go, M., Massie, B.M., Wisneski, J.A., & Gertz, E.W. (1985). Influence of R-wave amplitude on exercise-induced ST depression: Need for a "gain factor" correction when interpreting stress electrocardiograms. *American Journal of Cardiology*, **56**, 13-17.

Hollmann, W. (1991). Physical fitness: An introduction. In P. Oja & R. Telama (Eds.), *Sport for all* (pp. 77-80). Amsterdam: Elsevier.

Hollmann, W. (in press). Physical activity and the brain. In C. Bouchard, R.J. Shephard, & T. Stephens (Eds.), *Physical activity, fitness, and health*. Champaign, IL: Human Kinetics.

Hollmann, W., & Hettinger, T. (1976). *Sportmedizin-Arbeits-und Trainingsgrundlagen* [Basics of sports medicine, work and training]. Stuttgart: Schattauer Verlag.

Hollmann, W., & Venrath, H. (1963). Die Beinflussung von Herzgrösse, maximaler O_2-Aufnahme und Ausdauersgranze durch ein Ausdauerstraining mittlerer und hoher Intensität [The influence on heart size, maximal oxygen uptake and endurance time of endurance training at moderate and high intensity]. *Der Sportarzt, 9*, 189-193.

Holloszy, J.O. (1973). Biochemical adaptations to exercise: Aerobic metabolism. *Exercise and Sport Sciences Reviews, 1*, 45-71.

Holly, R.G., Baranard, R.J., Rosenthal, M., Applegate, E., & Pritikin, N. (1986). Triathlete characterization and response to prolonged strenuous competition. *Medicine and Science in Sports and Exercise, 18*, 123-127.

Holmdahl, D.E., & Ingelmark, B.E. (1948). Der Bau des Gelenkknorpels unter verschiedenen funktionellen Verhaltnis [The structure of cartilage with different functional proportions]. *Acta Anatomica, 6*, 309-375.

Holmér, I. (1972). Oxygen uptake during swimming in man. *Journal of Applied Physiology, 33*, 502-509.

Holmgren, A. (1967a). Cardio-respiratory determinants of cardiovascular fitness. *Canadian Medical Association Journal, 96*, 697-702.

Holmgren, A. (1967b). Vaso-regulatory asthenia. *Canadian Medical Association Journal, 96*, 853.

Holmgren, A., & Linderholm, H. (1958). Oxygen and carbon dioxide tensions of arterial blood during heavy and exhaustive exercise. *Acta Physiologica Scandinavica, 44*, 203-215.

Hortobagyi, T., Katch, F.I., & LaChance, P.F. (1991). Effects of simultaneous training for strength and endurance on upper and lower body strength and running performance. *Journal of Sports Medicine and Physical Fitness, 31*, 20-30.

Horvath, S.M., Raven, P.B., Dahms, T.E., & Gray, D.J. (1977). Maximal aerobic capacity at different levels of carboxyhemoglobin. *Journal of Applied Physiology, 38*, 300-303.

Hoummard, J.A. (1992). Impact of reduced training on performance in endurance athletes. *Sports Medicine, 12*, 380-393.

Houston, C.S., & Riley, R.L. (1947). Respiratory and circulatory changes during acclimatization to high altitude. *American Journal of Physiology, 149*, 565-588.

Howald, H. (1975). Ultrastructural adaptation of skeletal muscle to prolonged physical exercise. In H. Howald & J.R. Poortmans (Eds.), *Metabolic adaptations to prolonged exercise* (pp. 372-383). Basel: Birkhauser Verlag.

Howald, H. (1982). Training induced morphological and functional changes in skeletal muscle. *International Journal of Sports Medicine, 3*, 1-12.

Howell, M.L., & MacNab, R. (1968). *The physical working capacity of Canadian children 7-17 years*. Ottawa: Canadian Association for Health, Physical Education and Recreation.

Hoyt, R.W., Jones, T.E., Stein, T.P., McAninch, G.W., Lieberman, H.R., Askew, E.W., & Cymerman, A. (1991). Doubly labeled water measurement of human energy expenditure during strenuous exercise. *Journal of Applied Physiology, 71*, 16-22.

Hsieh, S., & Hermiston, R. (1983). The acute effects of controlled-breathing swimming on glycolytic parameters. *Canadian Journal of Applied Sport Sciences, 8*, 149-154.

Hubbard, R.W., & Armstrong, L.E. (1989). Hyperthermia: New thoughts on an old problem. *The Physician and Sportsmedicine, 17*(6), 97-113.

Huddleston, A.L., Rockwell, D., Kulund, D.N., & Harrison, R.B. (1980). Bone mass in lifetime tennis players. *Journal of the American Medical Association, 244*, 1107-1109.

Hughes, A.L., & Goldman, R.F. (1970). Energy cost of hard work. *Journal of Applied Physiology, 29*, 570-572.

Hughson, R.L. (1989). Ramp-work test with three different beta-blockers in normal human subjects. *European Journal of Applied Physiology, 58*, 710-716.

Hultman, E., & Greenhaff, P.L. (1992). Food stores and energy reserves. In R.J. Shephard & P.O. Åstrand (Eds.), *Endurance in sport* (pp. 129-137). Oxford: Blackwell Scientific.

Hultman, E., & Sahlin, K. (1980). Acid-base balance during exercise. *Exercise and Sport Sciences Reviews*, **8**, 41-128.

Husemann, B., Neubauer, M.G., & Duhme, C. (1980). Sitzende Tätigkeit und Rektum-Sigma-Karzinom [Sedentary activity and cancer of the rectum and sigmoid colon]. *Onkologie*, **3**, 168-171.

Ikegami, Y., Hiruta, S., Ikegami, H., & Miyamura, M. (1988). Development of a telemetry system for measuring oxygen uptake during sports activities. *European Journal of Applied Physiology*, **57**, 622-626.

Ilbäck, N.-G., Friman, G., Beisel, W.R., Johnson, A.L., & Berendt, R.F. (1984). Modifying effects of exercise on clinical course and biochemical response of the myocardium in influenza and tularaemia in mice. *Infection and Immunity*, **45**, 498-504.

Ilmarinen, J., & Rutenfranz, J. (1980). Longitudinal studies of the changes in habitual activity of schoolchildren and working adolescents. In K. Berg & B.O. Eriksson (Eds.), *Children and exercise IX* (pp. 149-159). Baltimore: University Park Press.

Ilsley, C., Canepa-Anson, R., Westgate, C., Webb, S., Rickards, A., & Poole-Wilson, P. (1982). Influence of R wave analysis upon diagnostic accuracy of exercise testing in women. *British Heart Journal*, **48**, 161-168.

Inbar, O., Gutin, B., Dotan, R., & Bar-Or, O. (1978). Conditioning vs. heat exposures as methods for acclimatizing 8-10 year old boys to dry heat. *Medicine and Science in Sports*, **10**, 62.

Ingjer, F. (1979). Capillary supply and mitochondrial content of different skeletal muscle fiber types in untrained and endurance trained men: A histochemical and ultrastructural study. *European Journal of Applied Physiology*, **40**, 197-209.

Innes, J.A., Campbell, I.W., Campbell, C.J., Needle, A.L., & Munroe, J.F. (1974). Long term follow-up of therapeutic starvation. *British Medical Journal*, (ii), 357-359.

International Committee. (1967). International committee on standardization in haematology. *British Journal of Haematology*, (Suppl. 13), 71.

Ishiko, T. (1967). Aerobic capacity and external criteria of performance. *Canadian Medical Association Journal*, **96**, 746-749.

Ishiko, T., Ikeda, N., & Enomoto, Y. (1968). Obese children in Japan. *Research Journal of Physical Education*, **12**, 168-174.

Issekutz, B., Blizzard, J.J., Birkhead, N.C., & Rodahl, K. (1966). Effect of prolonged bed rest on urinary calcium output. *Journal of Applied Physiology*, **21**, 1013-1020.

Jackson, A.S., Squires, W.G., Grimes, G., & Beard, E.F. (1983). Prediction of future resting hypertension from exercise blood pressure. *Journal of Cardiac Rehabilitation*, **3**, 263-268.

Jacobs, I. (1981). Lactate, muscle glycogen, and exercise performance in man. *Acta Physiologica Scandinavica*, **495**(Suppl.), 1-35.

Jacobs, S.J., & Berson, B.L. (1986). Injuries to runners: A study of entrants to a 10,000-meter race. *American Journal of Sports Medicine*, **14**, 151-155.

James, W.P.T. (1976). *Research on obesity: A report of the DHSS-MRC group*. London: Her Majesty's Stationery Office.

Jansson, E., & Kaijser, L. (1977). Muscle adaptation to extreme endurance training in man. *Acta Physiologica Scandinavica*, **62**, 364-379.

Järvholm, U., Styf, J., Suurkula, M., & Herberts, P. (1988). Intramuscular pressure and muscle blood flow in supraspinatus. *European Journal of Applied Physiology*, **58**, 219-224.

Jelinek, M.V. (1980). Exercise-induced arrhythmias: Their implications for cardiac rehabilitation programs. *Medicine and Science in Sports*, **15**, 223-230.

Jenkins, R.R. (1988). Free radical chemistry: Relationship to exercise. *Sports Medicine*, **5**, 156-170.

Jetté, M., Campbell, J., Mongeon, J., & Routhier, R. (1976). The Canadian Home Fitness Test as a predictor of aerobic capacity. *Canadian Medical Association Journal*, **114**, 680-682.

Jetté, M., Heller, R., Landry, F., & Blümchen, G. (1991). Randomized 4-week exercise program in patients with impaired left ventricular function. *Circulation*, **84**, 1561-1567.

Jetté, M., Landry, F., Sidney, K.H., & Blümchen, G. (1988). Exaggerated blood pressure response in the detection of hypertension. *Journal of Cardiopulmonary Rehabilitation*, **8**, 171-177.

Jetté, M., Mongeon, J., & Shephard, R.J. (1982). Demonstration of a training effect by the Canadian Home Fitness Test. *European Journal of Applied Physiology*, **49**, 143-150.

Johnson, H.E. (1946). Applied physiology. *Annual Reviews of Physiology*, **8**, 535-558.

Johnson, J.M. (1977). Regulation of skin circulation during prolonged exercise. *Annals of New York Academy of Sciences*, **301**, 195-212.

Johnson, J.M. (1987). Central and peripheral adjustments to long-term exercise in humans. *Canadian Journal of Sport Sciences*, **12**, S84-S88.

Johnson, J.M., Rowell, L.B., & Brengelmann, G.L. (1974). Modification of the blood flow-body temperature relationship by upright exercise. *Journal of Applied Physiology*, **37**, 880-886.

Johnson, L.R., & Van Liew, H.D. (1974). Use of arterial PO_2 to study convective and diffusive gas mixing in the lungs. *Journal of Applied Physiology*, **36**, 91-97.

Johnson, P.C., Driscoll, T.B., & Carpentier, W.R. (1971). Vascular and extravascular fluid changes during six days of bed rest. *Aerospace Medicine*, **42**, 875-878.

Johnson, P.C., Leach, C.S., & Rambaut, P.C. (1973). Estimates of fluid and energy balances of Apollo 17. *Aerospace Medicine*, **44**, 1227-1230.

Johnson, P.C., Nicogossian, A.E., Bergman, S.A., & Hoffler, G.W. (1976). Lower body negative pressure: The second manned Skylab mission. *Aviation, Space and Environmental Medicine*, **47**, 347-353.

Jokl, E. (1977). The immunological status of athletes. In D. Brunner & E. Jokl (Eds.), *The role of exercise in internal medicine* (pp. 129-134). Basel: Karger.

Jonason, T., Jonzon, B., Ringqvist, I., & Oman-Rydberg, A. (1979). Effect of physical training on different categories of patients with intermittent claudication. *Acta Medica Scandinavica*, **206**, 253-258.

Jones, D.A., Newham, D.J., Round, J.M., & Tolfree, S.E. (1986). Experimental human muscle damage: Morphological changes in relation to other indices of damage. *Journal of Physiology*, **375**, 435-448.

Jones, N.L. (1984). Dyspnea in exercise. *Medicine and Science in Sports and Exercise*, **16**, 14-19.

Jones, N.L. (1989). Exercise in chronic airway obstruction. In J. Torg, P. Welsh, & R.J. Shephard. *Current therapy in sports medicine 2* (pp. 31-34). Burlington, ON: Decker.

Jones, N.L., & Kane, M. (1979). Inter-laboratory standardization of methodology. *Medicine and Science in Sports*, **11**, 368-372.

Jones, N.L., & Killian, K.J. (1990). Exercise in chronic airway obstruction. In C. Bouchard, R.J. Shephard, T. Stephens, J. Sutton, & B. McPherson. *Exercise, fitness, and health* (pp. 547-559). Champaign, IL: Human Kinetics.

Jones, P.W., & Wakefield, J.M. (1984). Effect of hyperventilation during exercise on oxygen consumption and CO_2 production measured at the mouth. *Clinical Science*, **67**(Suppl. 9), 32P.

Jonsson, B.G., & Berggren, G. (1979). Physical work capacity of young men in Sweden. *Scandinavian Journal of Social Medicine*, **7**, 93-95.

Joos, S.K., Mueller, W.H., Hanis, C.L., & Schull, W.J. (1984). Diabetes alert study: Weight history and upper body obesity in diabetic and non-diabetic Mexican American adults. *Annals of Human Biology*, **11**, 167-171.

Jorgensen, C.R. (1972). Coronary blood flow and myocardial oxygen consumption in man. In J.F. Alexander, R.C. Serfass, & C.M. Tipton (Eds.), *Fitness and exercise* (pp. 39-50). Chicago: Athletic Institute.

José, A.D., Stitt, F., & Collison, D. (1970). The effects of exercise and changes in body temperature on the intrinsic heart rate in man. *American Heart Journal*, **79**, 488-497.

Josenhans, W.T. (1967). Muscular factors. *Canadian Medical Association Journal*, **96**, 761-763.

Jossa, D. (1985). *Smoking behaviour of Canadians 1983*. Ottawa: Minister of Supply and Services. (Cat. #H39-66/1985E)

Jost, J., Weiss, M., & Weicker, H. (1989). Comparison of sympatho-adrenergic regulation at rest and of the adrenoceptor system in swimmers, long-distance runners, weight-lifters, wrestlers, and untrained men. *European Journal of Applied Physiology*, **58**, 596-604.

Kaijser, L. (1970). Limiting factors for aerobic muscle performance. *Acta Physiologica Scandinavica*, **346**(Suppl.), 1-96.

Kanehisa, H., & Miyashita, M. (1983). Specificity of velocity in strength training. *European Journal of Applied Physiology*, **52**, 104-106.

Kanstrup, I.L., & Ekblöm, B. (1984). Blood volume and hemoglobin concentration as determinants of maximal aerobic power. *Medicine and Science in Sports and Exercise*, **16**, 256-262.

Kaplan, R. (1985). Quantifition of health outcomes for policy studies in behavioral epidemiology. In R. Kaplan & M.H. Criqui (Eds.), *Behavioral epidemiology and disease prevention* (pp. 31-56). New York: Plenum Press.

Kappagoda, C.T., Linden, R.J., & Newell, J.P. (1977). Validation of a submaximal exercise test. *Journal of Physiology*, **268**, 19P-20P.

Karpovich, P.V., & Sinning, W.E. (1971). *Physiology of muscular activity*. Philadelphia: Saunders.

Karpakka, J., Väänänen, K., Orava, S., & Takala, T.E.S. (1990). The effects of preimmobilization on collagen synthesis in rat skeletal muscle. *International Journal of Sports Medicine*, **11**, 484-488.

Karvonen, M.J., Klemola, H., Virkajarvi, J., & Kekkonen, A. (1974). Longevity of endurance skiers. *Medicine and Science in Sports*, **6**, 49-51.

Kasch, F.W., Wallace, J.P., Van Camp, S.P., & Verity, L. (1988). A longitudinal study of cardiovascular stability in active men aged 45 to 65 years. *The Physician and Sportsmedicine*, **16**(1), 117-126.

Kashiwazaki, H., Inaoka, T., Suzuki, T., & Kendo, Y. (1986). Correlations of pedometer readings with energy expenditure in workers during free living daily activities. *European Journal of Applied Physiology*, **54**, 585-590.

Katch, V.L., Martin, R., & Martin, J. (1979). Effects of exercise intensity on food consumption in the male rat. *American Journal of Clinical Nutrition*, **32**, 1401-1407.

Kattus, A., & Grollman, J. (1972). Patterns of coronary collateral circulation in angina pectoris: Relation to exercise training. In H.I. Russek & B.L. Zohman (Eds.), *Changing concepts in cardiovascular disease* (pp. 352-376). Baltimore: Williams & Wilkins.

Katz, V.L., McMurray, R., Berry, M.J., & Cefalo, R.C. (1988). Fetal and uterine responses to immersion and exercise. *Obstetrics and Gynecology*, **72**, 225-230.

Kavanagh, T. (1989). Does exercise training improve coronary collateralization? A new look at an old belief. *The Physician and Sportsmedicine*, **17**(1), 96-114.

Kavanagh, T. (1992). *Heart attack? Counter attack!* Toronto: Van Nostrand.

Kavanagh, T., Lindley, L.J., Shephard, R.J., & Campbell, R. (1988). Health and socio-demographic characteristics of the Masters competitor. *Annals of Sports Medicine*, **4**, 55-64.

Kavanagh, T., Mertens, D.J., Baigrie, R.S., Myers, M.G., & Shephard, R.J. (1991). Assessment of patients with chronic congestive heart failure: Ventilatory threshold or aerobic power determination? *Sports Training, Medicine and Rehabilitation*, **3**, 1-11.

Kavanagh, T., Myers, M.G., Baigrie, R.S., Mertens, D.J., Sawyer, P., & Shephard, R.J. (1992, July). Effectiveness of training in congestive failure. Paper presented at International Congress of Cardiac Rehabilitation, Bordeaux, France.

Kavanagh, T., & Shephard, R.J. (1975). Conditioning of post-coronary patients: Comparison of continuous and interval training. *Archives of Physical Medicine and Rehabilitation*, **56**, 72-76.

Kavanagh, T., & Shephard, R.J. (1977a). The effects of continued training on the aging process. *Annals of the New York Academy of Sciences*, **301**, 656-670.

Kavanagh, T., & Shephard, R.J. (1977b). On the choice of fluid for the middle-aged marathon runners. *British Journal of Sports Medicine*, **11**, 26-35.

Kavanagh, T., Shephard, R.J., Chisholm, A.W., Qureshi, S., & Kennedy, J. (1979). Prognostic indexes for patients with ischemic heart disease enrolled in an exercise-centered rehabilitation program. *American Journal of Cardiology*, **44**, 1230-1240.

Kavanagh, T., Shephard, R.J., Lindley, L.J., & Pieper, M. (1983). Influence of exercise and lifestyle variables upon high density lipoprotein cholesterol after myocardial infarction. *Arteriosclerosis*, **3**, 249-259.

Kavanagh, T., Shephard, R.J., & Pandit, V. (1974). Marathon running after myocardial infarction. *Journal of the American Medical Association*, **229**, 1602-1605.

Kavanagh, T., Shephard, R.J., Tuck, J.A., & Qureshi, S. (1977). Depression following myocardial infarction: The effects of distance running. *Annals of the New York Academy of Sciences*, **301**, 1029-1038.

Kavanagh, T., Yacoub, M.H., Mertens, D.J., Kennedy, J., & Campbell, R.B. (1988). Cardio-respiratory responses to exercise training after orthotopic cardiac transplantation. *Circulation*, **77**, 162-171.

Kavanagh, T., Shephard, R.J., & Mertens, D.J. (1992). The long-term health prospects of Masters competitors. Unpublished manuscript.

Kay, C., & Shephard, R.J. (1969). On muscle strength and the threshold of anaerobic work. *Internationale Zeitschrift für Angewandte Physiologie* **27**, 311-328.

Kearon, M.C., Summers, E., Jones, N.L., Campbell, E.J.M., & Killian, K.J. (1991). Effort and dyspnoea during work of varying intensity and duration. *European Respiratory Journal*, **4**, 917-925.

Keens, T.G., Krastins, J.R.B., Wannamaker, E.M., Levison, H., Crozier, D.N., & Bryan, A.C. (1977). Ventilatory muscle endurance training in normal subjects and patients with cystic fibrosis. *American Review of Respiratory Diseases*, **116**, 853-860.

Kelemen, M.H. (1989). Resistive training safety and assessment guidelines for cardiac and coronary prone patients. *Medicine and Science in Sports and Exercise*, **21**, 675-677.

Kelemen, M.H., Stewart, K.J., Gillilan, R.E., Ewart, K., Valenti, S.A., Manley, J.D., & Kelemen, M.D. (1986). Circuit weight training in cardiac patients. *Journal of the American College of Cardiology*, **7**, 38-42.

Kemper, H., Storm-van Essen, L., & Verschuur, R. (1989). Tracking of risk indicators for coronary heart disease from teenager to adult: The Amsterdam growth and health study. In S. Oseid & H-K Carlsen (Eds.), *Children and exercise XIII* (pp. 235-245). Champaign, IL: Human Kinetics.

Kemper, H., & Verschuur, R. (1977). Validity and reliability of pedometers in research on habitual physical activity. In H. Lavallée & R.J. Shephard (Eds.), *Frontiers of activity and child health* (pp. 83-92). Québec: Editions du Pélican.

Kemper, H.C.G., & Verschuur, R. (1982). Development of physical fitness of Dutch teenagers from 12 to 17 years of age. In *Youth and sport research*. Amsterdam: Institute of Sports Science & Physical Education Studies.

Kendrick, Z.B., Pollock, M.L., Hickman, T.N., & Miller, H.S. (1971). Effects of training and detraining on cardiovascular efficiency. *American Corrective Therapy Journal*, **25**, 79-83.

Kenyon, G.S. (1968). Six scales for assessing attitudes toward physical activity. *Research Quarterly*, **39**, 566-574.

Keys, A. (1980). *Seven countries: A multivariate analysis of death and coronary heart disease*. Cambridge, MA: Harvard University Press.

Keys, A., Anderson, J.T., & Grande, F. (1957). Prediction of serum cholesterol responses of man to changes in fats in the diet. *Lancet*, **2**, 959-966.

Keys, A., Aravanis, C., Blackburn, H., Van Buchem, F.S.P., Buzina, R., Djordevic, B.S., Fidanza, F., Karvonen, M.J., Menotti, A., Puddu, V., & Taylor, H.L. (1972). Coronary heart disease: Overweight and obesity. *Annals of Internal Medicine*, **77**, 15-27.

Keys, A., Brozek, J., Henschel, A., Mickelson, O., & Taylor, H.L. (1950). *Biology of human starvation*. Minneapolis: University of Minnesota Press.

Khosla, T., & Campbell, H. (1982). Resting pulse rate in marathon runners. *British Medical Journal*, **284**, 1444.

Kiens, B., Jorgensen, I., Lewis, S., Jensen, G., Lithell, H., Vessby, B., Hoe, S., & Schnor, P. (1980). Increased plasma HDL-cholesterol and apo A-I in sedentary middle-aged men after physical conditioning. *European Journal of Clinical Investigation*, **10**, 203-209.

Kiiskinen, A., & Heikkinen, E. (1975). Effect of prolonged physical training on the development of connective tissues in growing mice. In H. Howald & J.R. Poortmans (Eds.), *Metabolic adaptations to prolonged physical exercise* (pp. 253-261). Basel: Birkhauser Verlag.

Kilbom, A. (1971a). Physical training with submaximal intensities in women: 1. Reaction to exercise and orthostasis. *Scandinavian Journal of Clinical and Laboratory investigation*, **28**, 141-161.

Kilbom, A. (1971b). Physical training with submaximal intensities in women: 3. Effect on adaptation to professional work. *Scandinavian Journal of Clinical and Laboratory Investigation*, **28**, 331-343.

Kilbom, A. (1976). Circulatory adaptations during static muscular exercise. *Scandinavian Journal of Work and Environmental Health*, **2**, 1-13.

Killian, K.J. (1987). Limitation of exercise by dyspnea. *Canadian Journal of Sport Sciences*, **12**(Suppl.), 53S-60S.

Killian, K.J., Summers, E., & Basalygo, M. (1985). Effect of frequency on perceived magnitude of added loads to breathing. *Journal of Applied Physiology*, **58**, 1616-1621.

King, D.W., & Pengelly, R.G. (1973). Effect of running on the density of rat tibias. *Medicine and Science in Sports*, **5**, 68-69.

King, H., Zimmet, P., Raper, L.R., & Balkau, B. (1984). Risk factors for diabetes in three Pacific populations. *American Journal of Epidemiology*, **119**, 396-409.

Kirby, R.L., Nugent, S.T., Marlow, R.W., MacLeod, D.A., & Marble, A.E. (1989). Coupling of cardiac and locomotor rhythms. *Journal of Applied Physiology*, **66**, 323-329.

Kirby, R.L., Sacamano, J.T., Balch, D.E., & Kriellaars, D.J. (1983). Oxygen consumption during exercise in a heated pool. *Archives of Physical Medicine and Rehabilitation*, **65**, 21-23.

Kissling, G., & Jacob, R. (1973). Limitation of the stroke volume during increased myocardial performance. In J. Keul (Ed.), *Limiting factors of physical performance* (pp. 218-224). Stuttgart: Thieme.

Klausen, K., Andersen, L.B., & Pelle, I. (1981). Adaptive changes in work capacity, skeletal muscle capillarization, and enzyme levels during training and detraining. *Acta Physiologica Scandinavica*, **113**, 9-16.

Klausen, K., Secher, N.H., Clausen, J.P., Hartling, O., & Trap-Jensen, J. (1982). Central and regional circulatory adaptations to one-leg training. *Journal of Applied Physiology*, **52**, 976-983.

Klein, K.E., Wegmann, H.M., & Kuklinski, P. (1977). Athletic endurance training—advantage for space flight?: The significance of physical fitness for selection and training of Spacelab crews. *Aviation, Space and Environmental Medicine*, **48**, 215-222.

Kleinhauss, G., & Franke, W. (1971). Zum Aussagewert indirekter Blutdruckbestimmungen in Rühe und bei Kreislaufbelastung durch Ergometerarbeit [Indirect blood pressure estimation at rest and under the circulatory stress of ergometer work]. *Zeitschrift für Kreisslaufforschung*, **60**, 588-599.

Klimt, F. (1966). Telemotorische Herzschlagfrequenz: Registrierungen bei Kleinkindern wahrend einer körperlichen Tätigkeit [Telemetric registration of cardiac frequency in small children during physical activity]. *Deutsches Gesundheitwesen*, **21**, 599.

Klissouras, V. (1971). Heritability of adaptive variation. *Journal of Applied Physiology*, **31**, 338-344.

Knapik, J.J., Maudsley, R.H., & Rammos, N.V. (1983). Angular specificity and test mode specificity of isometric and isokinetic strength training. *Journal of Orthopedic Sports Physical Therapy*, **5**, 58-65.

Knuttgen, H.G., & Kraemer, W.J. (1987). Terminology and measurement in exercise performance. *Journal of Applied Sports Science Research*, **1**, 1-10.

Knuttgen, H.G., Nordesjø, L.O., Ollander, B., & Saltin, B. (1973). Physical conditioning through interval training with young male adults. *Medicine and Science in Sports*, **5**, 220-226.

Knuttgen, H.G., & Steendahl, K. (1963). Fitness of Danish school children during the course of one academic year. *Research Quarterly*, **34**, 34-40.

Kofranyi, E., & Michaelis, H.F. (1949). Ein tragbarer Apparat zur Bestimmung des Gasstoffwechsels [A portable apparatus for the estimation of gas exchange]. *Arbeitsphysiologie*, **11**, 148-150.

Kohl, H.W., LaPorte, R.E., & Blair, S.N. (1988). Physical activity and cancer: An epidemiological perspective. *Sports Medicine*, **6**, 222-237.

Kohl, J., Koller, E.A., & Jager, M. (1981). Relation between pedalling and breathing rhythm. *European Journal of Applied Physiology*, **47**, 223-237.

Kohn, R.M., Ibrahim, M.A., & Feldman, J.G. (1971). Premature ventricular beats and coronary heart disease risk factors. *American Journal of Epidemiology*, **94**, 556-563.

Kokkinos, P.F., & Hurley, B.F. (1990). Strength training and lipoprotein-lipid profiles: A critical analysis. *Sports Medicine*, **9**, 266-272.

Kokkinos, P.F., Hurley, B.F., Smutok, M.A., Farmer, C., Reece, C., Shulman, R., Charabogos, C., Patterson, J., Will, S., Devane-Bell, J., & Goldberg, A.P. (1991). Strength training does not improve lipoprotein-lipid profiles in men at risk for CHD. *Medicine and Science in Sports and Exercise*, **23**, 1134-1139.

Kollias, J., & Buskirk, E.R. (1974). Exercise and altitude. In W.R. Johnson & E.R. Buskirk (Eds.), *Science and medicine of exercise and sports* (pp. 211-227). New York: Harper & Row.

Koplan, J.P., Powell, K.E., Sikes, R.K., Shirley, R.W., & Campbell, C.C. (1982). An epidemiologic study of the benefits and risks of running. *Journal of the American Medical Association*, **248**, 3118-3121.

Kottke, B.A., Zinsmeister, A.R., Holmes, D.R., Kneller, R.W., Hallaway, B.J., & Mao, S.J. (1986). Apolipoproteins and coronary artery disease. *Proceedings of the Mayo Clinic*, **61**, 313-320.

Kral, J., Chrastek, J., & Adamirova, J. (1966). The hypotensive effect of physical activity in hypertensive subjects. In W. Raab (Ed.), *Prevention of ischemic heart disease: Principles and practice* (pp. 359-371). Springfield, IL: Charles C Thomas.

Kramsch, D.M., Aspen, A.J., Abramowitz, B.M., Kreimendahl, T., & Hood, W.B. (1981). Reduction of coronary atherosclerosis by moderate exercise in monkeys on an atherogenic diet. *New England Journal of Medicine*, **305**, 1483-1489.

Krebs, P., Zinkgraf, S., & Virgilio, S. (1983). The effects of training variables, maximal aerobic capacities, and body composition upon cycling performance time. *Medicine and Science in Sports and Exercise*, **15**, 133 (abstract).

Krølner, B., & Toft, B. (1983). Vertebral bone loss: An unheeded side effect of therapeutic bed rest. *Clinical Science*, **64**, 537-540.

Krølner, B., Toft, B., Pors-Nielsen, S., & Tondevold, E. (1983). Physical exercise as prophylaxis against involutional vertebral bone loss: A controlled trial. *Clinical Science*, **64**, 541-546.

Krotkiewski, M.K., Mandroukas, K., Sjöstrom, L., Sullivan, L., Wetterqvist, H., & Björntorp, P. (1979). Effects of long-term physical training on body fat, metabolism, and blood pressure in obesity. *Metabolism*, **28**, 650-658.

Krzeminski, K., Niewiadomski, W., & Nazar, K. (1989). Dynamics of changes in the cardiovascular response to submaximal exercise during low-intensity endurance training with particular reference to the systolic time intervals. *European Journal of Applied Physiology*, **59**, 377-384.

Kuipers, H., & Janssen, E. (1985). Exercise and muscle soreness. In P. Welsh & R.J. Shephard (Eds.), *Current therapy in sports medicine, 1985-1986* (pp. 276-278). Burlington, ON: Decker.

Kuipers, H., & Keizer, H.A. (1988). Over-training in elite athletes: Review and directions for the future. *Sports Medicine*, **6**, 79-92.

Kukkonen, K., Rauramaa, R., Siitonen, O., & Hanninen, O. (1982). Physical training of obese middle-aged persons. *Annals of Clinical Research*, **14**, 80-85.

Kullmer, T., Kindermann, W., & Singer, M. (1987). Effects on physical performance of intrinsic sympathomimetic activity (ISA) during selective beta-1 blockade. *European Journal of Applied Physiology*, **56**, 292-298.

Kulpa, P.J., White, B.M., & Visscher, R. (1987). Aerobic exercise in pregnancy. *American Journal of Obstetrics and Gynecology*, **156**, 1395-1403.

Kyle, C.R. (1979). Reduction of wind resistance and power output of racing cyclists and runners travelling in groups. *Ergonomics*, **22**, 387-397.

Laakso, L., & Telama, R. (1979). Sport activities of Finnish youth with special reference to young school leavers. *Jyväskylä Reports of Physical Culture and Health*, **24**, 27-36.

Lahiri, S., & Milledge, J.S. (1968). Relative respiratory insensitivity of Himalayan Sherpa altitude residents to hypoxia at 4,800 m and at sea level. In R.W. Torrance (Ed.), *Arterial chemoreceptors* (pp. 387-392). Oxford: Blackwell Scientific.

Laird, G.D., & Campbell, M.J. (1988). Exercise levels and resting pulse rate in the community. *British Journal of Sports Medicine*, **22**, 148-152.

Lalonde, M. (1974). *A new perspective on the health of Canadians*. Ottawa: Health and Welfare Canada.

Lammert, O. (1972). Maximal aerobic power and energy expenditure of Eskimo hunters in Greenland. *Journal of Applied Physiology*, **33**, 184-188.

Lamont, L.S. (1987). Sweat lactate secretion during exercise in relation to women's aerobic capacity. *Journal of Applied Physiology*, **62**, 194-198.

Landry, F., Bouchard, C., & Dumesnil, J. (1985). Cardiac dimension changes with endurance training: Indications of a genotype dependency. *Journal of the American Medical Association*, **254**, 77-80.

Landry, F., Carrière, S., Poirier, L., LeBlanc, C., Gaudreau, J., Moisau, A., Carrier, R., & Potvin, R. (1980). Observations sur la condition physique des Québecois [Observations on the physical condition of Québecois]. *Union Médicale*, **109**, 1-6.

Landt, K.W., Campaigne, B.N., James, F.W., & Sperling, M.A. (1985). Effects of exercise training on insulin sensitivity in adolescents with Type I diabetes. *Diabetes Care*, **8**, 461-465.

Lane, N.E., Bloch, D.A., Jones, H.H., Marshall, W.H., Wood, P.D., & Fries, J.F. (1986). Long-distance running, bone density, and osteoarthritis. *Journal of the American Medical Association*, **255**, 1147-1151.

LaPerriere, A., Schneiderman, H., Antoni, M.H., & Fletcher, M.A. (1990). Aerobic exercise training and psychoimmunology in AIDS research. In A. Baum & L. Temoshok (Eds.), *Psychological aspects of AIDS* (pp. 259-286). Hillsdale, NJ: Erlbaum.

Lapidus, L., Bengtsson, C., Larsson, B., Pennert, K., Rybo, E., & Sjöstrom, L. (1984). Distribution of adipose tissue and risk of cardiovascular disease and death: A 12-year follow-up of participants in the population study of women in Göthenburg, Sweden. *British Medical Journal*, **289**, 1257-1261.

LaPorte, W. (1966). The influence of a gymnastic pause upon recovery following post-office work. *Ergonomics*, **9**, 501-506.

Lapsley, D., Khuri, S., Patel, M., Strauss, W., & Sharma, G.V.R.K. (1991). Impact of coronary artery bypass surgery on the smoking habit: Implications for rehabilitation. *Journal of Cardiopulmonary Rehabilitation*, **11**, 315 (abstract).

Laughlin, H.R., & Armstrong, R.B. (1985). Muscle blood flow during locomotory exercise. *Exercise and Sport Science Reviews*, **13**, 95-136.

Laughlin, H.R., McAllister, R.M., & Delp, M.D. (in press). Physical activity and the microcirculation. In C. Bouchard, R.J. Shephard, & T. Stephens (Eds.), *Physical activity, fitness, and health*. Champaign, IL: Human Kinetics.

Lawrence, G. (1981). *Aqua fitness for women*. Toronto: Personal Library Publishers.

Leaf, D.A. (1989). Exercise during pregnancy: Guidelines and controversies. *Postgraduate Medicine*, **85**, 233-238.

LeBlanc, C., Bouchard, C., Godbout, P., & Mondor, J.C. (1981). Specificity of submaximal working capacity. *Journal of Sports Medicine and Physical Fitness*, **21**, 15-22.

LeBlanc, P., Bowie, D.M., Summers, E., Jones, N.L., & Killian, K.J. (1986). Factors contributing to the alleviation of breathlessness by exercise training in patients with cardiorespiratory disease. *American Review of Respiratory Diseases*, **133**, 21-25.

Léger, L. (1982). Energy cost of disco dancing. *Research Quarterly*, **53**, 46-49.

Leith, D.E., & Bradley, M. (1976). Ventilatory muscle strength and endurance training. *Journal of Applied Physiology*, **41**, 508-516.

LeJumtal, T.H., Maskin, C.S., Lucido, D., & Chadwicj, B.J. (1986). Failure to augment maximal limb blood flow in response to one-leg versus two-leg exercise in patients with severe heart failure. *Circulation*, **74**, 245-251.

Leon, A.S., Connett, J., Jacobs, D.R., & Rauramaa, R. (1987). Leisure-time physical activity levels and risk of coronary heart disease and death: The Multiple Risk Factor Intervention Trial. *Journal of the American Medical Association*, **258**, 2388-2395.

Lesage, R., Simoneau, J.A., Jobin, J., LeBlanc, J., & Bouchard, C. (1985). Familial resemblance in maximal heart rate, blood lactate, and aerobic power. *Human Heredity*, **35**, 182-189.

Leveille, G.A., & Romsos, D.R. (1974, Nov/Dec). Meal eating and obesity. *Nutrition Today*, **9**, 4-9.

Levison, H., & Cherniak, R.M. (1968). Ventilatory cost of exercise in chronic obstructive pulmonary disease. *Journal of Applied Physiology*, **25**, 21-27.

Lewis, S.F., Taylor, W.F., Bastian, B.C., Graham, R.M., Pattinger, W.A., & Blomqvist, C.G. (1983). Haemodynamic responses to static and dynamic handgrip before and after autonomic blockade. *Clinical Science*, **64**, 593-599.

Lie, H., Mundal, R., & Erikssen, J. (1985). Coronary risk factors and incidence of coronary death in relation to fitness: Seven year follow-up study of middle-aged and elderly men. *European Heart Journal*, **6**, 147-157.

Lieber, D.C., Lieber, R.L., & Adams, W.C. (1989). Effects of run-training and swim-training at similar absolute intensities on treadmill VO_2max. *Medicine and Science in Sports and Exercise*, **21**, 655-661.

Liesen, H., & Uhlenbruck, G. (1992). Sports immunology. *Sports Science Review*, **1**, 94-116.

Lind, A.R., & McNicol, G.W. (1967). Muscular factors which determine the cardiovascular response to sustained and rhythmic exercise. *Canadian Medical Association Journal*, **96**, 706-712.

Lindén, V. (1969). Absence from work and physical fitness. *British Journal of Industrial Medicine*, **26**, 47-53.

Linderholm, H. (1959). Diffusing capacity of the lungs as a limiting factor for physical work capacity. *Acta Medica Scandinavica*, **163**, 61-84.

Lipid Research Clinics Program. (1984). The Lipid Research Clinics primary prevention trial results: II. The relationship of reduction in incidence of coronary heart disease to cholesterol lowering. *Journal of the American Medical Association*, **251**, 365-374.

Loftin, M., Boileau, R.A., Massey, B.H., & Lohman, T.G. (1988). Effect of arm training on central and peripheral circulatory function. *Medicine and Science in Sports and Exercise*, **20**, 136-141.

Loke, D., Mahler, D.A., & Virgulto, J.A. (1982). Respiratory muscle fatigue after marathon running. *Journal of Applied Physiology*, **52**, 821-824.

Lokey, E.A., Tran, Z.V., Wells, C.L., Meyers, B.C., & Tran, A.C. (1989). The effects of physical exercise on pregnancy outcomes: A metaanalysis. *Medicine and Science in Sports and Exercise*, **21**, S31.

Londeree, B., & Moeschberger, M.L. (1984). Influence of age and other factors on heart rate. *Journal of Cardiac Rehabilitation*, **4**, 44-49.

Londeree, B.R., & Moeschberger, L. (1982). Effect of age and other factors on maximal heart rate. *Research Quarterly*, **53**, 297-304.

Lorlin, R.E., Beck, J.E., & Kinnear, G.R. (1979). Human erythrocyte response to training: Geometry and deformability. *Canadian Journal of Applied Sport Sciences*, **4**, 285-288.

Lortie, G., Simoneau, J.A., Hamel, P., Boulay, M.R., Landry, F., & Bouchard, C. (1984). Responses of maximal aerobic power and capacity to aerobic training. *International Journal of Sports Medicine*, **5**, 232-236.

Lotgering, F.K., & Longo, L.D. (1984). Exercise and pregnancy: How much is too much? *Contemporary Obstetrics and Gynecology*, **23**(1), 63-80.

Loucks, A.B. (in press). Physical activity, fitness, and menstrual cycles. In C. Bouchard, R.J. Shephard, & T. Stephens (Eds.), *Physical activity, fitness, and health*. Champaign, IL: Human Kinetics.

Lovell, R.R.H. (1967). Race and blood pressure, with special reference to Oceania. In J. Stamler, R. Stamler, & T.N. Pullman (Eds.), *The epidemiology of hypertension* (pp. 122-138). New York: Grune & Stratton.

MacDonald, R.A. (1983). Physiological changes after six weeks sequence training. *British Journal of Sports Medicine*, **17**, 76-83.

MacDougall, J.D., Tuxen, D., Sale, D.G., Moroz, J.R., & Sutton, J.R. (1985). Arterial blood pressure response to heavy resistance exercise. *Journal of Applied Physiology*, **58**, 785-790.

MacIntosh, D., Skrien, T., & Shephard, R.J. (1972). Physical activity and injury: A study of sports injuries at the University of Toronto, 1951-1968. *Journal of Sports Medicine*, **12**, 224-237.

Mackinnon, L.T. (1992). *Exercise and immunology*. Champaign, IL: Human Kinetics.

Magder, S.A., Daughters, G.T., Hung, J., Alderman, E.L., & Ingels, N.B. (1987). Adaptation of human left ventricular volumes at the onset of supine exercise. *European Journal of Applied Physiology*, **56**, 467-473.

Magel, J.R., Foglia, G.F., McArdle, W.D., Gutin, B., Pechar, G.S., & Katch, F.I. (1975). Specificity of swim training on maximum oxygen uptake. *Journal of Applied Physiology*, **38**, 151-155.

Magora, A., & Taustein, I. (1969). An investigation of the problem of sick-leave in the patient suffering from low back pain. *Industrial Medicine*, **38**, 80-90.

Mahlamarki, E., & Mahlamarki, S. (1988). Iron deficiency in adolescent female dancers. *British Journal of Sports Medicine*, **22**, 55-56.

Mainwood, G.W., & Renaud, J.M. (1985). The effect of acid-base balance on fatigue of skeletal muscle. *Canadian Journal of Physiology and Pharmacology*, **63**, 403-416.

Mairbäurl, H., Humpeler, E., Schwaberger, JG., & Pessenhofer, H. (1983). Training dependent changes of red cell density and erythrocyte oxygen transport. *Journal of Applied Physiology*, **55**, 1403-1407.

Malhotra, M.S., Sen Gupta, J., & Joseph, N.T. (1973). Comparative evaluation of different training programmes on physical fitness. *Indian Journal of Physiology and Pharmacology*, **17**, 356-364.

Malina, R.M. (in press). Physical activity: Relationship to growth, maturation, and fitness. In C. Bouchard, R.J. Shephard, & T. Stephens (Eds.), *Physical activity, fitness, and health*. Champaign, IL: Human Kinetics.

Mann, J.I., Lewis, B., Shepherd, J., Winder, A.F., Fenster, S., Rose, L., et al. (1988). Blood lipid concentrations and other cardiovascular risk factors: Distribution, prevalence, and detection in Britain. *British Medical Association*, **296**, 1702-1706.

Manohar, M. (1987). Transmural coronary vasodilator reserve and flow distribution during maximal exercise in normal and splenectomized ponies. *Journal of Physiology*, **387**, 425-440.

Manohar, M. (1988). Left ventricular oxygen extraction during submaximal and maximal exertion in ponies. *Journal of Physiology*, **404**, 547-556.

Marcus, B.H., Albrecht, A.E., Niaura, R.S., Abrams, D.B., & Thompson, P.D. (1991). Usefulness of physical exercise in maintaining smoking cessation in women. *American Journal of Cardiology*, **68**, 406-407.

Marcus, P. (1972). Heat acclimatization by exercise-induced elevation of body temperature. *Journal of Applied Physiology*, **33**, 283-288.

Marcus, R., & Carter, D.R. (1988). The role of physical activity in bone mass regulation. *Advances in Sports Medicine and Physical Fitness*, **1**, 63-82.

Margaria, R. (1966). An outline for setting significant tests of muscular performance. In H. Yoshimura & J.S. Weiner (Eds.), *Human adaptability and its methodology* (pp. 205-211). Tokyo: Society for the Promotion of Sciences.

Maron, M.B., Hamilton, L.H., & Maksud, M.G. (1979). Alterations in pulmonary function consequent to competitive marathon running. *Medicine and Science in Sports and Exercise*, **11**, 244-249.

Marshall, D.J., Conger, P., & Quinney, H.A. (1983). Exercise intensity in elementary school physical education classes. *Canadian Journal of Applied Sport Sciences*, **8**, 205 (abstract).

Martin, B.J. (1987). Limitations imposed by respiratory muscle fatigue. *Canadian Journal of Sport Sciences*, **12**(Suppl.), 61S-62S.

Martin, B.J., & Chen, H-I. (1982). Ventilatory endurance in athletes: A family study. *International Journal of Sports Medicine*, **3**, 100-104.

Martin, B.J., Chen, H-I., & Kolka, M.A. (1984). Anaerobic metabolism of the respiratory muscles during exercise. *Medicine and Science in Sports and Exercise*, **16**, 82-86.

Martin, B.J., Sparks, K.E., Zwillich, C.W., & Weil, J.V. (1979). Low exercise ventilation in endurance athletes. *Medicine and Science in Sports*, **11**, 181-185.

Martin, D.E., Vroom, D.E., May, D.F., & Pilbeam, S.P. (1986). Physiological changes in elite male distance runners training for Olympic competition. *The Physician and Sportsmedicine*, **14**(1), 152-171.

Martin, W.H., Coyle, E.F., Bloomfield, S.A., & Ehsani, A.A. (1986). Effects of physical deconditioning after intense training on left ventricular dimensions and stroke volume. *Journal of the American College of Cardiology*, **7**, 982-989.

Masironi, R., & Mansourian, P. (1974). Determination of habitual physical activity by means of a portable R-R wave interval distribution recorder. *Bulletin of the World Health Organisation*, **51**, 291-298.

Massie, J., Rode, A., Skrien, T., & Shephard, R.J. (1970). A critical review of the ''aerobics'' points system. *Medicine and Science in Sports*, **2**, 1-6.

Massie, J., & Shephard, R.J. (1971). Physiological and psychological effects of training. *Medicine and Science in Sports*, **3**, 110-117.

Matsuda, M., Sugishita, Y., Koseki, S., Ito, I., Akatsula, T., & Takamatsu, K. (1983). Effect of exercise on left ventricular diastolic filling in athletes and non-athletes. *Journal of Applied Physiology*, **55**, 323-328.

Mattfeldt, T., Krämer, K.L., Zeitz, R., & Mall, G. (1986). Stereology of myocardial hypertrophy induced by physical exercise. *Virchows Archiv [A]*, **409**, 473-484.

Mausner, J.S., & Bahn, A.K. (1974). *Epidemiology: An introductory text*. Philadelphia: Saunders.

May, G.S., Furberg, C.D., Eberlin, K.A., & Geraci, B.J. (1983). Secondary prevention after myocardial infarction: A review of long-term trials. *Progress in Cardiovascular Diseases*, **24**, 335-359.

Mayer, J. (1960). Exercise and weight control. In W.E. Johnson (Ed.), *Science and medicine of exercise and sports*(1st ed.) (pp. 301-310). New York: Harper.

McCole, S.D., Claney, K., Conte, J.C., Anderson, R., & Hagberg, J.M. (1990). Energy expenditure during bicycling. *Journal of Applied Physiology*, **68**, 748-753.

McCord, P., Nichols, J., & Patterson, P. (1989). The effect of low-impact dance training on aerobic capacity, submaximal heart rates, and body composition of college-aged females. *Journal of Sports Medicine and Physical Fitness*, **29**, 184-188.

McCoy, D.E., Wiley, R.L., Clayton, R.P., & Dunn, C.L. (1991). Cardiopulmonary responses to combined rhythmic and isometric exercise in humans. *European Journal of Applied Physiology*, **62**, 305-309.

McDowell, A.J. (1989). Cardiovascular endurance, strength, and lung function tests in the National Health and Nutrition Examination Surveys. In T. Drury (Ed.), *Assessing physical fitness and physical activity in population-based surveys* (pp. 21-77). Hyattsville, MD: U.S. Dept. of Health & Human Services.

McFadden, E.R. (1987). Respiratory thermal events and airway function. *Canadian Journal of Sport Sciences*, **12**(Suppl.), 63S-65S.

McGill, H.C. (1980). Morphologic development of atherosclerotic plaque. In R.M. Lauer & R.R. Shekelle (Eds.), *Childhood prevention of atherosclerosis and hypertension* (pp. 41-49). New York: Raven Press.

McGilvery, R.W. (1975). The use of fuels for muscular work. In H. Howald & J.R. Poortmans (Eds.), *Metabolic adaptations to prolonged physical exercise* (pp. 12-30). Basel: Birkhauser Verlag.

McKelvey, R.S., & McCartney, N. (1990). Weight-lifting training in cardiac patients: Considerations. *Sports Medicine*, **10**, 355-364.

McKenzie, D.C. (1992). Pregnant women and endurance exercise. In R.J. Shephard & P.O. Åstrand (Eds.), *Endurance in sport* (pp. 385-389). Oxford: Blackwell Scientific.

McLellan, T.M. (1987). The anaerobic threshold: Concept and controversy. *Australian Journal of Science and Medicine in Sport*, **19**, 3-8.

McMurray, R.G., & Katz, V.L. (1990). Thermoregulation in pregnancy: Implications for exercise. *Sports Medicine*, **10**, 146-158.

McNamara, P.S., Otto, R.M., & Smith, T.K. (1985). The acute response of simulated bicycle and rowing exercise on the elderly population. *Medicine and Science in Sports and Exercise*, **17**, 266.

McPherson, B.D., & Curtis, J.E. (1986). *Regional and community type differences in the physical activity patterns of Canadian adults*. Ottawa: Canadian Fitness and Lifestyle Research Institute.

Mead, J. (1980). Expiratory flow limitation: A physiologist's point of view. *Federation Proceedings*, **39**, 2771-2775.

Medbø, J-I., Mohn, A.C., Tabata, I., Bahr, R., Vaage, O., & Sejersted, O.M. (1988). Anaerobic capacity determined by maximal accumulated O_2 deficit. *Journal of Applied Physiology*, **64**, 50-60.

Meen, H.D., Holter, P.H., & Refsum, H.E. (1981). Changes in 2,3-diphosphoglycerate (2,3-DPG) after exercise. *European Journal of Applied Physiology*, **46**, 177-184.

Mertens, D.J., Shephard, R.J., & Kavanagh, T. (1978). Long-term exercise for chronic obstructive lung disease. *Respiration*, **35**, 96-107.

Metropolitan Life Insurance Company. (1983). *Nutrition and athletic performance: Values for ideal weight*. New York: Metropolitan Life Insurance.

Miall, W.E., Ashcroft, M.T., Lovell, H.G., & Moore, F. (1967). A longitudinal study of the decline of adult height with age in two Welsh communities. *Human Biology*, **39**, 445-454.

Michel, B.A., Block, D.A., & Fries, J.F. (1989). Weight-bearing exercise, overexercise, and lumbar bone density over age 50 years. *Archives of Internal Medicine*, **149**, 2325-2329.

Mickelson, J.K., Byrd, B.F., Bouchard, A., Botvinik, E.H., & Schiller, N.B. (1986). Left ventricular dimensions and mechanics in distance runners. *American Heart Journal*, **112**, 1251-1256.

Milburn, S., & Butts, N.K. (1983). A comparison of the training responses to aerobic dance and jogging in college females. *Medicine and Science in Sports and Exercise*, **15**, 510-513.

Miles, D.S., Enoch, A.D., & Grevey, S.C. (1986). Interpretation of changes in $D_{L,co}$ and pulmonary function after running five miles. *Respiratory Physiology*, **66**, 135-145.

Miles, D.S., Sawka, M.N., Glaser, R.M., & Petrofsky, J.S. (1983). Plasma volume shifts during progressive arm and leg exercise. *Journal of Applied Physiology*, **54**, 491-495.

Miller, F.R., & Manfredi, T.G. (1981). Physiological and anthropological predictors of 15-km cycling. *Research Quarterly*, **58**, 250-254.

Miller, G.J., & Miller, N.E. (1975). Plasma high-density lipoprotein concentrations and the development of ischemic heart disease. *Lancet*, **1**, 16-19.

Miller, N.E., Forde, O.H., Thelle, D.S., & Mjos, O.D. (1977). The Tromso Heart Study: High-density lipoprotein and coronary heart disease: A prospective case control study. *Lancet*, **1**, 965-967.

Millikan, G.A. (1937). Experiments on muscle haemoglobin *in vivo*: The instantaneous measurement of muscle metabolism. *Proceedings of the Royal Society (Biology)*, **123**, 218-241.

Milne, C.J. (1988). Rhabdomyolysis, myoglobinuria, and exercise. *Sports Medicine*, **6**, 93-106.

Mirwald, R.L., & Bailey, D.A. (1986). *Maximal aerobic power* (pp. 1-80). London, ON: Sports Dynamics.

Misner, J.E., Going, S.B., Massey, B.H., Ball, T.E., Bemben, M.G., & Essandoah, L.K. (1990). Cardiovascular responses to sustained maximal voluntary static muscle contraction. *Medicine and Science in Sports and Exercise*, **22**, 194-199.

Mitchell, J.H., & Schmidt, R.F. (1983). Cardiovascular reflex control by afferent fibers from skeletal muscle receptors. In J.T. Shepherd & F.M. Abboud (Eds.), *Handbook of physiology: Vol. 3. Circulation, part 2* (pp. 623-658). Bethesda, MD: American Physiological Society.

Miyamoto, Y., & Moll, W. (1971). Measurement of dimension and pathway of red cells in rapidly frozen lungs *in situ*. *Respiratory Physiology*, **12**, 141-156.

Miyamura, M., & Ishida, K. (1990). Adaptive changes in hypercapnic ventilatory response during traning and detraining. *European Journal of Applied Physiology*, **60**, 353-359.

Mocellin, R. (1985). Exercise in pediatric cardiology. In P. Welsh & R.J. Shephard (Eds.), *Current therapy in sports medicine 1985-1986* (pp. 72-76). Burlington, ON: Decker.

Moldover, J.R., & Downey, J.A. (1983). Cardiac response to exercise: Comparison of 3 ergometers. *Archives of Physical Medicine and Rehabilitation*, **64**, 155-159.

Molé, P. (1978). Increased contractile protein of papillary muscles from exercise-trained rat hearts. *American Journal of Physiology*, **234**, H421-H425.

Molé, P. (1990). Impact of energy intake and exercise on resting metabolic rate. *Sports Medicine*, **10**, 72-87.

Molé, P.A., & Coulson, R.L. (1985). Energetics of myocardial function. *Medicine and Science in Sports and Exercise*, **17**, 538-545.

Molé, P.A., Stern, J.S., Schultz, C.L., Bernauer, E.M., & Holcomb, B.J. (1989). Exercise reverses depressed metabolic rate produced by severe caloric restriction. *Medicine and Science in Sports and Exercise*, **21**, 29-33.

Montoye, H.J. (1975). *Physical activity and health: An epidemiologic study of an entire community*. Englewood Cliffs, NJ: Prentice Hall.

Montoye, H.J. (1984). Age and cardiovascular response to submaximal treadmill exercise in males. *Research Quarterly*, **55**, 85-88.

Montoye, H.J. (1985). Risk indicators for cardiovascular disease in relation to physical activity in youth. In R.A. Binkhorst, H.C.G. Kemper, & W.H.M. Saris (Eds.), *Children and exercise* XI (pp. 3-25). Champaign, IL: Human Kinetics.

Montoye, H.J., Metzner, H.L., & Keller, J.B. (1972). Habitual physical activity and blood pressure. *Medicine and Science in Sports*, **4**, 175-181.

Montoye, H.J., Van Huss, W.D., Olson, H.W., Pierson, W.O., & Hudec, A.J. (1957). *The longevity and morbidity of college athletes*. Lansing, MI: Michigan State University, Phi Epsilon Kappa Fraternity.

Montoye, H.J., Washburn, R., Servais, S., Ertl, A., Webster, J.G., & Nagle, F.J. (1983). Estimation of energy expenditure by a portable accelerometer. *Medicine and Science in Sports and Exercise*, **15**, 403-407.

Moore, R.L., & Gollnick, P.D. (1982). Response of the ventilatory muscles of the rat to endurance training. *Pflügers Archiv*, **392**, 268-271.

Morgan, D.W., Kohrt, W.M., Bates, B.J., & Skinner, J.S. (1987). Effects of respiratory muscle endurance training on ventilatory and endurance performance of moderately trained cyclists. *International Journal of Sports Medicine*, **8**, 88-93.

Morgan, P., Gildiner, M., & Wright, G. (1976). Smoking reduction in adults who take up exercise: A survey of running clubs for adults. *Canadian Association for Health, Physical Education and Recreation Journal*, **42**(5), 39-43.

Morgan, R.E., & Adamson, G.T. (1965). *Circuit training*. London: Bell.

Morganroth, J., & Maron, B.J. (1977). The athlete's-heart syndrome: A new perspective. *Annals of the New York Academy of Sciences*, **301**, 931-939.

Moroz, D.E., & Houston, M.E. (1987). The effects of replacing endurance-running training with cycling in female runners. *Canadian Journal of Sport Sciences*, **12**, 131-135.

Morris, G.S., Baldwin, K.M., Lash, J.M., Hamlin, R.L., & Sherman, W.M. (1990). Exercise alters cardiac myosin isozyme distribution in obese Zucker and Wistar rats. *Journal of Applied Physiology*, **69**, 380-383.

Morris, J.N. (1951). Recent history of coronary disease. *Lancet*, (1), 1-7.

Morris, J.N., Chave, S.P., Adam, C., Sirey, C., & Epstein, L. (1973). Vigorous exercise in leisure time and the incidence of coronary heart disease. *Lancet*, (i), 333-339.

Morris, J.N., Clayton, D.G., Everitt, M.G., Semmence, A.M., & Burgess, E.H. (1990). Exercise in leisure time: Coronary attack and death rates. *British Heart Journal*, **63**, 325-334.

Morris, J.N., & Crawford, M.D. (1958). Coronary heart disease and physical activity of work: Evidence of a national necropsy study. *British Medical Journal*, (ii), 1485-1496.

Morris, J.N., Everitt, M.G., Pollard, R., Chave, S.P.W., & Semmence, A.M. (1980). Vigorous exercise in leisure time: Protection against coronary heart disease. *Lancet*, (ii), 1207-1210.

Morris, J.N., Heady, J., & Raffle, P. (1956). Physique of London busmen. *Lancet*, (ii), 569-570.

Morris, J.N., Heady, J., Raffle, P., Roberts, C., & Parks, J. (1953). Coronary heart disease and physical activity of work. *Lancet*, (ii), 1053-1057, 1111-1120.

Morris, J.N., Kagan, A., Pattison, D.C., Gardner, M.J., & Raffle, P.A.B. (1966). Incidence and prediction of ischaemic heart disease in London busmen. *Lancet*, (ii), 553-559.

Morris, W.H.M. (1967). Heart disease in farm workers. *Canadian Medical Association Journal*, **96**, 821-824.

Morrison, J.F., Van Malsen, F., & Noakes, T. (1983). Evidence for an inverse relationship between the ventilatory response to exercise and the maximum whole-body oxygen consumption value. *European Journal of Applied Physiology*, **50**, 265-272.

Morse, B.S. (1968). Erythrokinetic changes in man associated with rest. *Clinical Research*, **16**, 240-254.

Morton, A.R., & Fitch, K.D. (1989). Exercise-induced bronchial obstruction. In J. Torg, P. Welsh, & R.J. Shephard (Eds.), *Current therapy in sports medicine 2* (pp. 53-59). Burlington, ON: Decker.

Murray, S.J., & Shephard, R.J. (1988). Possible anthropometric alternatives to skinfold measurements. *Human Biology*, **60**, 273-282.

Murray, S.J., Shephard, R.J., Greaves, S., Allen, C., & Radomski, M. (1986). Effects of cold stress and exercise on fat loss in females. *European Journal of Applied Physiology*, **55**, 610-618.

Musch, T.I. (1988). Skeletal muscle blood flow in exercising dogs. *Medicine and Science in Sports and Exercise*, **20**, S104-S109.

Musch, T.I., Haidet, G.C., Ordway, G.A., Longhurst, J.C., & Mitchell, J.H. (1987). Training effects on regional blood flow response to maximal exercise in foxhounds. *Journal of Applied Physiology*, **62**, 1724-1732.

Myerson, M., Gutin, B., Warren, M.P., May, M.T., Contento, I., Lee, M., Pi-Sunyer, F.X., Pierson, R.N., & Brooks-Gunn, J. (1991). Resting metabolic rate and energy balance in amenorrheic and eumenorrheic runners. *Medicine and Science in Sports and Exercise*, **23**, 15-22.

Nagel, D., Seiler, D., Franz, H., & Kung, K. (1990). Ultra-long-distance running and the liver. *International Journal of Sports Medicine*, **11**, 441-445.

Nagle, F.J., Seals, D.R., & Hanson, P. (1989). Time to fatigue during isometric exercise using different muscle masses. *International Journal of Sports Medicine*, **9**, 313-315.

Naimark, B.J., Morris, A., Sigurdsson, S.B., Tate, R.B., Axelsson, J., & Stephens, N.L. (1991). Echocardiographic assessment of cardiac abnormalities and their relationship to exercise blood pressure in two Icelandic populations. In B. Postl, P. Gilbert, J. Goodwill, M.E.K. Moffatt, J.D. O'Neil, P.A. Sarsfield, & T.K. Young (Eds.), *Circumpolar health 90* (pp. 436-438). Winnipeg: Canadian Society for Circumpolar Health.

Narici, M.V., Roi, G.S., Landoni, L., Minetti, A.E., & Cerretelli, P. (1989). Changes in force, cross-sectional area, and neural activation during strength training and detraining of the human quadriceps. *European Journal of Applied Physiology*, **59**, 310-319.

Narvaez-Pérez, G.E., D'Angelo, C.P., & Zabala, R.D. (1991). Physical fitness in children and adolescents from differing socioeconomic strata. In R.J. Shephard & J. Pařízková (Eds.), *Human growth, physical fitness and nutrition* (pp. 80-98). Basel: S. Karger.

National Institutes of Health. (1987). Consensus Development Conference on diet and exercise in non-insulin dependent diabetes mellitus. *Diabetes Care*, **10**, 639-643.

Nauss, K.N., Jacobs, L.R., & Newperne, R.M. (1987). Dieting, fat and fiber relationship to caloric intake, body growth, and colon tumorigenesis. *American Journal of Clinical Nutrition*, **45**, 243-251.

Neijens, H.J., Duiverman, E.J., & Kerrebijn, K.F. (1985). Exercise-induced bronchial obstruction. In P. Welsh & R.J. Shephard (Eds.), *Current therapy in sports medicine 1985-1986* (pp. 95-97). Burlington, ON: Decker.

Nelson, M.E., Fisher, E.C., Catsos, P.D., Meredith, C.N., Turksoy, R.N., & Evans, W.J. (1986). Diet and bone status in amenorrheic runners. *American Journal of Clinical Nutrition*, **43**, 910-916.

Nemeth, P.M., Chi, M.M-L., Hintz, C.S., & Lowry, O.H. (1982). Myoglobin content of normal and trained human muscle fibers. In H.G. Knuttgen, J.A. Vogel, & J. Poortmans (Eds.), *Biochemistry of exercise* (pp. 826-831). Champaign, IL: Human Kinetics.

Neufer, P.D. (1989). The effect of detraining and reduced training on the physiological adaptations to aerobic exercise training. *Sports Medicine*, **8**, 302-320.

Neumann, G. (1992). Cycling. In R.J. Shephard & P.O. Åstrand (Eds.), *Endurance in sport* (pp. 582-596). Oxford: Blackwell Scientific.

Newhouse, I.J., & Clement, D.B. (1988). Iron status in athletes: An update. *Sports Medicine*, **5**, 337-352.

Newsholme, E.A. (1990). Psychoimmunology and cellular nutrition: An alternative hypothesis. *Biological Psychiatry*, **27**, 1-3.

Newsholme, E.A. (in press). Effects of exercise and overtraining on the immune response. In C. Bouchard, R.J. Shephard, & T. Stephens (Eds.), *Physical activity, fitness, and health*. Champaign, IL: Human Kinetics.

Nicholl, J.P., Coleman, P., & Williams, B.T. (1991). Pilot study of the epidemiology of sports injuries and exercise-related morbidity. *British Journal of Sports Medicine*, **25**, 61-66.

Niederman, M.S., Clemente, P.H., Fein, A.M., Feinsilver, S.H., Robinson, D.A., Ilowite, J.S., & Bernstein, M.G. (1991). Benefits of a multidisciplinary pulmonary rehabilitation program: Improvements are independent of lung function. *Chest*, **99**, 798-804.

Nieman, D.C., Johanssen, L.M., Lee, J.W., & Arabatzis, K. (1990). Infectious episodes in runners before and after the Los Angeles marathon. *Journal of Sports Medicine and Physical Fitness*, **30**, 316-328.

Niinimaa, V., Cole, P., Mintz, S., & Shephard, R.J. (1980). The switching point from nasal to oronasal breathing. *Respiration Physiology*, **42**, 61-71.

Niinimaa, V., Shephard, R.J., & Dyon, M. (1979). Determination of performance and mechanical efficiency in Nordic skiing. *British Journal of Sports Medicine*, **13**, 62-65.

Niinimaa, V., Woch, Z., & Shephard, R.J. (1978). Intensity of physical effort during a free figure skating program. Proceedings, Pan American Sports Science Congress, Edmonton.

Niinimaa, V.M.J., & Shephard, R.J. (1978). Training and oxygen conductance in the elderly: II. The cardiovascular system. *Journal of Gerontology*, **33**, 362-367.

Niinimaa, V.M.J., Wright, G., Shephard, R.J., & Clarke, A.J. (1977). Characteristics of the successful dinghy sailor. *Journal of Sports Medicine and Physical Fitness*, **17**, 83-96.

Nilsson, B.E., & Westlin, N.E. (1971). Bone density in athletes. *Clinical Orthopedics*, **77**, 179-182.

Noakes, T.D. (1987). Effects of exercise on serum enzyme activities in humans. *Sports Medicine*, **4**, 245-267.

Noakes, T.D., Kotzenburg, G., McArthur, P.S., & Dykman, T. (1983). Elevated serum creatine kinase MB and creatine kinase BB isozyme fractions after ultramarathon running. *European Journal of Applied Physiology*, **52**, 75-79.

Noreau, L., & Shephard, R.J. (1992). Physical activity and productivity of paraplegics. *Sports Training, Rehabilitation and Medicine*, **24**, 165-181.

North, T.C., McCullagh, P., & Tran, Z.V. (1990). Effect of exercise on depression. *Exercise and Sport Sciences Reviews*, **18**, 379-416.

Northcote, R.J., McKillop, G., Todd, I.C., & Canning, G.P. (1990). The effect of habitual sustained endurance exercise on cardiac structure and function. *European Heart Journal*, **11**, 17-22.

Norwegian Confederation of Sport. (1984). *Physical activity in Norway, 1983*. Oslo: Author.

Nygaard, E., Bentzen, H., Houston, M., Larsen, H., Nielsen, H., & Saltin, B. (1977). Capillary supply and morphology of trained human skeletal muscle. *Proceedings of 27th International Congress of Physiological Sciences, Paris*, **XIII**, 557.

Nylander, E., Sigvardsson, K., & Kilbom, A. (1982). Training-induced bradycardia and intrinsic heart rate in rats. *European Journal of Applied Physiology*, **48**, 189-199.

Oberst, F.W. (1961). Factors affecting inhalation and retention of toxic vapors. In C.N. Davies (Ed.), *Inhaled particles and vapours* (pp. 249-266). Oxford: Pergamon Press.

O'Brien, M., Davies, B., & Daggett, A. (1982). Women in sport. In B. Davies & G. Thomas (Eds.), *Science and sporting performance: Management or manipulation?* (pp. 52-67). Oxford: Clarendon Press.

O'Brodovich, H. (1992). Lung fluid movement. In R.J. Shephard & P.O. Åstrand (Eds.), *Endurance in sport* (pp. 459-463). Oxford: Blackwell Scientific.

O'Hara, W.J., Allen, C., & Shephard, R.J. (1978). Loss of body fat during an arctic winter expedition. *Canadian Journal of Physiology*, **55**, 1235-1241.

O'Hara, W.J., Allen, C., Shephard, R.J., & Allen, G. (1979). Fat loss in the cold: A controlled study. *Journal of Applied Physiology*, **46**, 872-877.

Oja, P. (1991). Elements and assessment of fitness in sport for all. In P. Oja & R. Telama (Eds.) *Sport for all* (pp. 103-110). Amsterdam: Elsevier.

Okin, P.M., Kligfield, P.L., Ameisen, O., Goldberg, H.L., & Borer, J.S. (1988). Identification of anatomically extensive coronary artery disease by the exercise ST segment/heart rate slope. *American Heart Journal*, **115**, 1002-1112.

Oldridge, N. (1979). The problem of compliance. *Medicine and Science in Sports*, **11**, 373-375.

Oldridge, N.B. (1990). Discussion: Exercise, fitness, and recovery from surgery, disease, or trauma. In C. Bouchard, R.J. Shephard, T. Stephens, J. Sutton, & B. McPherson (Eds.), *Exercise, fitness, and health* (pp. 601-606). Champaign, IL: Human Kinetics.

Oldridge, N.B., Guyatt, G., Fischer, M., & Rimm, A.A. (1988). Randomized trials of cardiac rehabilitation: Combined experience of randomized clinical trials. *Journal of the American Medical Association*, **260**, 945-950.

Orban, W.R. (1962). *The Royal Canadian Air Force 5BX plan for physical fitness* (2nd ed.). Ottawa: Queen's Printer.

Orchard, T.J., Donahue, R.P., Kuller, L.H., Hodge, P.N., & Drash, A.L. (1983). Cholesterol screening in childhood: Does it predict adult hypercholesterolemia? The Beaver County experience. *Journal of Pediatrics*, **103**, 687-691.

Orenstein, D.M., Franklin, B.A., Doershuk, C.F., Hellerstein, H.K., Germann, K.J., Horowitz, J.G., & Stern, R.G. (1981). Exercise conditioning and cardiopulmonary fitness in cystic fibrosis. *Chest*, **80**, 392-398.

Orenstein, D.M., & Nixon, P.A. (1989). Exercise in cystic fibrosis. In J. Torg, P. Welsh, & R.J. Shephard (Eds.), *Current therapy in sports medicine 2* (pp. 26-31). Burlington, ON: Decker.

Orlander, J., Kiessling, K.H., Karlsson, J., & Ekblom, B. (1977). Low-intensity training, inactivity, and resumed training in sedentary men. *Acta Physiologica Scandinavica*, **101**, 351-362.

Otis, A.B. (1964). The work of breathing. In W.O. Fenn & H. Rahn (Eds.), *Handbook of physiology, Section 3: Respiration, Vol. 1* (pp. 463-476). Washington, DC: American Physiological Society.

O'Toole, M., Hiller, W.D., Roalstad, M.S., & Douglas, P.S. (1988). Hemolysis during triathlon races: Its relation to race distance. *Medicine and Science in Sports and Exercise*, **20**, 272-275.

Owens, S.G., al-Ahmed, A., & Moffat, R.J. (1989). Physiological effects of walking and running with hand-held weights. *Journal of Sports Medicine and Physical Fitness*, **29**, 384-387.

Ozolin, P. (1986). Blood flow in the extremities of athletes. *International Journal of Sports Medicine*, **7**, 117-122.

Paffenbarger, R. (1977). Physical activity and fatal heart attack: Protection or selection? In E.A. Amsterdam, J.H. Wilmore, & A.N. deMaria (Eds.), *Exercise in cardiovascular health and disease* (pp. 35-49). New York: Yorke Medical Books.

Paffenbarger, R. (1988). Contributions of epidemiology to exercise science and cardiovascular health. *Medicine and Science in Sports and Exercise*, **20**, 426-438.

Paffenbarger, R.S., Hyde, R.T., & Wing, A.L. (1987). Physical activity and incidence of cancer in diverse populations: A preliminary report. *American Journal of Clinical Nutrition*, **45**, 312-317.

Paffenbarger, R. S., Hyde, R.T., Wing, A.L., & Hsieh, C.C. (1986). Physical activity, all-cause mortality, and longevity of college athletes. *New England Journal of Medicine*, **314**, 605-613.

Paffenbarger, R., Hyde, R., Wing, A., Jung, D., & Kampert, J. (1991). Influence of changes in physical activities and other characteristics on all-cause mortality. *Medicine and Science in Sports and Exercise*, **23**, S82.

Page, L.B., Damon, A., & Moelleriag, R.C. (1974). Antecedents of cardiovascular disease in six Solomon Island societies. *Circulation*, **49**, 1132-1146.

Painter, P., & Hanson, P. (1984). Isometric exercise: Implications for the cardiac patient. *Cardiovascular Reviews and Reports*, **5**, 261-279.

Paivio, M. (1967). Commentary. *Canadian Medical Association Journal*, **96**, 768.

Palmore, E. (1970). Health practices and illness among the aged. *Gerontologist*, **10**, 313-316.

Panush, R.S., & Brown, D.G. (1987). Exercise and arthritis. *Sports Medicine*, **4**, 54-64.

Panush, R.S., Schmidt, C., Caldwell, J.R., Edwards, N.L., Longley, S., Yonker, R., Webster, E., Naumann, J., Stork, J., & Petterson, H. (1986). Is running associated with degenerative joint disease? *Journal of the American Medical Association*, **255**, 1152-1154.

Panzram, G. (1987). Mortality and survival in Type 2 (non-insulin dependent) diabetes mellitus. *Diabetologia*, **30**, 123-132.

Paolone, A.M., & Worthington, S. (1985). Cautions and advice on exercise during pregnancy. *Contemporary Obstetrics and Gynecology*, **25**(5), 150-162.

Pappenheimer, J. C. (1950). Chairman of Committee on Standardization of Definitions and Symbols in Respiratory Physiology. *Federation Proceedings*, **9**, 602-605.

Pardy, R.L., & Leith, D.E. (1985). Ventilatory muscle training. In C. Roussos & P.T. Macklem (Eds.), *The thorax* (pp. 1353-1372). New York: Marcel Dekker.

Pařízková, J. (1977). *Body fat and physical fitness*. The Hague: Martin Nijhoff.

Pařízková, J. (1982). Physical training in weight reduction of obese adolescents. *Annals of Clinical Research*, **34**, 63-68.

Pařízková, J., Merhautova, J., & Prokopec, M. (1972). Comparaison entre la croissance des jeunes Tunisiennes et celle des jeunes Tchèques âgés de 11 et 12 ans. [Comparison between the growth of young Tunisians and that of young Czechs aged 11 and 12 years.] *Biométrie Humaine*, **7**, 1-10.

Parker, J.O., diGiorgi, S., & West, R.O. (1966). A hemodynamic study of acute coronary insufficiency precipitated by exercise: With observations on the effects of nitroglycerin. *American Journal of Medicine*, **17**, 470-483.

Parkhouse, W.S., McKenzie, D.S., Rhodes, E.C., Dunwoody, D., & Wiley, P. (1982). Cardiac frequency and anaerobic threshold: Implications for prescriptive exercise programs. *European Journal of Applied Physiology*, **50**, 117-123.

Pascale, M., & Grana, W.A. (1989). Does running cause osteoarthritis? *The Physician and Sportsmedicine*, **17**(3), 157-166.

Pate, R.R., & Shephard, R.J. (1989). Characteristics of physical fitness in youth. In C.V. Gisolfi & D.R. Lamb (Eds.), *Youth, exercise, and sport* (pp. 1-46). Indianapolis: Benchmark Press.

Paterson, D.H., Cunningham, D.A., & Bumstead, L.A. (1986). Recovery O_2 and blood lactic acid: Longitudinal analysis in boys aged 11 to 15 years. *European Journal of Applied Physiology*, **55**, 530-537.

Patton, R.W., Corry, J.M., Gettman, L.R., Schovee, G.J. (1986). *Implementing health and fitness programs*. Champaign, IL: Human Kinetics.

Pavlou, K.N., Steffe, W.P., Lerman, R.H., & Burrows, B.A. (1985). Effects of dieting and exercise on lean body mass, oxygen uptake, and strength. *Medicine and Science in Sports and Exercise*, **17**, 466-471.

Pearce, N.D. (1989). General population surveys: An overview. In T. Drury (Ed.), *Assessing physical fitness and physical activity*. Hyattsville, MD: U.S. Dept. of Health & Human Services.

Pearl, P. (1987). The effects of exercise on the development and function of the coronary collateral circulation. *Sports Medicine*, **4**, 86-94.

Pearson, L. (1978). Jogging and cancer. *Medicine and Sport*, **12**, 126-127.

Pechar, G.S., McArdle, W.D., Katch, F.I., Magel, J.R., & deLucca, J. (1974). Specificity of cardio-respiratory adaptation to bicycle and treadmill training. *Journal of Applied Physiology*, **36**, 753-756.

Pekkanen, J., Marti, B., Nissinen, A., Tuomilehto, J., Punsar, S., & Karvonen, M.J. (1987). Reduction of premature mortality by high physical activity: A 20-year follow-up of middle-aged Finnish men. *Lancet*, (i), 1473-1477.

Pelosi, G., & Agliate, G. (1968). The heart muscle in functional overload and hypoxia: A biochemical and ultrastructural study. *Laboratory Investigation*, **18**, 86-93.

Pels, A.E., Pollock, M.L., Dohmeier, T.E., Lemberger, K.A., & Oehrlein, B.F. (1987). Effects of leg press training on cycling, leg press, and running peak cardiorespiratory measures. *Medicine and Science in Sports and Exercise*, **19**, 66-70.

Péronnet, F., & Thibault, G. (1989). Mathematical analysis of running performances and world running records. *Journal of Applied Physiology*, **67**, 453-465.

Perrier. (1979). *The Perrier study: Fitness in America*. New York: Author.

Persky, V., Dyer, A.R., Leonas, J., Stamler, J., Berkson, D.M., Lindberg, H.A., Oglesby, P., Shekelle, R.B., Lepper, M.H., & Schoenberger, J.A. (1981). Heart rate: A risk factor for cancer? *American Journal of Epidemiology*, **114**, 477-487.

Pérusse, L., Després, J-P., Tremblay, A., LeBlanc, C., Talbot, J., Allard, C., & Bouchard, C. (1989). Genetic and environmental determinants of serum lipids and lipoproteins in French-Canadian families. *Arteriosclerosis*, **9**, 308-318.

Pérusse, L., LeBlanc, C., & Bouchard, C. (1988). Inter-generation transmission of physical fitness in the Canadian population. *Canadian Journal of Sport Sciences*, **13**, 8-14.

Pérusse, L., Lortie, G., LeBlanc, C., Tremblay, A., Thériault, G., & Bouchard, C. (1987). Genetic and environmental sources of variation in physical fitness. *Annals of Human Biology*, **14**, 425-434.

Pérusse, L., Tremblay, A., LeBlanc, C., & Bouchard, C. (1989). Genetic and familial environmental influences on level of habitual physical activity. *American Journal of Epidemiology*, **129**, 1012-1022.

Peters, R.K., Cady, L.D., Bischoff, D.P., Bernstein, L., & Pike, M.C. (1983). Physical fitness and subsequent myocardial infarction in healthy workers. *Journal of the American Medical Association*, **249**, 3052-3056.

Pett, L.B., & Ogilvie, G.F. (1956). The report on Canadian average weights, heights, and skinfolds. *Human Biology*, **28**, 177-188.

Phair, J., Carey, G.C.R., & Shephard, R.J. (1958). Measuring human reactions to air pollution. In *Monograph 4: Journal of the Franklin Institute* (pp. 37-49). Philadelphia.

Pirnay, F., Deroanne, R., & Petit, J.M. (1970). Maximal oxygen consumption in a hot environment. *Journal of Applied Physiology*, **28**, 642-645.

Pirnay, F., Lamy, M., Dujardin, J., Deroanne, R., & Petit, J.M. (1972). Analysis of femoral venous blood during maximum muscular exercise. *Journal of Applied Physiology*, **33**, 289-292.

Platt, L.D., Artal, R., Semel, J., Sipos, L., & Kammula, R.K. (1983). Exercise in pregnancy: II. Fetal responses. *Obstetrics and Gynecology*, **147**, 487-491.

Polednak, A.P. (1978). *The longevity of athletes*. Springfield, IL: Charles C. Thomas.

Pollitt, E., & Amante, P. (1984). *Energy intake and activity*. New York: Liss.

Pollock, M.L., Carroll, J.F., Graves, J.A., Leggett, S.H., Braith, R.W., Limacher, M., & Hagberg, J.M. (1991). Injuries and adherence to walk/jog and resistance training programs in the elderly. *Medicine and Science in Sports and Exercise*, **23**, 1194-1200.

Pollock, M.L. (1973). The quantification of endurance training. *Exercise and Sport Sciences Reviews*, **1**, 155-188.

Pollock, M.L., Dawson, G.A., Miller, H.S., Ward, A., Cooper, D., Headley, W., Linnerud, A.C., & Nomeir, M-M. (1976). Physiologic responses of men 49 to 65 years of age to endurance training. *Journal of the American Geriatric Society*, **24**, 97-104.

Pollock, M.L., Dimmick, J., Miller, H.S., Kendrick, Z., & Linnerud, A.C. (1975). Effects of mode of training on cardiovascular function and body composition of middle-aged men. *Medicine and Science in Sports*, **7**, 139-145.

Pollock, M.L., Foster, C., Knapp, D., Rod, J.S., & Schmidt, D.H. (1987). Effect of age and training on aerobic capacity and body composition of master athletes. *Journal of Applied Physiology*, **62**, 725-731.

Pollock, M.L., Gettman, L.B., Milesis, C.A., Bah, M.D., Durstine, L., & Johnson, R.B. (1977). Effects of frequency and duration of training on attrition and incidence of injury. *Medicine and Science in Sports*, **9**, 31-36.

Pomerance, J.J., Gluck, L., & Lynch, V.A. (1974). Maternal exercise as a screening test for utero-placental insufficiency. *Obstetrics and Gynecology*, **44**, 383-387.

Poole, D.C., & Gasser, G.A. (1985). Response of ventilatory and lactate thresholds to continuous and interval training. *Journal of Applied Physiology*, **58**, 1115-1121.

Poortmans, J.R. (1978). Protein turnover during exercise. In F. Landry & W.A.R. Orban (Eds.), *Third international symposium of exercise biochemistry* (pp. 159-184). Miami, FL: Symposia Specialists.

Poortmans, J.R. (1984). Exercise and renal function. *Sports Medicine*, **1**, 125-153.

Poortmans, J.R., Rampaer, L., & Wolfs, J-C. (1989). Renal protein excretion after exercise in man. *European Journal of Applied Physiology*, **58**, 476-480.

Porcari, J., McCarron, R., Kline, G., Freedson, P.S., Ward, A., Ross, J.A., & Rippe, J.M. (1987). Is fast walking an adequate aerobic training stimulus for 30- to 69-year old men and women? *The Physician and Sportsmedicine*, **15**(2), 119-129.

Powell, K.E., Kohl, H.W., Caspersen, C.J., & Blair, S.N. (1986). An epidemiologic perspective on the causes of running injuries. *The Physician and Sportsmedicine*, **14**(6), 100-114.

Powell, K.E., Stephens, T., Marti, B., Heinemann, L., & Kreuter, M. (1991). Progress and problems in the promotion of physical activity. In P. Oja & R. Telama (Eds.), *Sport for all* (pp. 55-73). Amsterdam: Elsevier.

Powell, K.E., Thompson, P.D., Caspersen, C.J., & Kendrick, J.S. (1987). Physical activity and the incidence of coronary heart disease. *Annual Review of Public Health*, **8**, 253-287.

Powers, S.K., Dodd, S., Deason, R., Byrd, J., & McKnight, T. (1983). Ventilatory threshold, running economy, and distance running performance of trained athletes. *Research Quarterly*, **54**, 179-182.

Powers, S.K., Dodd, S., Lawler, J., Landry, G., Kirtley, M., McKnight, T., & Grinton, S. (1988). Incidence of exercise-induced hypoxemia in elite endurance athletes at sea level. *European Journal of Applied Physiology*, **58**, 298-302.

Powers, S.K., Dodd, S., Woodyard, J., Beadle, R.E., & Church, G. (1984). Haemoglobin saturation during incremental arm and leg exercise. *British Journal of Sports Medicine*, **18**, 212-216.

Powles, A.C.P., Sutton, J.R., & Jones, N.L. (1974). The prediction of maximal working capacity from sub-maximal exercise testing in persons with ischaemic heart disease. *Medicine and Science in Sports*, **6**, 70 (abstract).

Prahl-Andersen, B., Lowalski, C.J., & Heyendael, P. (1979). *A mixed longitudinal interdisciplinary study of growth and development*. London: Academic Press.

Pravosudov, V.P. (1978). Effects of physical exercises on health and economic efficiency. In F. Landry & W.A.R. Orban (Eds.), *Physical activity and human well-being* (pp. 261-271). Miami, FL: Symposia Specialists.

Preece, M.A., & Baines, M.J. (1978). A new family of mathematical models describing the human growth curve. *Annals of Human Biology*, **5**, 1-24.

Prior, J-L. (1990). Reproduction: Exercise-related adaptations and the health of men and women. In C. Bouchard, R.J. Shephard, T. Stephens, J. Sutton, & B. McPherson. *Exercise, fitness, and health* (pp. 661-675). Champaign, IL: Human Kinetics.

Prud'homme, D., Bouchard, C., LeBlanc, C., Landry, F., & Fontaine, E. (1984). Sensitivity of maximal aerobic power to training is genotype dependent. *Medicine and Science in Sports and Exercise*, **16**, 489-493.

Pugh, L.G.C.E. (1962). Physiological and medical aspects of the Himalayan Scientific and Mountaineering Expedition 1960-61. *British Medical Journal*, **2**, 621-627.

Pugh, L.G.C.E., Corbett, J.L., & Johnson, R.H. (1967). Rectal temperatures, weight losses, and sweat rates in marathon runners. *Journal of Applied Physiology*, **23**, 347-372.

Puhl, J.L., Runyan, W.S., & Kruse, S.J. (1981). Erythrocyte changes during training in high school women cross-country runners. *Research Quarterly*, **52**, 484-494.

Purvis, J.W., & Cureton, K.J. (1981). Ratings of perceived exertion at the anaerobic threshold. *Ergonomics*, **24**, 295-300.

Pyke, F.S., Ewing, A.S., & Roberts, A.D. (1978). Physiological adjustments to continuous and interval running training. In F. Landry & W.A.R. Orban (Eds.), *Proceedings of the International Congress of Physical Activity Sciences, Vol. 4* (pp. 369-377). Miami: Symposia Specialists.

Quinney, H.A. (1990). Sport on ice. In T. Reilly, N. Secher, P. Snell, & C. Williams. *Physiology of sports* (pp. 311-336). London: E. & F. Spon.

Quirk, J.E., & Sinning, W.E. (1982). Anaerobic and aerobic responses of males and females to rope skipping. *Medicine and Science in Sports*, **14**, 26-29.

Raab, W., & Krzywanek, H.J. (1966). Cardiac sympathetic tone and stress response related to personality patterns and exercise habit. In W. Raab (Ed.), *Prevention of ischemic heart disease: Principles and practice*. Springfield, IL: Charles C Thomas.

Rakusan, K., Wicker, P., Abdul-Samad, M., Healy, B., & Turez, Z. (1987). Failure of swimming exercise to improve capillarization in cardiac hypertrophy of renal hypertensive rats. *Circulation Research*, **61**, 641-647.

Rall, J.A. (1985). Energetic aspects of skeletal muscle contraction: Implications of fiber types. *Exercise and Sport Sciences Reviews*, **13**, 33-74.

Rashkis, H.A. (1952). Systemic stress as an inhibitor of experimental tumors in Swiss mice. *Science*, **116**, 169-171.

Rauramaa, R., & Salonen, J.T. (in press). Physical activity, fibrinolysis, and platelet aggregability. In C. Bouchard, R.J. Shephard, & T. Stephens (Eds.), *Physical activity, fitness, and health*. Champaign, IL: Human Kinetics.

Rautaharju, P.M., Friedrich, H., & Wolf, H. (1971). Measurement and interpretation of exercise electrocardiograms. In R.J. Shephard (Ed.), *Frontiers of fitness*. Springfield, IL: Charles C Thomas.

Ray, C.A., Cureton, K.J., & Ouzts, H.G. (1990). Postural specificity of cardiovascular adaptations to exercise training. *Journal of Applied Physiology*, **69**, 2202-2208.

Reading, J.L., Goodman, J., Plyley, M., Floras, J., Liu, P., McLaughlin, P.R., & Shephard, R.J. (1993). Relationship of skeletal muscle vascular conductance to aerobic power and left ventricular function: Data for sedentary patients, endurance athletes, and patients with congestive heart failure. *Journal of Applied Physiology*. **74**, 567-573.

Reaven, G.M. (1980). Insulin-dependent diabetes mellitus: Metabolic characteristics. *Metabolism*, **29**, 445-454.

Rebuck, A.S., D'Urzo, A.D., & Chapman, K.R. (1985). Exercise in chronic obstructive lung disease. In P. Welsh & R.J. Shephard (Eds.), *Current therapy in sports medicine, 1985-1986* (pp. 101-105). Burlington, ON: Decker.

Reichley, K.B., Mueller, W.H., Harris, C.L., Tulloch, B.R., Barton, S., & Schull, W.J. (1987). Centralized obesity and cardiovascular disease risk in Mexican-Americans. *American Journal of Epidemiology*, **125**, 373-386.

Reiff, G. (1980). Physical fitness guidelines for schoolage youth. In *Proceedings of the National Conference on Physical Fitness and Sports for All* (pp. 25-31). Washington, DC: President's Council on Physical Fitness and Sports.

Reijnen, J., & Velthuijsen, J.W. (1989). Economic aspects of health through sport. In British Sports Council (Ed.), *Economic impact of sport in Europe* (pp. 1-31). London: British Sports Council.

Reilly, T., & Secher, N. (1990). Physiology of sports: An overview. In T. Reilly, N. Secher, P. Snell, & C. Williams (Eds.), *Physiology of sports* (pp. 465-486). London: E. & F. Spon.

Reindell, H., König, K., & Roskamm, H. (1966). *Funktionsdiagnostik des gesunden und kranken Herzens* [Functional diagnosis of healthy and diseased hearts]. Stuttgart: Thieme.

Reindell, H., Roskamm, H., & Gerschler, W. (1962). *Interval training*. Munich: Barth.

Reinhart, W.H., Stäubli, M., & Straub, P.W. (1983). Impaired red cell filterability with elimination of old red blood cells during a 100-km race. *Journal of Applied Physiology*, **54**, 827-830.

Reitman, J.S., Vasquez, B., Klimes, I., & Nagulesparan, M. (1984). Improvement of glucose homeostasis after exercise training in non-insulin dependent diabetes. *Diabetes Care*, **7**, 434-441.

Rennie, M.J., Bowtell, J.L., & Millward, D.J. (in press). The effects of exercise on protein and amino acid metabolism. In C. Bouchard, R.J. Shephard, & T. Stephens (Eds.), *Physical activity, fitness, and health*. Champaign, IL: Human Kinetics.

Renold, A.E. (1981). Epidemiological considerations of overweight and obesity. In G. Enzi, G. Crepaldi, G. Pozza, & A.E. Renold (Eds.), *Obesity: Pathogenesis and treatment* (pp. 1-6). London: Academic Press.

Reybrouck, T., Ghesquiere, J., Cattaert, A., Fagard R., & Amery A. (1983). Ventilatory thresholds during short- and long-term exercise. *Journal of Applied Physiology*, **55**, 1694-1700.

Ribeiro, J.P., Fielding, R.A., Hughes, V., Black, A., Bochese, M.A., & Knuttgen, H.G. (1985). Heart rate break-point may coincide with the anaerobic and not the aerobic threshold. *International Journal of Sports Medicine*, **6**, 220-224.

Ribeiro, J.P., Ibanez, J.M., & Stein, R. (1991). Autonomic nervous control of the heart rate response to dynamic incremental exercise: Evaluation of the Rosenblueth-Simeone model. *European Journal of Applied Physiology*, **62**, 140-144.

Ricci, G., Lajoie, D., Petitclerc, R., Perronet, F., Ferguson, R.J., Fournier, M., & Taylor, A.W. (1982). Left ventricular size following endurance, sprint, and strength training. *Medicine and Science in Sports*, **14**, 344-347.

Richter, E.A., & Sutton, J. (in press). Hormonal adaptation to physical activity. In C. Bouchard, R.J. Shephard, & T. Stephens (Eds.), *Physical activity, fitness, and health*. Champaign, IL: Human Kinetics.

Rifkind, B.M., & Segal, P. (1983). Lipid research clinics' program reference values for hyperlipidemia and hypolipidemia. *Journal of the American Medical Association*, **250**, 1869-1879.

Robb-Nicholson, L.C., Daltroy, L., Eaton, H., Gall, V., Wright, E., Hartley, L.H., Schur, P.H., & Liang, M.H. (1989). Effects of aerobic conditioning on lupus fatigue: A pilot study. *British Journal of Rheumatology*, **28**, 500-505.

Robergs, R.A., Chwalbiaska-Moneta, J., Mitchell, J.B., Pascoe, D.D., Houmard, J., & Costill, D.L. (1990). Blood lactate threshold differences between arterial and venous blood. *International Journal of Sports Medicine*, **11**, 446-451.

Roberts, N.J. (1979). Temperature and host defence. *Microbiological Reviews*, **43**, 241-259.

Roberts, W.O. (1989). Exercise-associated collapse in endurance events: A classification system. *The Physician and Sportsmedicine*, **17**(5), 49-55.

Robertson, J.D., Maughan, R.J., & Davidson, R.J. (1987). Faecal blood loss in response to exercise. *British Medical Journal*, **295**, 303-305.

Robinson, E.P., & Kjellgaard, J.M. (1982). Improvement in ventilatory muscle function with running. *Journal of Applied Physiology*, **52**, 1400-1406.

Rode, A., Ross, R., & Shephard, R.J. (1972). Smoking withdrawal program. *AMA Archives of Environment Health*, **24**, 27-36.

Rode, A., & Shephard, R.J. (1971). The influence of cigarette smoking upon the work of breathing in near-maximal exercise. *Medicine and Science in Sports*, **3**, 51-55.

Rode, A., & Shephard, R.J. (1973). Fitness of the Canadian Eskimo: The influence of season. *Medicine and Science in Sports*, **5**, 170-173.

Rode, A., & Shephard, R.J. (1992). *Fitness and health of an Inuit community: 20 years of cultural change*. Ottawa: Circumpolar and Scientific Affairs.

Rogers, M.A., Stull, G.A., & Apple, F.S. (1985). Creatine kinase isoenzyme activities in men and women following a marathon race. *Medicine and Science in Sports and Exercise*, **17**, 679-682.

Rogers, M.A., Yamamoto, C., Hagberg, J.M., Martin, W.H., Ehsani, A.A., & Holloszy, J.O. (1988). Effect of 6 days of exercise training on responses to maximal and submaximal exercise in middle-aged men. *Medicine and Science in Sports and Exercise*, **20**, 260-264.

Rose, G. (1970). Current developments in Europe. In R.J. Jones (Ed.), *Atherosclerosis II* (pp. 310-314). Berlin: Springer-Verlag.

Rosenbaum, P.D., & Bursten, J. (1988). *Canada's Health Promotion Survey: Special study on labour force groups*. Ottawa: Ministry of Supply and Services.

Roskamm, H. (1967). Optimum patterns of exercise for healthy adults. *Canadian Medical Association Journal*, **96**, 895-899.

Roskamm, H. (1973). Limits and age dependency in the adaptation of the heart to physical stress. In O. Grüpe, D. Jurz, & J.M. Teipel (Eds.), *Sport in the modern world: Chances and problems*. Berlin: Springer-Verlag.

Rösler, K., Conley, K.E., Howald, H., Gerber, C., & Hoppeler, H. (1986). Specificity of leg-power changes to velocities used in bicycle endurance training. *Journal of Applied Physiology*, **61**, 30-36.

Rösler, K., Hoppeler, H., Conley, K.E., Claassen, H., Gehr, P., & Howald, H. (1985). Transfer effects in endurance exercise: Adaptations in trained and untrained muscle. *European Journal of Applied Physiology*, **54**, 355-362.

Ross, J.A. (1950). Hypertrophy of the little finger. *British Medical Journal*, (ii), 987.

Ross, J.C. (1989). Evaluating fitness and activity assessments from the National Children and Youth Fitness Studies I and II. In T. Drury (Ed.), *Assessing physical fitness and physical activity in population-based surveys* (pp. 229-259). Hyattsville, MD: U.S. Dept. of Health & Human Services.

Ross, J.H., & Attwood, E.C. (1984). Severe repetitive exercise and haematological status. *Postgraduate Medical Journal*, **60**, 454-457.

Rost, R., & Hollmann, W. (1983). Athlete's heart: A review of its historical assessment and new aspects. *International Journal of Sports Medicine*, **4**, 147-165.

Rost, R., & Hollmann, W. (1992). Cardiac problems in endurance sports. In R.J. Shephard & P.O. Åstrand (Eds.), *Endurance in sport* (pp. 438-452). Oxford: Blackwell Scientific.

Rothwell, N.J., & Stocks, M.J. (1983). Luxuskonsumption, diet-induced thermogenesis: The case in favour. *Clinical Science*, **64**, 19-23.

Rotter, J.B. (1975). Some problems and misconceptions related to the construct validity of internal versus external control of reinforcement. *Journal of Consulting and Clinical Psychology*, **43**, 56-67.

Rovere, G.D., & Nichols, A.W. (1985). Frequency, associated factors, and treatment of breast-stroker's knee in competitive swimmers. *American Journal of Sports Medicine*, **13**, 99-104.

Rowell, L.B. (1974). Human cardiovascular adjustments to exercise and thermal stress. *Physiological Reviews*, **54**, 75-159.

Rowell, L.B. (1985). Cardiovascular adjustments to thermal stress. In J.T. Shepherd & F.M. Abboud (Eds.), *Handbook of physiology, Circulation, Part 2*, 967-1023.

Rowell, L.B. (1986). *Human circulation during physical stress*. New York: Oxford.

Rowell, L.B. (1988). Muscle blood flow in humans: How high can it go? *Medicine and Science in Sports and Exercise*, **20**, S97-S103.

Rowell, L.B., Brengelmann, G.L., Blackmon, J.R., Bruce, R.A., & Murray, J.A. (1968). Disparities between aortic and peripheral pulse pressures induced by upright exercise and vasomotor changes in man. *Circulation*, **37**, 954-964.

Rowland, T. (1985). Aerobic response to endurance training in prepubescent children: A critical analysis. *Medicine and Science in Sports and Exercise*, **17**, 493-497.

Rowland, T. (1992). Aerobic responses to physical training in children. In R.J. Shephard & P.O. Åstrand (Eds.), *Endurance in sport* (pp. 377-384). Oxford: Blackwell Scientific.

Royce, J. (1958). Isometric fatigue curves in human muscle with normal and occluded circulation. *Research Quarterly*, **29**, 204-212.

Rubal, B.J., Moody, J.M., Damore, S., Bunker, S.R., & Diaz, N.M. (1986). Left ventricular performance of the athletic heart during upright exercise: A heart-rate-controlled study. *Medicine and Science in Sports and Exercise*, **18**, 134-140.

Rummel, J.A., Michel, E.L., & Berry, C.A. (1973). Physiological response to exercise after space flight: Apollo 7 to Apollo 11. *Aerospace Medicine*, **44**, 235-238.

Rummel, J.A., Sawin, C.F., Buderer, M.C., Mauldin, D.G., & Michel, E.L. (1975). Physiological response to exercise after space flight: Apollo 14 through Apollo 17. *Aviation, Space and Environmental Medicine*, **46**, 679-683.

Ruskin, H. (1978). Physical performance of schoolchildren in Israel. In R.J. Shephard & H. Lavallée (Eds.), *Physical fitness assessment* (pp. 273-320). Springfield, IL: Charles C Thomas.

Rusko, H., & Rahkila, P. (1983). Effect of training on aerobic capacity of female athletes differing in muscle fibre composition. *Journal of Sports Science*, **1**, 185-194.

Rylander, R. (1968). Pulmonary defence mechanisms to airborne bacteria. *Acta Physiologica Scandinavica*, (Suppl.), 306.

Ryschon, T.W., & Stray-Gunderson, J. (1991). The effect of body position on the energy cost of cycling. *Medicine and Science in Sports and Exercise*, **23**, 949-953.

Sachs, M.L. (1982). Compliance and addiction to exercise. In R. Cantu (Ed.), *The exercising adult* (pp. 19-28). Lexington, MA: Collamore Press.

Safran, M.R., Seaber, A.V., & Garrett, W.E. (1989). Warm-up and muscular injury prevention. *Sports Medicine*, **8**, 239-249.

Salans, L.B., Horton, E.S., & Sims, E.A.H. (1971). Experimental obesity in man: Cellular character of the adipose tissue. *Journal of Clinical Investigation*, **50**, 1005-1011.

Saltin, B. (1964). Circulatory response to submaximal and maximal exercise after thermal dehydration. *Journal of Applied Physiology*, **19**, 1125-1132.

Saltin, B. (1973). Oxygen transport by the circulatory system during exercise. In J. Keul (Ed.), *Limiting factors of physical performance* (pp. 235-252). Stuttgart: Thieme.

Saltin, B. (1977). The interplay between peripheral and central factors in the adaptive response to exercise and training. *Annals of the New York Academy of Sciences*, **301**, 234-231.

Saltin, B. (1992). Training-induced physiological adjustments. In *Proceedings, International Symposium: Montagne et Sport* (p. 32). Chamonix, France, February 1992.

Saltin, B., Blomqvist, G., Mitchell, J.H., Johnson, R.L., Wildenthal, K., & Chapman, C.B. (1968). Response to exercise after bed rest and after training: A longitudinal study of adaptive changes in oxygen transport and body composition. *Circulation*, VII-1–VII-78.

Saltin, B., Gagge, A.P., Bergh, V., & Stolwijk, J.A.J. (1972). Body temperature and sweating during exhaustive exercise. *Journal of Applied Physiology*, **32**, 635-643.

Saltin, B., & Grimby, G. (1968). Physiological analysis of middle-aged and old former athletes: Comparison with still active athletes of the same ages. *Circulation*, **38**, 1104-1115.

Saltin, B., Hartley, L.H., Kilbom, Å., & Åstrand, I. (1969). Physical training in sedentary middle-aged and older men: II. Oxygen uptake, heart rate, and blood lactate concentration at submaximal and maximal exercise. *Scandinavian Journal of Clinical and Laboratory Investigation*, **24**, 323-334.

Saltin, B., Henriksson, J., Nygaard, E., & Andersen, P. (1977). Fiber types and metabolic potentials of skeletal muscles in sedentary men and endurance runners. *Annals of the New York Academy of Sciences*, **301**, 3-29.

Saltin, B., & Karlsson, J. (1971). Muscle ATP, CP, and lactate during exercise after physical conditioning. In B. Pernow & B. Saltin (Eds.), *Muscle metabolism during exercise* (pp. 395-399). New York: Plenum Press.

Saltin, B., Nazar, K., Costill, D.L., Stein, E., Jansson, B., Essén, B., & Gollnick, P.D. (1976). The nature of the training response: Peripheral and central adaptations to one-legged exercise. *Acta Physiologica Scandinavica*, **96**, 289-305.

Sargeant, A.J., & Dolan, P. (1987). Human muscle function following prolonged eccentric exercise. *European Journal of Applied Physiology*, **56**, 704-711.

Sarvotham, S.G., & Berry, J.N. (1968). Prevalence of coronary heart disease in an urban population in Northern India. *Circulation*, **37**, 939-953.

Savard, P., Kiens, B., & Saltin, B. (1987). Limited blood flow in prolonged exercise: Magnitude and implication for cardiovascular control during muscular work in man. *Canadian Journal of Sport Sciences*, **12**, S89-S101.

Sawin, C.F., Rummel, J.A., & Michel, E.L. (1975). Instrumented personal exercise during long-duration space flights. *Aviation, Space and Environmental Medicine*, **46**, 394-400.

Schaper, W. (1982). Influence of physical exercise on coronary collateral blood flow in chronic, experimental two-vessel occlusion. *Circulation*, **65**, 905-912.

Schettler, G. (1977). Atherosclerosis: The main problem of industrialized societies. In G. Schettler, Y. Goto, Y. Hata, & G. Klose (Eds.), *Atherosclerosis* IV. Berlin: Springer-Verlag.

Scheuer, J., & Tipton, C.M. (1977). Cardiovascular adaptations in training. *Annual Reviews of Physiology*, **39**, 221-251.

Schilling, J.A., & Molen, M.T. (1984). Physical fitness and its relationship to postoperative recovery in abdominal hysterectomy patients. *Heart and Lung*, **13**, 639-644.

Schmidt, W., Maasen, N., Trost, F., & Böning, D. (1988). Training-induced effects on blood volume, erythrocyte turnover, and haemoglobin oxygen-binding properties. *European Journal of Applied Physiology*, **57**, 490-498.

Schnabel, A., & Kinderman, W. (1983). Assessment of anaerobic capacity in runners. *European Journal of Applied Physiology*, **52**, 42-46.

Schneider, S.H., Amorosa, L.F., Khachadurian, A.K., & Ruderman, N.B. (1984). Studies on the mechanism of improved glucose control during regular exercise in Type II (noninsulin-dependent) diabetes. *Diabetologia*, **25**, 355-360.

Schnor, P., & Hansen, A.T. (1976). A blood pressure information campaign including mass screening for hypertension in Copenhagen supermarkets. *Acta Medica Scandinavica*, **199**, 269-272.

Schoenfield, Y., Keren, G., Birnfield, Ch., & Sohar, E. (1981). Age, weight, and heart rate at rest as possible predictors of aerobic fitness. *Journal of Sports Medicine and Physical Fitness*, **21**, 377-382.

Schols, A.M.W.J., Mostert, R., Soeters, P.B., & Wouters, E.F.M. (1991). Body composition and exercise performance in patients with chronic obstructive pulmonary disease. *Thorax*, **46**, 695-699.

Schull, W.J. (1990). Heredity, fitness, and health. In C. Bouchard, R.J. Shephard, T. Stephens, J. Sutton, & B. McPherson (Eds.), *Exercise, fitness, and health* (pp. 137-146). Champaign, IL: Human Kinetics.

Schuster, K.D. (1987). Diffusion limitation and limitation by chemical reactions during alveolar-capillary transfer of oxygen-labeled CO_2. *Respiratory Physiology*, **67**, 13-22.

Schwane, J.A., Williams, J.S., & Sloan, J.H. (1987). Effects of training on delayed muscle soreness and serum creatine kinase activity after running. *Medicine and Science in Sports and Exercise*, **19**, 584-590.

Schwartz, R.S., Shuman, W.P., Larson, V., Cain, K.C., Fellingham, G.W., Beard, J.C., Kahn, S.E., Stratton, J.R., Cerqueria, M.D., & Abrass, I.B. (1991). The effect of intensive endurance exercise training on body fat distribution in young and older men. *Metabolism*, **40**, 545-551.

Scott, J.C. (1967). Physical activity and the coronary circulation. *Canadian Medical Association Journal*, **96**, 853-859.

Scragg, R., Stewart, A., Jackson, R., & Beaglehole, R. (1987). Alcohol and exercise in myocardial infarction and sudden coronary death in men and women. *American Journal of Epidemiology*, **126**, 77-85.

Seals, D.R., Hagberg, J.M., Hurley, B.F., Ehsani, A.A., & Holloszy, J.O. (1984). Endurance training in older men and women: I. Cardiovascular responses to exercise. *Journal of Applied Physiology*, **57**, 1024-1029.

Seals, D.R., Rogers, M.A., Hagberg, J.M., Yamamoto, C., Cryer, P.E., & Ehsani, A.A. (1988). Left ventricular dysfunction after prolonged strenuous exercise in healthy subjects. *American Journal of Cardiology*, **61**, 875-879.

Secher, N. (1990). Rowing. In T. Reilly, N. Secher, P. Snell, & C. Williams (Eds.), *Physiology of sports* (pp. 259-286). London: E. & F. Spon.

Secher, N. (1992). Rowing. In R.J. Shephard & P.O. Åstrand (Eds.), *Endurance in sport* (pp. 563-569). Oxford: Blackwell Scientific.

Secher, N.H., & Vaage, O. (1983). Rowing performance: A mathematical model based on analysis of body dimensions as exemplified by body weight. *European Journal of Applied Physiology*, **52**, 88-93.

Sedlock, D.A., Knowlton, R.G., & Fitzgerald, P.I. (1988). The effects of arm crank training on the physiological responses to submaximal wheelchair ergometry. *European Journal of Applied Physiology*, **57**, 55-59.

Segersted, M., Hargens, A.R., Kardel, K.R., Blom, P., Jensen, O., & Hermansen, L. (1984). Intramuscular fluid pressure during isometric contraction of human skeletal muscle. *Journal of Applied Physiology*, **56**, 287-295.

Sejersen, P., & Tonnesen, K.H. (1972). Shunting by diffusion of inert gas in skeletal muscle. *Acta Physiologica Scandinavica*, **86**, 82-91.

Seliger, V. (1970). Physical fitness of Czechoslovak children at 12 and 15 years of age: International Biological Programme results of investigations. *Acta Universitas Carolinska Gymnica, Prague*, **5**, 6-169.

Seliger, V., Bartunek, Zd., & Trefny, Zd. (1974). Comparison of the habitual activity in two groups of boys. *International Congress of Pediatric Work Physiology*, Seč, Czechoslovakia.

Selye, H. (1978). On the real benefits of eustress. *Psychology Today*, **11**, 60-70.

Sexton, W.L., Korthuis, R.J., & Laughlin, M.H. (1988). High-intensity exercise training increases vascular transport capacity of rat hindquarters. *American Journal of Physiology*, **254**, H274-H278.

Shah, V.V., Shah, S.R., & Panse, V.N. (1968). Nutritional and physical factors in coronary heart disease. *Geriatrics*, **23**, 99-103.

Shaper, A.G. (1970). Current developments in atherosclerosis in Africa. In R.J. Jones (Ed.), *Atherosclerosis* II (pp. 314-320). Berlin: Springer-Verlag.

Shapiro, L.M. (1987). Left ventricular hypertrophy in athletes in relation to the type of sport. *Sports Medicine*, **4**, 239-244.

Shaw, J.H., & Cordts, H.J. (1960). Athletic participation and academic performance. In W.R. Johnson (Ed.), *Science and medicine of sports* (pp. 620-632). New York: Harper.

Sheffield, L.T. (1974). The meaning of exercise test findings. In S. Fox (Ed.), *Coronary heart disease: Prevention, detection, rehabilitation with emphasis on exercise testing.* (pp. 9-1–9-35). Denver: International Medical.

Sheldahl, L.M. (1986). Special ergometric techniques and weight reduction. *Medicine and Science in Sports and Exercise*, **18**, 25-30.

Shepard, R.H. (1958). Effect of pulmonary diffusing capacity on exercise tolerance. *Journal of Applied Physiology*, **12**, 487-488.

Shephard, R.J. (1957). Some factors affecting the open-circuit determination of breathing capacity. *Journal of Physiology*, **135**, 98-113.

Shephard, R.J. (1962). The ergonomics of the respirator. In C.N. Davies (Ed.), *Design and use of respirators* (pp. 51-66). New York: Macmillan.

Shephard, R.J. (1965). The development of cardiorespiratory fitness. *Medical Services Journal of Canada, 21,* 533-544.

Shephard, R.J. (1966a). Oxygen cost of breathing during vigorous exercise. *Quarterly Journal of Experimental Physiology, 51,* 336-350.

Shephard, R.J. (1966b). World standards of cardiorespiratory performance. *Archives of Environmental Health, 13,* 664-672.

Shephard, R.J. (1967). Normal levels of activity in Canadian city dwellers. *Canadian Medical Association Journal, 96,* 912-914.

Shephard, R.J. (1968a). Exercise and physical fitness. *Ontario Medical Review, 35,* 77-82.

Shephard, R.J. (1968b). Intensity, duration, and frequency of exercise as determinants of the response to a training regimen. *Internationale Zeitschrift für Angewandte Physiologie, 26,* 272-278.

Shephard, R.J. (1968c). Practical indices of metabolic activity: An experimental comparison of pulse rate and ventilation. *Internationale Zeitschrift für Angewandte Physiologie, 25,* 13-24.

Shephard, R.J. (1968d). Rapporteur: Meeting of investigators on exercise tests in relation to cardiovascular function. *WHO Technical Report,* 388.

Shephard, R.J. (1969). Learning, habituation, and training. *Internationale Zeitschrift für Angewandte Physiologie, 28,* 38-48.

Shephard, R.J. (1971a). The oxygen conductance equation. In R.J. Shephard (Ed.), *Frontiers of fitness* (pp. 129-154). Springfield, IL: Charles C Thomas.

Shephard, R.J. (1971b). The working capacity of schoolchildren. In R.J. Shephard (Ed.), *Frontiers of fitness* (pp. 319-344). Springfield, IL: Charles C Thomas.

Shephard, R.J. (1972). An integrated approach to cardio-respiratory performance at sea level and at an altitude of 7,350 ft. In G.R. Cumming, A.W. Taylor, & D. Snidal (Eds.), *Environmental effects on work performance* (pp. 87-100). Ottawa: Canadian Association of Sport Sciences.

Shephard, R.J. (1974, August). Physical fitness from the viewpoint of the physiologist. Keynote address to the International Committee on Physical Fitness Research, Jerusalem.

Shephard, R.J. (1974a). Altitude training camps. *British Journal of Sports Medicine, 8,* 38-45.

Shephard, R.J. (1974b). Sudden death: A significant hazard of exercise? *British Journal of Sports Medicine, 8,* 101-110.

Shephard, R.J. (1974c). What causes second wind? *The Physician and Sportsmedicine, 2*(11), 36-42.

Shephard, R.J. (1975). Future research on the quantifying of endurance training. *Journal of Human Ergology, 3,* 163-181.

Shephard, R.J. (1976). Exercise and chronic obstructive lung disease. *Exercise and Sport Sciences Reviews, 4,* 263-296.

Shephard, R.J. (1977a). *Endurance fitness* (2nd ed.). Toronto: University of Toronto Press.

Shephard, R.J. (1977b). Exercise-induced bronchospasm: A review. *Medicine and Science in Sports, 9,* 1-10.

Shephard, R.J. (1978). *Human physiological work capacity.* London: Cambridge University Press.

Shephard, R.J. (1979a). Exercise for the asthmatic: A brief historical review. *Journal of Sports Medicine and Physical Fitness, 18,* 301-307.

Shephard, R.J. (1979b). Recurrence of myocardial infarction in an exercising population. *British Heart Journal, 42,* 133-138.

Shephard, R.J. (1980). Work physiology and activity patterns. In F. Milan (Ed.), *The human biology of circumpolar populations* (pp. 305-338). London: Cambridge University Press.

Shephard, R.J. (1981). *Ischemic heart disease and exercise*. London: Croom Helm.

Shephard, R.J. (1982a). *Physical activity and growth*. Chicago: Year Book.

Shephard, R.J. (1982b). *Physiology and biochemistry of exercise*. New York: Praeger.

Shephard, R.J. (1983a). *Biochemistry of exercise*. Springfield, IL: Charles C Thomas.

Shephard, R.J. (1983b). *Carbon monoxide: The silent killer*. Springfield, IL: Charles C Thomas.

Shephard, R.J. (1983c). The workload of the postal carrier. *Journal of Human Ergology*, **11**, 151-164.

Shephard, R.J. (1985a). Adaptation to exercise in the cold. *Sports Medicine*, **2**, 59-71.

Shephard, R.J. (1985b). Exercise in coronary heart disease. *Sports Medicine*, **3**, 26-49.

Shephard, R.J. (1985c). Physical activity for the senior: A role for pool exercises? *Canadian Association for Health, Physical Education and Recreation Journal*, **50**(6), 2-5, 20.

Shephard, R.J. (1986a). *The economic benefits of enhanced fitness*. Champaign, IL: Human Kinetics.

Shephard, R.J. (1986b). *Fitness and health in industry*. Basel: Karger.

Shephard, R.J. (1986c). *Fitness of a nation: Lessons from the Canada Fitness Survey*. Basel: Karger.

Shephard, R.J. (1987a). *Physical activity and aging* (2nd ed.). London: Croom Helm.

Shephard, R.J. (1987b). Respiratory factors limiting prolonged effort. *Canadian Journal of Sport Sciences*, **12**, 45S-52S.

Shephard, R.J. (1987c). Science and medicine of canoeing and kayaking. *Sports Medicine*, **4**, 19-33.

Shephard, R.J. (1988a). The aging of cardiovascular function. In W.W. Spirduso & H.M. Eckert (Eds.), *The Academy papers: Physical activity and aging* (pp. 175-185). Champaign, IL: Human Kinetics.

Shephard, R.J. (1988b). Fitness boom or bust: The Canadian perspective. *Research Quarterly*, **59**, 265-269.

Shephard, R.J. (1988c). Sport, leisure, and well-being: An ergonomic perspective. *Ergonomics*, **31**, 1501-1517.

Shephard, R.J. (1989a). Current perspectives on the economics of fitness and sport with particular reference to worksite programmes. *Sports Medicine*, **7**, 286-309.

Shephard, R.J. (1989b). Exercise and lifestyle change. *British Journal of Sports Medicine*, **23**, 11-22.

Shephard, R.J. (1989c). Exercise in secondary and tertiary rehabilitation: Costs and benefits. *Journal of Cardiopulmonary Rehabilitation*, **9**, 188-194.

Shephard, R.J. (1989d). Exercise in the tertiary prevention of ischemic heart disease: Experimental proof. *Canadian Journal of Sport Sciences*, **14**, 74-84.

Shephard, R.J. (1990a). Assessment of occupational fitness in the context of Human Rights Legislation. *Canadian Journal of Sport Sciences*, **15**, 89-95.

Shephard, R.J. (1990b). Exercise for the frail elderly. *Sports Training, Medicine, and Rehabilitation*, **1**, 263-277.

Shephard, R.J. (1990c). *Fitness in special populations*. Champaign, IL: Human Kinetics.

Shephard, R.J. (1990d). Measuring physical activity in the elderly: Some implications for nutrition. *Canadian Journal on Aging*, **9**, 188-203.

Shephard, R.J. (1990e). Physical activity and cancer. *International Journal of Sports Medicine*, **11**, 413-420.

Shephard, R.J. (1991a). Acute and chronic effects of exercise upon immune function. *Canadian Journal of Sport Sciences*, **16**, 163-185.

Shephard, R.J. (1991b). *Body composition in biological anthropology*. London: Cambridge University Press.

Shephard, R.J. (1991c). Fitness and aging. In C. Blais (Ed.), *Aging into the twenty-first century* (pp. 22-35). Downsview, ON: Captus University Publications.

Shephard, R.J. (1991d). Responses to acute exercise and training after cardiac transplantation: A review. *Canadian Journal of Sport Sciences*, **16**, 9-22.

Shephard, R.J. (1992a). Effectiveness of training programmes for prepubescent children. *Sports Medicine*, **13**, 194-213.

Shephard, R.J. (1992b). General considerations. In R.J. Shephard & P.O. Åstrand (Eds.), *Endurance in sport* (pp. 21-33). Oxford: Blackwell Scientific.

Shephard, R.J. (1992c). Muscular endurance and blood lactate. In R.J. Shephard & P.O. Åstrand (Eds.), *Endurance in sport* (pp. 217-227). Oxford: Blackwell Scientific.

Shephard, R.J. (1992d). Problems of high altitude. In R.J. Shephard & P.O. Åstrand. *Endurance in sport* (pp. 477-484). Oxford: Blackwell Scientific.

Shephard, R.J. (1992e). A critical analysis of work-site fitness programs and their postulated economic benefits. *Medicine and Science in Sports and Exercise*, **24**, 354-370.

Shephard, R.J. (1992f). Does exercise reduce all-cancer death rates? *British Journal of Sports Medicine*, **26**, 125-128, 1992.

Shephard, R.J. (1992g). Fat metabolism, exercise and cold. *Canadian Journal of Sport Sciences*, **17**, 83-90.

Shephard, R.J. (1992h). Vehicle injuries to joggers: Case report and review. *Journal of Sports Medicine and Physical Fitness*, **32**, 321-331.

Shephard, R.J., Allcn, C., Bar-Or, O., Davies, C.T.M., Degré, S., Hedman, R., Ishii, K., Kaneko, M., LaCour, R., diPrampero, P.E., & Seliger, V. (1968). The working capacity of Toronto schoolchildren. *Canadian Medical Association Journal*, **100**, 560-566, 705-714.

Shephard, R.J., Allen, C., Benade, A.J.S., Davies, C.T.M., diPrampero, P.E., Hedman, R., Merriman, J.E., Myhre, K., & Simmons, R. (1968a). The maximum oxygen intake: An international reference standard of cardiorespiratory fitness. *Bulletin of the World Health Organisation*, **38**, 757-764.

Shephard, R.J., Allen, C., Benade, A.J.S., Davies, C.T.M., diPrampero, P.E., Hedman, R., Merriman, J.E., Myhre, K., & Simmons, R. (1968b). Standardization of submaximal exercise tests. *Bulletin of the World Health Organisation*, **38**, 765-776.

Shephard, R.J., & Bar-Or, O. (1970). Alveolar ventilation in near-maximum exercise: Data on pre-adolescent children and young adults. *Medicine and Science in Sports*, **2**, 83-92.

Shephard, R.J., Berridge, M., & Montelpare, W. (1990). On the generality of the sit-and-reach test. *Research Quarterly*, **61**, 326-330.

Shephard, R.J., Bouhlel, E., Vandewalle, H., & Monod, H. (1988). Muscle mass as a factor limiting physical work. *Journal of Applied Physiology*, **64**, 1472-1479.

Shephard, R.J., & Callaway, S. (1966). Principal component analysis of the responses to standard exercise training. *Ergonomics*, **9**, 141-154.

Shephard, R.J., Corey, P., & Cox, M.H. (1982). Health hazard appraisal—The influence of an employee fitness programme. *Canadian Journal of Public Health*, **73**, 183-187.

Shephard, R.J., Corey, P., & Kavanagh, T. (1981). Exercise compliance and the prevention of a recurrence of myocardial infarction. *Medicine and Science in Sports and Exercise*, **13**, 1-5.

Shephard, R.J., Corey, P., Renzland, P., & Cox, M.H. (1982). The influence of an industrial fitness programme upon medical care costs. *Canadian Journal of Public Health*, **73**, 259-263.

Shephard, R.J., Cox, M., & Simper, K. (1981). An analysis of PAR-Q responses in an office population. *Canadian Journal of Public Health*, **72**, 37-40.

Shephard, R.J., Godin, G., & Valois, P. (1989). Exercise-induced injury and current exercise behavior. *Clinical Sports Medicine*, **1**, 197-204.

Shephard, R.J., & Kavanagh, T. (1975). What exercise to prescribe for the post MI patient. *The Physician and Sportsmedicine*, **3**(8), 56-63.

Shephard, R.J., Kavanagh, T., & Moore, R. (1978). Fluid and mineral balance of post-coronary distance runners: Studies on the 1975 Boston marathon. In G. Ricci & A. Venerando (Eds.), *Nutrition, dietetics, and sport* (pp. 217-228). Turin: Minerva Medica.

Shephard, R.J., Kavanagh, T., Tuck, J., & Kennedy, J. (1983). Marathon jogging in postmyocardial infarction patients. *Journal of Cardiopulmonary Rehabilitation*, **3**, 321-329.

Shephard, R.J., & Lavallée, H. (1978). *Physical fitness assessment: Principles, practice, and applications*. Springfield, IL: Charles C Thomas.

Shephard, R.J., Lavallée, H., Beaucage, C., Pérusse, M., Rajic, M., Brisson, G., Jéquier, J-C, Lariviére, G., & LaBarre, R. (1975). La capacité physique des enfants canadiens: Une comparaison entre les enfants canadiens français, canadiens anglais, et esquimaux. III. Psychologie et sociologie des enfants canadiens français [Physical work capacity of Canadian children—a comparison of French Canadian children, English Canadian children, and Eskimos (3). Psychology and sociology of French Canadian children]. *Union Médicale*, **104**, 1131-1136.

Shephard, R.J., Lavallée, H., Jéquier, J-C., et al. (1977). Un programme complémentaire d'éducation physique: Etude préliminaire de l'expérience pratiquée dans le district de Trois Rivières [A complementary program of physical education: Preliminary study of the experiment undertaken in the Trois Rivieres region]. In J.R. LaCour (Ed.), *Facteurs limitant l'endurance Humaine: Les techniques d'amélioration de la performance* [Limiting factors in human endurance—techniques of improving performance] (pp. 43-54). Université de St. Etienne, France.

Shephard, R.J., Lavallée, H., Jéquier, J-C., LaBarre, R., Rajic, M., & Beaucage, C. (1978). Seasonal differences in aerobic power. In R.J. Shephard & H. Lavallée (Eds.), *Physical activity assessment: Principles, practice, and applications* (pp. 194-210). Springfield, IL: Charles C Thomas.

Shephard, R.J., Lavallée, H., Jéquier, J-C., Rajic, M., & LaBarre, R. (1980). On the basis of data standardization in prepubescent children. In M. Ostyn, G. Beunen, & J. Simons (Eds.), *Kinanthropometry* II (pp. 306-316). Baltimore: University Park Press.

Shephard, R.J., Lavallée, H., LaBarre, R., Rajic, M., Jéquier, J-C., & Volle, M. (1984a). Body dimensions of Québecois children. *Annals of Human Biology*, **11**, 243-252.

Shephard, R.J., Lavallée, H., & LaRivière, G. (1978). Competitive selection among age-class ice-hockey players. *British Journal of Sports Medicine*, **12**, 11-13.

Shephard, R.J., Lavallée, H., LaRivière, G., Rajic, M., Brisson, G., Beaucage, C., Jéquier, J-C., & LaBarre, R. (1974). La capacité physique des enfants canadiens: Une comparaison entre les enfants canadiens français, canadiens anglais, et esquimaux. I. Consommation maximale d'oxygène et débit cardiaque [Physical work capacity of Canadian children—a comparison of French Canadian children, English Canadian children, and Eskimos (1). Maximal oxygen consumption and cardiac output]. *Union Médicale*, **103**, 1131-1136.

Shephard, R.J., Lavallée, H., Rajic, M., Jéquier, J-C., Brisson, G., & Beaucage, C. (1978). Radiographic age in the interpretation of physiological and anthropological data. In J. Borms & M. Hebbelinck (Eds.), *Pediatric work physiology* (pp. 124-133). Basel: S. Karger.

Shephard, R.J., & McClure, R.L. (1965). The prediction of cardiorespiratory fitness. *Internationale Zeitschrift für Angewandte Physiologie*, **21**, 212-223.

Shephard, R.J., & Montelpare, W. (1988, July). Geriatric benefits of exercise as an adult. *Journal of Gerontology: Medical Sciences*, **43**(4), M86-M90.

Shephard, R.J., & Pařízková, J. (1991). *Human growth, physical fitness, and nutrition.* Basel: Karger.

Shephard, R.J., & Plyley, M. (1992). Peripheral circulation. In R.J. Shephard & P.O. Åstrand (Eds.), *Endurance in sport* (pp. 80-95). Oxford: Blackwell Scientific.

Shephard, R.J., & Rode, A. (1985). Acculturation and the biology of aging. In R. Fortuine (Ed.), *Circumpolar health '84* (pp. 45-48). Seattle: University of Washington Press.

Shephard, R.J., & Sidney, K.H. (1975). Effects of physical exercise on plasma growth hormone and cortisol levels in human subjects. *Exercise and Sport Sciences Reviews*, **3**, 1-30.

Shephard, R.J., Thomas, S., & Weller, I. (1991). The Canadian home fitness test: 1991 update. *Sports Medicine*, **11**, 358-366.

Shephard, R.J., Verde, T.J., Thomas, S.G., & Shek, P. (1991). Physical activity and the immune system. *Canadian Journal of Sport Sciences*, **16**, 163-185.

Shephard, R.J., Youldon, P.E., Cox, M., & West, C. (1979). Effect of a 6-month industrial fitness programme on serum lipid concentrations. *Atherosclerosis*, **35**, 277-286.

Sherif, C., & Rattray, G.D. (1976). Psychological development and activity in middle childhood (5-12 years). In J.G. Albinson & G.M. Andrew (Eds.), *Child in sport and physical activity* (pp. 97-132). Baltimore: University Park Press.

Shinkai, S., Shore, S., Shek, P.N., & Shephard, R.J. (1992). Acute exercise and immune function change: I. Relationship between lymphocyte activity and subset. *International Journal of Sports Medicine*, **13**, 452-461.

Shvartz, E., & Reibold, R.C. (1990). Aerobic fitness norms for males and females aged 6 to 75 years: A review. *Aviation, Space and Environmental Medicine*, **61**, 3-11.

Sidney, K.H. (1975). *Responses of elderly subjects to a program of progressive exercise training.* Ph.D. thesis, University of Toronto.

Sidney, K.H., & Shephard, R.J. (1973). Physiological characteristics and performance of the white-water paddler. *Internationale Zeitschrift für Angewandte Physiologie*, **32**, 55-70.

Sidney, K.H., & Shephard, R.J. (1977a). Training and ECG abnormalities in the elderly. *British Heart Journal*, **39**, 1114-1120.

Sidney, K.H., & Shephard, R.J. (1977b). Activity patterns of elderly men and women. *Journal of Gerontology*, **32**, 25-32.

Sidney, K.H., & Shephard, R.J. (1978). Frequency and intensity of exercise training for elderly subjects. *Medicine and Science in Sports*, **10**, 125-131.

Sidney, K.H., Shephard, R.J., & Harrison, J. (1977). Endurance training and body composition of the elderly. *American Journal of Clinical Nutrition*, **30**, 326-333.

Siegel, A.J., Silverman, L.M., & Evans, W.J. (1983). Elevated skeletal muscle creatine kinase MB isoenzyme levels in marathon runners. *Journal of the American Medical Association*, **250**, 2835-2837.

Siiteri, P.K. (1987). Adipose tissue as a source of hormones. *American Journal of Clinical Nutrition*, **45**, 277-282.

Silber, D., McLaughlin, D., & Sinoway, L. (1991). Leg exercise conditioning increases peak forearm blood flow. *Journal of Applied Physiology*, **71**, 1568-1573.

Silverman, F., Urch, B., Corey, P., & Shephard, R.J. (1990). *Dose response for selected environmental air pollutants: A study on runners* (pp. 1-69). Final Report. Toronto: Ontario Ministry of the Environment, project 219RR.

Simmons, R., & Shephard, R.J. (1971a). Effect of physical conditioning upon the central and peripheral circulatory responses to arm work. *Internationale Zeitschrift für Angewandte Physiologie*, **30**, 73-84.

Simmons, R., & Shephard, R.J. (1971b). Measurement of cardiac output in maximum exercise. *Internationale Zeitschrift für Angewandte Physiologie*, **29**, 159-172.

Simoneau, J.A., Lortie, G., Boulay, M.R., Marcotte, M., Thibault, M.C., & Bouchard, C. (1987). Effects of two high-intensity intermittent training programs interspaced by detraining on human skeletal muscle and performance. *European Journal of Applied Physiology*, **56**, 516-521.

Simopoulos, A.P. (1987). Obesity and carcinogenesis: Historical perspective. *American Journal of Clinical Nutrition*, **45**, 271-276.

Sinoway, L.I., Sheberger, J., Wilson, J., McLaughlin, D., Musch, T., & Zelis, R. (1987). A 30-day forearm work protocol increases maximal forearm blood flow. *Journal of Applied Physiology*, **62**, 1063-1067.

Sinzinger, H., & Virgolini, I. (1988). Effects of exercise on parameters of blood coagulation, platelet function, and the prostaglandin system. *Sports Medicine*, **6**, 238-245.

Siscovick, D.S. (1990). Risks of exercising: Sudden cardiac death and injuries. In C. Bouchard, R.J. Shephard, T. Stephens, J. Sutton, & B. McPherson (Eds.), *Exercise, fitness, and health* (pp. 707-713). Champaign, IL: Human Kinetics.

Siscovick, D.S., Weiss, N.S., Fletcher, R.H., & Lasky, T. (1984). The incidence of primary cardiac arrest during vigorous exercise. *New England Journal of Medicine*, **311**, 874-877.

Skrobak-Kaczynski, J., & Lewin, T. (1976). Secular changes in Lapps of northern Finland. In R.J. Shephard & S. Itoh (Eds.), *Circumpolar health* (pp. 239-247). Toronto: University of Toronto Press.

Slack, J., Noble, N., Meade, T.W., & North, W.R.S. (1977). Lipid and lipoprotein concentrations in 1,604 men and women in working populations in northwest London. *British Medical Journal*, (2), 353-356.

Slattery, M.L., & Jacobs, D.R. (1988). Physical fitness and cardiovascular disease mortality: the US railroad study. *American Journal of Epidemiology*, **127**, 571-580.

Smalley, K.A., Runyan, W.S., & Puhl, J.L. (1981). Effect of training on erythrocyte 2,3-diphosphoglycerate in two groups of women cross-country runners. *Journal of Sports Medicine and Physical Fitness*, **21**, 352-358.

Smith E.L., Raab, D.M., Zook, S.K., & Gilligan, C. (1989). Bone changes with aging and exercise. In R. Harris & S. Harris (Eds.), *Physical activity and sports* (pp. 287-294). Albany, NY: Center for the Study of Aging.

Smith, E.L., Smith, K.A., & Gilligan, C. (1990). Exercise, fitness, osteoarthritis, and osteoporosis. In C. Bouchard, R.J. Shephard, T. Stephens, J. Sutton, & B. McPherson (Eds.), *Exercise, fitness, and health* (pp. 517-528). Champaign, IL: Human Kinetics.

Smith, E.L., Smith, P.E., Ensign, C.J., & Shea, M.M. (1984). Bone involution decrease in exercising middle-aged women. *Calciferous Tissue International*, **36**, S129-S138.

Smith, J.F., & Bishop, P.F. (1988). Rebounding exercise: Are the training effects sufficient for cardiorespiratory fitness? *Sports Medicine*, **5**, 6-10.

Smith, M.J., Hudson, D.L., Gratitzer, H.M., & Raven, P.B. (1989). Exercise training bradycardia: The role of autonomic balance. *Medicine and Science in Sports and Exercise*, **21**, 40-44.

Snell, P. (1990). Middle-distance running. In T. Reilly, N. Secher, P. Snell, & C. Williams (Eds.), *Physiology of sports* (pp. 101-120). London: E. & F. Spon.

Snell, P., & Mitchell, J.H. (1984). The role of maximal oxygen consumption in exercise performance. *Clinics in Chest Medicine*, **5**, 51-62.

Snoeckx, L.H.E.H., Abeling, H.F.M., Lambregts, J.A., Schmitz, J.J., Verstappen, F.T., & Renemann, R.S. (1983). Cardiac dimensions in athletes in relation to variations in their training program. *European Journal of Applied Physiology*, **52**, 20-28.

Snoeckx, L.H.E.H., Abeling, H.F.M., Lambregts, J.A.C., Schmitz, J.J.F., Verstappen, F.T.J., & Renemann, R.S. (1982). Echocardiographic dimensions in athletes in relation to their training programs. *Medicine and Science in Sports*, **14**, 428-434.

Sobel, B.E., & Kaufman, S. (1970). Enhanced RNA polymerase activity in skeletal muscle undergoing hypertrophy. *Archives of Biochemistry and Biophysics*, **137**, 469-476.

Society of Actuaries. (1959). *Build and blood pressure study*. Chicago: Society of Actuaries.

Soh, R.S., & Micheli, L. (1985). The effect of running on the pathogenesis of osteoarthritis of the hips and knees. *Clinical Orthopedics and Related Research*, **198**, 106-109.

Sohar, E., & Sneh, E. (1973). Follow-up of obese patients: 14 years after a successful reducing diet. *American Journal of Clinical Nutrition*, **26**, 845-848.

Southgate, D.A.T., & Shirling, D. (1970). The energy expenditure and food intake of the ship's company of a submarine. *Ergonomics*, **13**, 777-782.

Spasoff, R.A. (1987). *Report of the panel on health goals for Ontario*. Toronto: Ontario Ministry of Health.

Spasoff, R.A., McDowell, I., Wright, P.A., & Ounkeley, G. (1980). Reviewing health hazard appraisal. *Chronic Disease in Canada*, **1**, 16-17.

Spirduso, W.W. (1980). Physical fitness, aging, and psychomotor speed: A review. *Journal of Gerontology*, **30**, 550-565.

Spitler, D.L., Alexander, W.C., Hoffler, G.W., Doerr, D.F., & Buchanan, P. (1984). Haptoglobin and serum enzymatic response to maximal exercise in relation to physical fitness. *Medicine and Science in Sports and Exercise*, **16**, 366-370.

Spurr, G.B., Barac-Nieto, M., & Reina, J.C. (1991). Growth, maturation, body composition, and maximal aerobic power of nutritionally normal and marginally malnourished school-aged Colombian children. In R.J. Shephard & J. Pařízková (Eds.), *Human growth, physical fitness, and nutrition* (pp. 41-60). Basel: S. Karger.

Staab, J.S., Agnew, J.W., & Sicinolfi, S.F. (1992). Metabolic and performance responses to uphill and downhill running in distance runners. *Medicine and Science in Sports and Exercise*, **24**, 124-127.

Stainsby, W.N. (1986). Biochemical and physiological bases for lactate production. *Medicine and Science in Exercise and Sports*, **18**, 341-343.

Stainsby, W.N., Snyder, B., & Welch, H.G. (1988). A pictograph essay on blood and tissue oxygen transport. *Medicine and Science in Sports and Exercise*, **20**, 213-221.

Stamler, H.J. (1973). *High blood pressure in the United States: An overview of the problem and a challenge* (NIH Publication No. 73-486). Bethesda, MD: U.S. Dept. of Health, Education, & Welfare.

Staniloff, H.M., Diamond, G.A., & Pollock, B.H. (1984). Probabilistic diagnosis and prognosis of coronary artery disease. *Journal of Cardiac Rehabilitation*, **4**, 518-529.

Stanley, W.C., & Connett, R.J. (1991). Regulation of muscle carbohydrate metabolism during exercise. *FASEB Journal*, **5**, 2155-2159.

Stark, R.D., Gambles, S.A., & Lewis, J.A. (1981). Methods to assess breathlessness in healthy subjects: A critical evaluation and application to analyze the acute effects of diazepam and promezathine on breathlessness induced by exercise or exposure to raised levels of carbon dioxide. *Clinical Science*, **61**, 429-439.

Staten, M.A. (1991). The effect of exercise on food intake in men and women. *American Journal of Clinical Nutrition*, **53**, 27-31.

Staub, N.C., & Schultz, E.L. (1968). Pulmonary capillary length in dog, cat, and rabbit. *Respiratory Physiology*, **5**, 371-378.

Stäubli, M., Roessler, B., Köchli, H.P., Peheim, E., & Straub, P.W. (1985). Creatine kinase and creatine kinase MB in endurance runners and in patients with myocardial infarction. *European Journal of Applied Physiology*, **54**, 40-45.

Stefanik, M.L., & Wood, P.D. (in press). Physical activity, lipid metabolism, and lipid transport. In C. Bouchard, R.J. Shephard, & T. Stephens (Eds.), *Physical activity, fitness, and health*. Champaign, IL: Human Kinetics.

Stefanik, P.A., Heald, F.P., & Mayer, J. (1959). Caloric intake in relation to energy output of obese and nonobese adolescent boys. *American Journal of Clinical Nutrition*, **7**, 55-62.

Stephens, T. (1987). Secular trends in physical activity. Exercise boom or bust? *Research Quarterly*, **58**, 94-105.

Stephens, T. (1989). Fitness and activity measurements in the 1989 Canada fitness survey. In T. Drury (Ed.), *Assessing physical fitness and physical activity* (pp. 401-432). Hyattsville, MD: U.S. Dept. of Health & Human Services.

Stephens, T., & Caspersen, C.J. (in press). The demography of physical activity. In C. Bouchard, R.J. Shephard, & T. Stephens (Eds.), *Physical activity, fitness, and health*. Champaign, IL: Human Kinetics.

Stephens, T., & Craig, C.L. (1990). *The well-being of Canadians: The 1988 Campbell's survey*. Ottawa: Canadian Fitness and Lifestyle Research Institute.

Steplock, D.A., Veicsteinas, A., & Mariani, M. (1971). Maximal aerobic and anaerobic power and stroke volume of the heart in a subalpine population. *Internationale Zeitschrift für Angewandte Physiologie*, **29**, 203-214.

Stevenson, J.A.F. (1967). Exercise, food intake, and health in experimental animals. *Canadian Medical Association Journal*, **96**, 862-866.

Stewart, J.G., Ahlqvist, D.A., McGill, D.B., Ilstrup, D.M., Schwartz, S., & Owen, R.A. (1984). Gastrointestinal blood loss and anemia in runners. *Annals of Internal Medicine*, **100**, 843-845.

Stewart, K.J., Mason, M., & Kelemen, M.H. (1988). Three-year participation in circuit weight training improves muscular strength and self efficacy in cardiac patients. *Journal of Cardiopulmonary Rehabilitation*, **8**, 292-296.

Stick, C., Heinemann, W., & Witzleb, E. (1990). Slow volume changes in calf and thigh during cycle ergometer exercise. *European Journal of Applied Physiology*, **61**, 428-432.

Stundl, H. (1977). *Freizeit und Erhölungssport in der DDR*. Schorndorf: Karl Hofmann.

Sullivan, M.J., Binkley, P.F., Unverferth, D.V., Ren, J-H., Boudoulas, H., Bashore, T.M., Merola, A.J., & Leier, C.V. (1985). Prevention of bed rest-induced physical deconditioning by daily dobutamine infusions: Implications for drug-induced physical conditioning. *Journal of Clinical Investigation*, **76**, 1632-1642.

Sullivan, M.J., Merola, J., Timmerman, A.P., Unverferth, D.V., & Leier, C.V. (1986). Drug-induced aerobic enzyme activity of human skeletal muscle during bed-rest deconditioning. *Journal of Cardiopulmonary Rehabilitation*, **6**, 232-237.

Suominen, H., & Heikkinen, E. (1975). Effect of physical training on collagen. *Italian Journal of Biochemistry*, **24**, 64-65.

Superko, H.R., Berbauer, E., & Voss, J. (1983). Effects of a mandatory job performance test and voluntary remediation program on law enforcement personnel. *Medicine and Science in Sports and Exercise*, **15**, 149-150.

Surgeon General. (1986). *The health consequences of involuntary smoking*. Rockville, MD: U.S. Dept. of Health & Human Services, Public Health Service, pp. 1-359.

Sutton, J.S., Sutton, J.R., Reeves, J.T., Groves, B.M., Wagner, P.D., Alexander, J.K., Hultgren, H.N., Cymerman, A., & Houston, C.S. (1992). Oxygen transport and cardiovascular function at extreme altitude: Lessons from Operation Everest II. *International Journal of Sports Medicine*, **13**(Suppl. 1), S13-S17.

Svedenhag, J., & Sjödin, B. (1984). Maximal and submaximal oxygen uptakes and blood lactate levels in elite male middle- and long-distance runners. *International Journal of Sports Medicine*, **5**, 255-261.

Swain, D.P., Coast, J.R., Clifford, P.S., Milliken, M.C., & Stray-Gunderson, J. (1987). Influence of body size on oxygen consumption during bicycling. *Journal of Applied Physiology*, **62**, 668-672.

Swartman, J.R., Cook, E.A., & Taylor, P.B. (1978). Effects of exhaustive exercise and recovery on the (^{3}H) PHE incorporation into contractile proteins of the rat myocardium. *Canadian Journal of Applied Sport Sciences*, **3**, 194 (abstract).

Swinburn, C.R., Wakefield, J.M., & Jones, P.W. (1984). Relationship between ventilation and breathlessness during exercise in chronic obstructive airways disease is not altered by prevention of hypoxaemia. *Clinical Science*, **67**, 515-519.

Systrom, D.M., Kanarck, D.J., Kohler, S.J., & Kazemi, H. (1990). ^{31}P nuclear magnetic resonance spectroscopy study of the anaerobic threshold in humans. *Journal of Applied Physiology*, **68**, 2060-2066.

Szathmary, E.J.E., & Holt, N. (1983). Hyperglycemia in Dogrib Indians of the North West Territories, Canada: Association with age and a centripetal distribution of body fat. *Human Biology*, **55**, 493-515.

Szygula, Z. (1990). Erythrocytic system under the influence of physical exercise and training. *Sports Medicine*, **10**, 181-197.

Talmage, R.V., Stinnett, S.S., Landwehr, J.T., Vincent, L.M., & McCartney, W.H. (1986). Age-related loss of bone mineral density in non-athletic and athletic women. *Bone and Mineral*, **1**, 115-125.

Tamaki, N. (1987). Effect of endurance training on muscle-fiber type composition and capillary supply in rat diaphragm. *European Journal of Applied Physiology*, **56**, 127-131.

Taunton, J.E., McKenzie, D.C., Clement, D.B., & Cook, G.J. (1986). Physiological and metabolic changes associated with the ultramarathon. *Exercise Physiology*, **2**, 49-61.

Taylor, A.W. (1979). The effects of different feeding regimens and endurance exercise programs on carbohydrate and lipid metabolism. *Canadian Journal of Applied Sport Sciences*, **4**, 126-130.

Taylor, H.L., Henschel, A., Brozek, J., & Keys, A. (1949). Effects of bed rest on cardiovascular function and work performance. *Journal of Applied Physiology*, **2**, 223-239.

Taylor, H.L., Klepetar, E., Keys, A., Parlin, W., Blackburn, H., & Puchner, T. (1962). Death rates among physically active employees of the railroad industry. *American Journal of Public Health*, **52**, 1697-1707.

Telama, R. (1978). Pupil's interest and motivation for sport in Finland. *Jyväskylä Reports of Physical Culture and Health*, **20**, 26-49.

Telama, R. (1991). Nature as motivation for physical activity. In P. Oja & R. Telama (Eds.), *Sport for all* (pp. 607-616). Amsterdam: Elsevier.

Terjung, R.L., & Winder, W.W. (1975). Exercise and thyroid function. *Medicine and Science in Sports*, **7**, 20-26.

Tesch, P.A. (1983). Physiological characteristics of elite kayak paddlers. *Canadian Journal of Applied Sport Sciences*, **8**, 87-91.

Tesch, P.A. (1985). Exercise performance and beta-blockade. *Sports Medicine*, **2**, 389-412.

Tharp, G.D., Thorland, W.G., Johnson, G.O., & Peter, J.B. (1986). Cardiac dimensions in elite young track athletes. *Research Quarterly*, **57**, 139-143.

Thomas, D.P. (1985). Effects of acute and chronic exercise on myocardial ultrastructure. *Medicine and Science in Sports and Exercise*, **17**, 546-553.

Thomas, J.R., Salazar, W., & Landers, D.M. (in press). Physical activity and intellectual performance. In C. Bouchard, R.J. Shephard, & T. Stephens (Eds.), *Physical activity, fitness, and health*. Champaign, IL: Human Kinetics.

Thompson, H.J., Ronan, A.M., Ritacco, K.A., & Tagliafero, A.R. (1989). Effect of type and amount of dietary fat on the enhancement of rat mammary tumorigenesis by exercise. *Cancer Research*, **49**, 1904-1908.

Tibbits, G.F. (1985). Regulation of myocardial contractility in exhaustive exercise. *Medicine and Science in Sports and Exercise*, **17**, 529-537.

Timmons, B.A., Araujo, J., & Thomas, T.R. (1985). Fat utilization enhanced by exercise in a cold environment. *Medicine and Science in Sports and Exercise*, **17**, 673-678.

Tipton, C.M. (1984). Exercise, training, and hypertension. *Exercise and Sport Sciences Reviews*, **12**, 245-306.

Tipton, C.M. (1991). Exercise, training, and hypertension: An update. *Exercise and Sport Sciences Reviews*, **19**, 447-506.

Tipton, C.M., Matthes, R.D., & Vailas, A.C. (1977). Influence de l'exercice sur les structures ligamentaires [Influence of exercise on ligamentous structures]. In J.R. LaCour (Ed.), *Facteurs limitant l'endurance humaine: Les techniques d'amélioration de la performance* [Factors limiting human endurance: Techniques of improving performance] (pp. 103-114). France: Université de St. Etienne.

Todero, A., Pigorini, F., Rossi, F., & Venerando, A. (1979). A scintigraphic study of the pulmonary blood flow in endurance athletes at rest and after exercise. *Journal of Sports Medicine and Physical Fitness*, **19**, 327-340.

Tomporowski, P.D., & Ellis, N.R. (1986). Effects of exercise on cognitive processes: A review. *Psychological Bulletin*, **99**, 338-346.

Toner, M.H., Glickman, E.L., & McArdle, W.D. (1990). Cardiovascular adjustments to exercise distributed between the upper and lower body. *Medicine and Science in Sports and Exercise*, **22**, 773-778.

Torre-Buono, J.R., Wagner, P.D., Saltzman, H.A., Gale, G.E., & Moon, R.E. (1985). Diffusion limitation in normal humans during exercise at sea level and simulated altitude. *Journal of Applied Physiology*, **58**, 989-995.

Tremblay, A. (in press). Physical activity and adipose tissue. In C. Bouchard, R.J. Shephard, & T. Stephens (Eds.), *Physical activity, fitness, and health*. Champaign, IL: Human Kinetics.

Tremblay, A., Coté, J., & LeBlanc, J. (1984). Diminished dietary thermogenesis in exercise-trained human subjects. *European Journal of Applied Physiology*, **52**, 1-4.

Tremblay, A., Després, J-P, & Bouchard, C. (1985). The effects of exercise training on energy balance and adipose tissue morphology and metabolism. *Sports Medicine*, **2**, 223-233.

Tripathi, A., Mack, G.W., & Nadel, E.R. (1990). Cutaneous vascular reflexes during exercise in the heat. *Medicine and Science in Sports and Exercise*, **22**, 796-803.

Tucker, L.A. (1990). Television viewing and physical fitness in adults. *Research Quarterly*, **61**, 315-320.

United States Department of Health & Human Services. (1981). National Center for Health Statistics. Highlights from wave I of the National Survey of Personal Health Practices and Consequences. *Vital Health Statistics*, **15**.

United States President's Council on Physical Fitness and Sports. (1973). National Adult Physical Fitness Survey. *Physical Fitness Research Digest*, **4**, 1-27.

United States President's Council on Physical Fitness and Sports. (1985). *National School Population Fitness Survey*. Ann Arbor: University of Michigan.

Vaccaro, P., Clarke, D.H., Morris, A.F., & Gray, P.R. (1984). Physiological characteristics of the world champion whitewater slalom team. In N. Bachl, L. Prokop, & R. Suckert (Eds.), *Current topics in sports medicine* (pp. 637-647). Vienna: Urban & Schwarzenburg.

Vaccaro, P., & Clinton, M. (1981). The effects of aerobic dance conditioning on the body composition and maximal oxygen uptake of college women. *Journal of Sports Medicine and Physical Fitness*, **21**, 291-294.

Vaccaro, P., & Mahon, A. (1987). Cardiorespiratory responses to endurance training in children. *Sports Medicine*, **4**, 352-363.

Vailas, A.C., & Vailas, J.C. (in press). Physical activity and connective tissue. In C. Bouchard, R.J. Shephard, & T. Stephens (Eds.), *Physical activity, fitness, and health*. Champaign, IL: Human Kinetics.

Van Camp, S., & Peterson, R.A. (1986). Cardiovascular complications of outpatient cardiac rehabilitation programs. *Journal of the American Medical Association*, **256**, 1160-1163.

Van Citters, R.L., & Franklin, D.L. (1969). Cardiovascular performance of Alaska sled dogs during exercise. *Circulation Research*, **24**, 33-42.

Van Dale, D., Saris, W.H.M., Schoffelen, P.F.M., & ten Hoor, F. (1987). Does exercise give an additional effect in weight reduction regimens? *International Journal of Obesity*, **11**, 367-375.

Vander, L.B., Franklin, B.A., Wrisley, D., & Rubenfire, M. (1986). Acute cardiovascular responses to Nautilus exercise in cardiac patients: Implications for exercise training. *Annals of Sports Medicine*, **2**, 165-169.

Vandewalle, H., Pérès, G., & Monod, H. (1987). Standard anaerobic exercise tests. *Sports Medicine*, **4**, 268-289.

Veicsteinas, A., Ferretti, G., Margonato, V., Rosa, G., & Tagliabue, D. (1984). Energy cost of and energy sources for alpine skiing in top athletes. *Journal of Applied Physiology*, **57**, 52-58.

Vellar, O.D., & Hermansen, L. (1971). Physical performance and haematological parameters with special reference to hemoglobin and maximal oxygen uptake. *Acta Medica Scandinavica*, **190**(Suppl. 522), 1-40.

Vena, J.E., Graham, S. Zielezny, M., Brasure, J., & Swanson, M.K. (1987). Occupational exercise and risk of cancer. *American Journal of Clinical Nutrition*, **45**, 318-327.

Vena, J.E., Graham, S., Zielezny, M., Swanson, M.K., Barnes, R.E., & Nolan, J. (1985). Lifetime occupational exercise and colon cancer. *American Journal of Epidemiology*, **122**, 357-365.

Verabioff, L.J. (1981). Physical education: An activity subject. *Canadian Association for Health, Physical Education and Recreation Journal*, **47**(5), 31-34.

Verde, T., Shephard, R.J., Corey, P., & Moore, R. (1984). Sweat composition in exercise and heat. In N. Bachl, L. Prokop, & R. Suckert (Eds.), *Current topics in sports medicine* (pp. 1057-1065). Baltimore: Urban & Schwarzenburg.

Verde, T., Thomas, S., Shek, P., & Shephard, R.J. (1992). Immune responses and increased training of the athlete. *Journal of Applied Physiology*, **73**, 1494-1499.

Verde, T., Thomas, S., & Shephard, R.J. (1992). Potential markers of over-training in the distance athlete. *British Journal of Sports Medicine*, **26**, 167-175.

Verschuur, R. (1987). *Daily physical activity and health: Longitudinal changes during the teenage period*. Haarlem: Uitgeverij de Vrieseborch.

Viidik, A. (1973). Functional properties of collagenous tissues. *International Reviews of Connective Tissue Research*, **6**, 127-217.

Vogel, J.A., & Gleser, M.A. (1972). Effect of carbon monoxide on oxygen transport during exercise. *Journal of Applied Physiology*, **32**, 234-239.

Vogel, J.M., & Whittle, M.W. (1976). Bone mineral changes: The second manned Skylab mission. *Aviation, Space and Environmental Medicine*, **47**, 396-400.

Volle, M., Shephard, R.J., Lavallée, H., LaBarre, R., Jéquier, J-C., & Rajic, M. (1982). Influence of a program of required physical activity upon academic performance. In H. Lavallée & R.J. Shephard (Eds.), *Croissance et développement de l'enfant* [Growth and development of the child.] (pp. 91-109). Trois Rivières: Université de Québec à Trois Rivières.

Volle, M., Tisal, H., LaBarre, R., Lavallée, H., Shephard, R.J., Jéquier, J-C., & Rajic, M. (1982). Influence d'un programme expérimental d'activités physiques intégrés à l'école primaire sur le développement de quelques éléments psychomoteurs [Influence of a program of required physical activities on the development of certain elements of psychomotor function in primary school children]. In H. Lavallée & R.J. Shephard (Eds.), *Croissance et développement de l'enfant* [Growth and development of the child] (pp. 201-222). Trois Rivières: Université de Québec àe Trois Rivières.

Von Döbeln, W. (1966). Kroppstorlek, Energieomsättning och Kondition. In U. Aberg & N. Lundgren (Eds.), *Handbok i ergonomi*. Stockholm: Almqvist & Wiksell.

Vranic, M., & Berger, M. (1979). Exercise and diabetes mellitus. *Diabetes*, **28**, 147-167.

Vranic, M., & Wasserman, D. (1990). Exercise, fitness, and diabetes. In C. Bouchard, R.J. Shephard, T. Stephens, J. Sutton, & B. McPherson (Eds.), *Exercise, fitness, and health* (pp. 467-490). Champaign, IL: Human Kinetics.

Vuori, I., Suurnakki, L., & Suurnakki, T. (1982). Risk of sudden cardiovascular death (SCVD) in exercise. *Medicine and Science in Sports and Exercise*, **14**, 114-115.

Wadden, T.A., Foster, G.D., Letizia, K.A., & Mullen, J.L. (1990). Long-term effects of dieting on resting metabolic rate in obese outpatients. *Journal of the American Medical Association*, **264**, 707-711.

Wade, O.L., & Bishop, J.M. (1962). *Cardiac output and regional blood flow*. Oxford: Blackwell Scientific.

Walberg, J. (1986). Weight control and the athlete. In F.I. Katch (Ed.), *Sport, health, and nutrition* (pp. 11-20). Champaign, IL: Human Kinetics.

Wallberg-Henriksson, H., Gunnarsson, R., Henriksson, J., Ostman, J., & Wahren, J. (1984). Influence of physical training on formation of muscle capillaries in Type I diabetes. *Diabetes*, **33**, 851-857.

Ward, S.A., Poon, C-S., & Whipp, B. (1980). Does turbulent airflow constrain compensatory hyperpnea during metabolic acidosis in exercise? *Medicine and Science in Sports*, **12**, 123 (abstract).

Warren, M. (1985). Effect of exercise and physical training on menarche. *Seminars in Reproductive Endocrinology*, **3**(1), 17-26.

Warren, M. (in press). Physical activity, fitness, and reproductive health in women. In C. Bouchard, R.J. Shephard, & T. Stephens (Eds.), *Physical activity, fitness, and health*. Champaign, IL: Human Kinetics.

Warren, M., Brooks-Gunn, J., Hamilton, L.H., Warren, L.F., & Hamilton, W.G. (1986). Scoliosis and fractures in young ballet dancers. *New England Journal of Medicine*, **314**, 1348-1353.

Wasserman, D.H., Lickley, H.L.A., & Vranic, M. (1985). Role of beta-adrenergic mechanisms during exercise in poorly controlled, insulin deficient diabetes. *Journal of Applied Physiology*, **59**, 1282-1289.

Waterlow, J.C. (1986). Global nutritional status. *Bulletin of the World Health Organisation*, **64**, 929-941.

Watkins, J., Farrally, M.R., & Powley, A. (1983). *The anthropometry and physical fitness of secondary schoolgirls in Strathclyde*. Glasgow: Jordanhill College of Education.

Watt, P.W., Kelly, F.J., Goldspink, D.F., & Goldspink, G. (1982). Exercise-induced morphological and biochemical changes in skeletal muscles of the rat. *Journal of Applied Physiology*, **53**, 1144-1151.

Webb, K.A., Wolfe, L.A., Hall, P., Tranmer, J.E., & McGrath, M.J. (1989). Fetal heart rate (FHR) responses to maternal aerobic exercise and physical conditioning. *Medicine and Science in Sports and Exercise*, **21**, S32.

Webber, L.S., Cresanta, J.L., Voors, A.W., & Berenson, C.S. (1983). Tracking of cardiovascular disease risk factor variables in school-age children. *Journal of Chronic Diseases*, **36**, 647-660.

Weibel, E.R. (1973). A simplified morphometric method for estimating diffusing capacity in normal and emphysematous lungs. *American Review of Respiratory Diseases*, **107**, 579-588.

Weight, L.M., & Noakes, T.D. (in press). Iron balance in exercise. In C. Bouchard, R.J. Shephard, & T. Stephens (Eds.), *Physical activity, fitness, and health*. Champaign, IL: Human Kinetics.

Weiner, J.S. (1964). *Proposals for International Research: Human Adaptability Project, Document 5*. London: Royal Anthropological Institute.

Weiner, J.S., & Lourie, J.A. (1969). *Human biology: A guide to field methods*. Oxford: Blackwell Scientific.

Weiner, J.S., & Lourie, J.A. (1981). *Practical human biology*. London: Academic Press.

Weisfeldt, M.L., Gerstenblith, G., & Lakatta, E.G. (1985). Alterations in circulatory function. In R. Andres, E.L. Bierman, & W.R. Hazzard (Eds.), *Principles of geriatric medicine* (pp. 248-279). New York: McGraw-Hill.

Weiss, R.A., & Karpovich, P.V. (1947). Energy cost of exercises for convalescents. *Archives of Physical Medicine*, **28**, 447-454.

Wells, C.L., Hecht, L.H., & Krahlenbuhl, G.S. (1981). Physical characteristics and oxygen utilization of male and female marathon runners. *Research Quarterly*, **52**, 281-285.

Wenger, H.A., & Bell, G.J. (1986). The interactions of intensity, frequency, and duration of exercise training in altering cardio-respiratory fitness. *Sports Medicine*, **3**, 346-356.

West, J.B. (1977). *Regional differences in the lung*. New York: Academic Press.

Westerterp, K.R., Saris, W.H.M., van Es, M., & ten Hoor, F. (1986). Use of the doubly labeled water technique in humans during heavy sustained exercise. *Journal of Applied Physiology*, **61**, 2162-2167.

Whelton, P.K. (1985). Hypertension in the elderly. In R. Andres, E.L. Bierman, & W.R. Hazzard (Eds.), *Principles of geriatric medicine* (pp. 536-551). New York: McGraw-Hill.

White, J.A., Quinn, G., Al-Dawabi, M., & Mulhall, J. (1982). Seasonal changes in cyclists' performance: Part I. The Great Britain Olympic road race squad. *British Journal of Sports Medicine*, **16**, 4-12.

White, J.R. (1980). Changes following ten weeks of exercise using a minitrampoline in overweight women. *Medicine and Science in Sports*, **12**, 103 (abstract).

White, M.K., Martin, R.B., Yeater, R.A., Butcher, R.L., & Radin, E.L. (1984). The effects of exercise on the bones of post-menopausal women. *International Orthopaedics*, **7**, 209-214.

Whittaker, J.L., Baracos, V.E., Haennel, R.G., Brown, B.E., Humen, D.P., & Urtasun, R.C. (1991, October). Exercise training in the post-treatment remission period of patients with limited small cell lung cancer (SCLC). In *Proceedings of Annual Meeting, Canadian Association of Sport Sciences*, Kingston, ON.

Wilhelmsen, L., Tibblin, G., & Werkö, L. (1972). A primary preventive study in Göteborg, Sweden. *Preventive Medicine*, **1**, 153-160.

Wilkes, D., Gledhill, N., & Smyth, R. (1983). Effect of acute induced metabolic alkalosis on 800-m racing time. *Medicine and Science in Sports and Exercise*, **15**, 277-280.

Williams, J.H., Powers, S.K., & Stuart, M.K. (1986). Hemoglobin desaturation in highly trained athletes during heavy exercise. *Medicine and Science in Sports and Exercise*, **18**, 168-173.

Williams, M.H. (1974). *Drugs and athletic performance*. Springfield, IL: Charles C Thomas.

Williams, P.T., Wood, P.D., Haskell, W.L., & Vranizan, K. (1982). The effects of running mileage and duration on plasma lipoprotein levels. *Journal of the American Medical Association*, **247**, 2672-2679.

Williford, H.N., Blessing, D.L., Scharff, M., Keith, R.E., & Barksdale, J.M. (1990). The physiological characteristics of female aerobic dance instructors. *Journal of Applied Sport Science Research*, **4**, 27-30.

Wilmore, J.H. (1983). Body composition in sport and exercise: Directions for future research. *Medicine and Science in Sports and Exercise*, **15**, 21-31.

Wilmore, J.H., Davis, J.A., O'Brien, R.S., Vodak, P.A., Walder, G.R., & Amsterdam, E.A. (1980). Physiological alterations consequent to 20-week conditioning programs of bicycling, tennis, and jogging. *Medicine and Science in Sports*, **12**, 1-8.

Wilmore, J.H., & McNamara, J.J. (1974). Prevalence of coronary heart disease risk factors in boys 8 to 12 years of age. *Journal of Pediatrics*, **84**, 527-533.

Wilmore, J.H., Wambsgans, K.C., Kunkel, R.C., Baron, S.B., Ewy, G.A., Goolsby, J.P., Morris, D.L., Robinson, W.A., Strauss, M., & Kalis, J.K. (1990). Effect of beta-adrenergic blockade on achievement of the trained state in post-MI patients: Non-selective vs. beta$_1$-selective blockers. *Journal of Cardiopulmonary Rehabilitation*, **10**, 50-57.

Wilt, F. (1968). Training for competitive running. In H. Falls (Ed.), *Exercise physiology* (pp. 395-414). New York: Academic Press.

Withers, R.T., Sherman, W.M., Miller, J.M., & Costill, D.L. (1981). Specificity of the anaerobic threshold in endurance-trained cyclists and runners. *European Journal of Applied Physiology*, **47**, 93-104.

Wohlfart, B., Pahlm, O., Sörnmo, L., Albrechtsson, U., & Lárusdottir, H. (1990). ST changes in relation to heart rate during bicycle exercise in patients with coronary artery disease. *Clinical Physiology*, **10**, 561-572.

Wolfe, L.A., & Cunningham, D.A. (1978). Effects of jogging on left ventricular performance during exercise. *Canadian Journal of Sport Sciences*, **3**, 181 (abstract).

Wolfe, L.A., Cunningham, D.A., & Boughner, D.R. (1986). Physical conditioning effects on cardiac dimensions: A review of echocardiographic studies. *Canadian Journal of Applied Sport Sciences*, **11**, 66-79.

Wolfe, L.A., Ohtake, P.J., Mottola, M.F., & McGrath, M.J. (1989). Physiological interactions between pregnancy and aerobic exercise. *Exercise and Sport Sciences Reviews*, **17**, 295-351.

Wolff, H. (1958). The integrating pneumotachograph: A new instrument for the measurement of energy expenditures by indirect calorimetry. *Quarterly Journal of Experimental Physiology*, **43**, 270-283.

Womersley, J., & Durnin, J.V.G.A. (1973). An experimental study of the variability of measurements of skinfold thicknesses in young adults. *Human Biology*, **45**, 281-292.

Womersley, J., & Durnin, J.V.G.A. (1977). A comparison of the skinfold method with the extent of overweight and various weight-height relationships in the assessment of obesity. *British Journal of Nutrition*, **38**, 271-284.

Wong, S.C., & McKenzie, D.C. (1987). Cardiorespiratory fitness during pregnancy and its effects on outcome. *International Journal of Sports Medicine*, **8**, 79-83.

Wood, C.D., Shreck, R., Tommey, R., Towsley, K., Guess, C.W., Werth, R., & Pollard, M. (1985). Relative value of glucose and amino acids in preserving exercise capacity in the postoperative period. *American Journal of Surgery*, **149**, 383-386.

Wood, P.D., Haskell, W.L., Blair, S.N., Williams, P.T., Krauss, R.M., Lindgren, F.T., Albers, J.J., Ho, P.H., & Farquhar, J.W. (1983). Increased exercise level and plasma lipoprotein concentrations: A one-year, randomized, controlled study in sedentary, middle-aged men. *Metabolism*, **32**, 31-39.

Wood, P.D., & Stefanik, M.L. (1990). Exercise, fitness, and atherosclerosis. In C. Bouchard, R.J. Shephard, T. Stephens, J. Sutton, & B. McPherson (Eds.), *Exercise, fitness, and health* (pp. 409-423). Champaign, IL: Human Kinetics.

Woolf, C., & Suero, J.T. (1969). Alterations in lung mechanics following training in chronic obstructive lung disease. *Diseases of the Chest*, **55**, 37-44.

Work, J.A. (1989). Is weight training safe during pregnancy? *The Physician and Sportsmedicine*, **17**(3), 257-259.

World Health Organization. (1948). *Official Records, #2*. Geneva: Author.

Worthington, E.B. (1978). *The evolution of IBP*. London: Cambridge University Press.

Wright, G.R., Bompa, T., & Shephard, R.J. (1976). Physiological evaluation of winter training programme for oarsmen. *Journal of Sports Medicine and Physical Fitness*, **16**, 22-37.

Wright, G.R., Sidney, K.H., & Shephard, R.J. (1978). Variance of direct and indirect measurements of aerobic power. *Journal of Sports Medicine and Physical Fitness*, **18**, 33-42.

Wronski, T.J., & Morey, E.R. (1983). Alterations in calcium homeostasis and bone during actual and simulated space flight. *Medicine and Science in Sports and Exercise*, **15**, 410-414.

Wronski, T.J., Morey-Holton, E.R., Doty, S.B., Maese, A.C., & Walsh, C.C. (1987). Histomorphometric analysis of rat skeleton following space flight. *American Journal of Physiology*, **252**, R252-R255.

Wyndham, C.H., & Strydom, N.B. (1972). Körperliche Arbeit bei hoher Temperatur [Bodywork at high temperatures]. In W. Hollmann (Ed.), *Zentrale Themen der Sportmedizin* [Central themes of sport medicine] (pp. 131-149). Berlin: Springer-Verlag.

Wyndham, C.H., Strydom, N.B., Benade, A.J.S., & Van Rensberg, A.J. (1973). Limiting rates of work for acclimatization at high wet-bulb temperatures. *Journal of Applied Physiology*, **35**, 454-458.

Wyshak, G., Frisch, R.E., Albright, N., Albright, T., & Schiff, I. (1986). Lower prevalence of benign diseases of the breast and benign tumors of the reproductive system among former college athletes compared to non-athletes. *British Journal of Cancer*, **54**, 841-845.

Yamaji, K., Greenly, M., Northey, D.R., & Hughson, R.L. (1990). Oxygen uptake and heart rate responses to treadmill and water running. *Canadian Journal of Sport Sciences*, **15**, 96-98.

Yamaji, K., & Shephard, R.J. (1987). Grouping of runners during marathon competition. *British Journal of Sports Medicine*, **21**, 166-167.

Yang, J-C., Wesley, R.C., & Froelicher, V.F. (1991). Ventricular tachycardia during routine treadmill testing. *Archives of Internal Medicine*, **151**, 349-353.

Ylä-Herttula, S. (1985). Development of atherosclerotic plaques. *Acta Medica Scandinavica*, **701** (Suppl.), 7-14.

Ylitalo, V. (1981). Treatment of obese schoolchildren. *Acta Paediatrica Scandinavica*, **290** (Suppl.), 1-108.

Yoshida, T., Takeuchi, N., & Suda, Y. (1982). Arterial versus venous blood lactate increase in the forearm during incremental bicycle exercise. *European Journal of Applied Physiology*, **50**, 87-93.

Younes, M., & Bshoutzy, Z. (1989). Effect of high blood flow, ventilation, and breathing patterns on alveolar hypoxia and lung fluid flux. In J.R. Sutton, G. Coates, & J. Remmers (Eds.), *Hypoxia: The adaptations* (pp. 155-162). Philadelphia: Decker.

Young, A. (1990). Exercise, fitness, and recovery from surgery, disease or infection. In C. Bouchard, R.J. Shephard, T. Stephens, J. Sutton, & B. McPherson (Eds.), *Exercise, fitness, and health* (pp. 589-600). Champaign, IL: Human Kinetics.

Young, D.C., Bonen, A., Campagna, P., & Beresford, P. (1988, June). Fetal biophysical response to moderate maternal exercise in pregnancy. *Paper presented to 44th Annual Meeting of the Society of Obstetricians and Gynecologists*, Vancouver.

Young, M.A., Rowlands, D.B., Stallard, T.J., Watson, R.D., & Littler, W.A. (1983). Effect of environment on blood pressure. *British Medical Journal*, **286**, 1235-1236.

Zach, M.S., Oberwaldner, B., & Hausler, F. (1982). Cystic fibrosis: Physical exercise versus chest physiotherapy. *Archives of Disease in Childhood*, **57**, 587-589.

Zackin, M.J., & Meredith, C.N. (1989). Protein metabolism in aging: Effects of exercise and training. In R. Harris & S. Harris (Eds.), *Physical activity, sports, and aging* (pp. 271-286). Albany, NY: Center for the Study of Aging.

Zager, P.G., Melada, G.A., Goldman, R.H., Gonzales, C.M., & Luetscher, J.A. (1974). Increased plasma renin activity in prolonged bed rest. *Journal of Clinical Endocrinology*, **53**, 87a.

Zaharieva, E. (1972). Olympic participation by women: Effects on pregnancy and childbirth. *Journal of the American Medical Association*, **221**, 992-995.

Zitnik, R.S., Ambrosioni, E., & Shepherd, J.T. (1971). Effect of temperature on cutaneous venomotor reflexes in man. *Journal of Applied Physiology*, **31**, 507-512.

Zouloumian, P., & Freund, H. (1981). Lactate after exercise in man: III. Properties of the compartment model. *European Journal of Applied Physiology and Occupational Physiology*, **46**, 149-160.

Zuti, W.B., & Golding, L.A. (1976). Comparing diet and exercise as weight reduction tools. *The Physician and Sportsmedicine*, **4**(1), 49-53.

Zylstra, S., Hopkins, A., Erk, M., Hreshchyshyn, M.M., & Anbar, M. (1989). Effect of physical activity on lumbar spine and femoral neck bone densities. *International Journal of Sports Medicine*, **10**, 181-186.

Index

About the Author

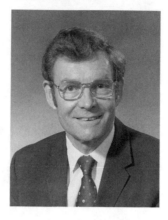

Roy J. Shephard, MD, PhD, DPE, is a professor of applied physiology at the University of Toronto. He has spent over three decades as an administrator, researcher, consultant, and teacher exploring the relationships among regular physical activity, aerobic function, and health.

Dr. Shephard has held many distinguished positions and been the recipient of many honors. He has served as the president of the American College of Sports Medicine (ACSM), president of the Canadian Association of Sports Sciences (CASS—now known as the Canadian Society of Exercise Physiology), and vice president of the International Committee for Physical Fitness Research. In 1985, he was given the CASS Honor Award, and in 1991 he received a Citation from ACSM. He is also a two-time recipient of the Philip Noel Baker Research Prize, and he has received honorary doctorates from the University of Gent (Belgium) and the University of Montreal.

Dr. Shephard is the author of more than 1,000 publications, including nearly 50 books, and he has served as editor-in-chief of the *Canadian Journal of Sport Sciences* (now known as the *Canadian Journal of Applied Physiology*). In his leisure time, Dr. Shephard enjoys stamp collecting, choral singing, walking, and reading French literature.